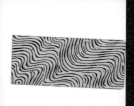

Comprehensive Care of the Transgender Patient

Comprehensive Care of the Transgender Patient

First Edition

Cecile A. Ferrando, MD, MPH
Obstetrics, Gynecology & Women's Health Institute
Center for Urogynecology & Pelvic Reconstructive Surgery
Center for LGBT Care
Cleveland Clinic
Cleveland, OH

ELSEVIER

1600 John F. Kennedy Blvd.
Ste 1800
Philadelphia, PA 19103-2899

COMPREHENSIVE CARE OF THE TRANSGENDER PATIENT, FIRST EDITION   ISBN: 978-0-323-49642-1

Notices

Practitioners and researchers must always rely on their own experience and knowledge in evaluating and using any information, methods, compounds or experiments described herein. Because of rapid advances in the medical sciences, in particular, independent verification of diagnoses and drug dosages should be made. To the fullest extent of the law, no responsibility is assumed by Elsevier, authors, editors or contributors for any injury and/or damage to persons or property as a matter of products liability, negligence or otherwise, or from any use or operation of any methods, products, instructions, or ideas contained in the material herein.

ISBN: 978-0-323-49642-1

Content Strategist: Sarah Barth
Content Development Manager: Katie DeFrancesco
Content Development Specialist: Angie Breckon
Publishing Services Manager: Shereen Jameel
Project Manager: Nadhiya Sekar
Design Direction: Ryan cook

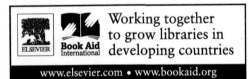

www.elsevier.com • www.bookaid.org

To my patients, thank you for the inspiration.
Only you can write your story the way it was meant to
be told.

CONTRIBUTORS

Benjamin Abelson, MD
Glickman Urological and Kidney Institute
Cleveland Clinic
Cleveland, Ohio

Paurush Babbar, MD
Chief Resident
Glickman Urological and Kidney Institute
Cleveland Clinic
Cleveland, Ohio

Stefan Baral, MD, MPH, CCFP, FRCPC
Director, Key Populations Program
Center for Public Health and Human Rights
Associate Professor
Department of Epidemiology
Johns Hopkins School of Public Health
Baltimore, Maryland

Marta R. Bizic, MD, PhD
University Children's Hospital
School of Medicine
University of Belgrade
Belgrade, Serbia

Marci Bowers, MD
Physician/Surgeon
Ob/gyn
Mills-Peninsula Hospital
Burlingame, California
Icahn school of Medicine
Mount Sinai Beth Israel
New York, New York

David Call, MD
Instructor of Psychiatry and Behavioral Sciences
Children's National Health System
Washington, DC

James Murphy, MD
Assistant Professor
University of Colorado
Denver, Colorado

Luis Capitán, MD, PhD
Director and Head Surgeon
FACIALTEAM Surgical Group
HC Marbella International Hospital
Marbella, Spain

Fermín Capitán-Cañadas, PhD
Director of Research and Development
FACIAL TEAM Surgical Group
HC Marbella International Hospital
Marbella, Spain

Jeremi Carswell, MD
Director, Gender Management Service
Division of Endocrinology
Boston Children's Hospital
Boston, Massachusetts

Gene DeHaan, MD
Kaiser Permanente – Northwest
East Interstate Medical Office
Obstetrics and Gynecology
Portland, Oregon

Miroslav L. Djordjevic, MD, PhD
Professor of Urology/Surgery
Belgrade Center for Genitourinary Reconstructive Surgery
Faculty of Medicine
University of Belgrade
Belgrade, Serbia

Cecile A. Ferrando, MD, MPH
Director, Transgender Surgery & Medicine Program
Center for Urogynecology & Pelvic Reconstructive Surgery
Center for LGBT Care
Cleveland Clinic
Cleveland, Ohio

Dan H. Karasic, MD
Health Sciences Clinical Professor
Psychiatry
University of California San Francisco
San Francisco, California

Gail Knudson, MD, MEd
Clinical Professor
Psychiatry
University of British Columbia
Vancouver, Canada

Juno Obedin-Maliver, MD, MPH, MAS
Assistant Professor
Obstetrics and Gynecology
Stanford University School of Medicine
Palo Alto, California

Parisa A. Samimi, MD
Clinical Fellow, Female Pelvic Medicine and Reconstructive Surgery
Department of Obstetrics and Gynecology
Vanderbilt University Medical Center
Nashville, Tennessee

Cherie Quesenberry Marfori, MD
Assistant Professor
Obstetrics and Gynecology
George Washington University
Washington, DC

Ray Qian, MD
Resident
Internal Medicine
Boston University Medical Center
Boston, Massachusetts

Sari L. Reisner, ScD
Assistant Professor of Pediatrics
Harvard Medical School and Boston Children's Hospital
Assistant Professor
Department of Epidemiology
Harvard T.H. Chan School of Public Health
Affiliated Research Scientist
The Fenway Institute
Fenway Health
Boston, Massachusetts

Audrey Rhee, MD
Assistant Professor
Urology
Cleveland Clinic Foundation
Cleveland, Ohio

Stephanie Roberts, MD
Attending
Endocrinology
Boston Children's Hospital
Boston, Massachusetts

Joshua D. Safer, MD, FACP
Executive Director
Center for Transgender Medicine and Surgery
Icahn School of Medicine at Mount Sinai
Mount Sinai Health System
New York, New York

Loren S. Schechter, MD
Clinical Professor of Surgery
University of Illinois at Chicago
Director, The Center for Gender Confirmation Surgery
Weiss Memorial Hospital
Chicago, Illinois

Rebecca B. Schechter, MD
Endocrinologist
Highland Park, Illinois

Anup Shah
Glickman Urological and Kidney Institute
Cleveland Clinic
Cleveland, Ohio

Matthew Siedhoff, MD, MSCR
Associate Professor
Minimally Invasive Gynecologic Surgery
Cedars-Sinai Medical Center
University of California
Los Angeles, California

Daniel Simon, DMD, MSc
Director and Head Surgeon
FACIALTEAM Surgical Group
HC Marbella International Hospital
Marbella, Spain

Tonya N. Thomas, MD
Associate Staff
Center for Urogynecology and Pelvic Reconstructive Surgery
Obstetrics, Gynecology & Women's Health Institute
Cleveland Clinic
Cleveland, Ohio

Carolyn Wolf-Gould, MD
Family Physician, Medical Director
The Gender Wellness Center/Susquehanna Family Practice
A.O. Fox Hospital/The Bassett Health Care Network
Oneonta, New York

Christopher Wolf-Gould, MD
Family Physician
The Gender Wellness Center/Susquehanna Family Practice
A.O. Fox Hospital/The Bassett Health Care Network
Oneonta, New York

Kevan Wylie, MD, FRCP, FRCPsych, FRCOG, FECSM
Honorary Professor of Sexual Medicine (Retired)
Neurosciences
University of Sheffield
Sheffield, United Kingdom

Sam Winter, B.Sc., P.G.D.E., M.Ed., Ph.D
Team leader, Human Sexuality
Associate Professor
School of Public Health
Faculty of Health Sciences
Curtin University
Perth, Australia

PREFACE

Transgender health and care now seem to be at the forefront of the medical conversation. Over the last decade, transgender individuals have become more visible, and their health-care needs are being addressed. Multidisciplinary teams of providers are being created in many prominent medical centers across the country, and care of this patient community continues to improve. Even better, outcomes of this type of care are now being studied, and the literature is starting to become more robust.

The intent of this textbook is to create a comprehensive overview of transgender health and care so that all providers caring for patients may use it as a reference to understand the health-care needs of transgender individuals. While the focus is mainly on transgender adults, two chapters on pediatric and adolescent management of transgender youth are included. Also included is an in-depth review of transition-specific services, including hormone therapy and surgical options for patients, in addition to an overview of routine health maintenance care that is integral to the overall care of the transgender patient.

More light is also being shed on transgender patients' reproductive needs as they relate to gynecologic care for both men and women, as well as their fertility health. In this book, these topics are explored, and up-to-date literature is provided.

The surgical chapters are meant to provide an overview of the basic techniques used to assist patients in affirming their genders through facial, chest, and/or genital surgery. These chapters include descriptions of each surgery, as well as illustrations or images depicting outcomes for each type of surgery described.

All authors of this textbook are dedicated providers who render care to transgender patients within their specialty of medicine. All authors are experts in their fields, and I was very fortunate to have each and every one graciously accept their invitation to contribute to this project. This is the first edition of this book, and I look forward to updating it as we continue to innovate this very extraordinary specialty.

ACKNOWLEDGMENTS

I would like to acknowledge Dr. Mark Walters, who provided me with a lot of guidance in the development of this textbook, allowing me to use one of his as a beautiful template. I would like to also acknowledge Natalie Weigand and the FPMRS fellows at Cleveland Clinic, who have and continue to take care of my transgender patients. Lastly, I would like to acknowledge Tina Reed, who has gone above and beyond to serve the transgender community and continues to be an integral part of my team.

CONTENTS

1

An Introduction to Gender Diversity

GAIL KNUDSON | SAM WINTER | STEFAN BARAL | SARI REISNER | KEVAN WYLIE

Introduction

Transsexual, transgender, and gender nonconforming individuals have been a part of all cultures historically, yet the emergence of, and advocacy for, transgender individuals in the Western world have become prominent only in recent decades.

The majority of clinical experience related to transgender care is derived from higher-income settings. Therefore local adaptation of clinical care protocols is required, in view of varying cultures and social norms across low- and middle-income countries. Gender roles are culturally stereotyped in most societies where men and women are supposed to participate in masculine and feminine roles specific to their assigned sex at birth.[1]

Deviation from normative gender roles often results in devaluation of social status and experiences of stigma.[2,3] Although transgender people exist across cultures throughout the world, transgenderism and transsexualism are considered abnormal in most societies, because they transgress the normative sex-gender binary system.[4-6] Perceptions of transgender people are affected by the profound differences in culture, religion, and history that exist between countries, and presentation and acceptance of gender diversity can vary widely even within regions of the world. For example, the variation in acceptance of gender diversity across Asia is independent of religion, economic level, and even subregion, with some countries having broader acceptance (such as Thailand, Laos, and Indonesia) and other countries (including Malaysia) having less acceptance.[7-12] Although many transgender people struggle to establish a separate gender category beyond the male-female binary system, only a few countries have acknowledged transgender as a "third" gender. In December of 2007, the Supreme Court of Nepal issued a groundbreaking verdict in favor of gender minorities and recognition of a third gender. In November 2013, two remarkable developments took place in the gender debate and legal and human rights framework: Germany became the first European country to officially recognize a third gender for babies born with ambiguous genitalia, through a new legislation by the country's constitutional court[13]; and the Government of Bangladesh officially approved a proposal by the social welfare ministry to identify transgender women (also known as *hijra*) within a separate gender category.[14] In April 2014, India's Supreme Court recognized transgender people as members of a third gender in a landmark ruling.[15] In 2015, the Nepalese authorities decided to issue passports to gender minorities, adding a third gender category.[16]

Although transgender people across cultures are known by various indigenous terms, the increased visibility in many settings of transgender women, compared with transgender men, has resulted in increased social awareness of these women. Transgender women across many settings share some commonalities, such as preferences for feminine attire and body gestures, a sense of community, and, because of their gender incongruence, a status that has traditionally not been socioculturally, religiously, politically, and legally acknowledged. Because of such pervasive nonacceptance, many transgender women seek social or medical transition.[1,17] Nevertheless, scientific information about transition-related issues is scarce. Access to transition-related health services is often limited, especially in many low- and middle-income countries. Many transgender women seek clinical or surgical procedures, or both, by taking hormones, removal of genitals, or other gender-affirming surgery.[18-20] For example, hijras in south Asian countries often seek social and psychological fulfillment by partial or complete removal of the male genital organs (castration) by modern or traditional caregivers, and some even seek modern gender affirmation surgery that is unavailable in their home countries.[21,22] The limited numbers of clinically skilled providers and high costs of medical interventions in most Asian countries have encouraged access to providers who are unskilled in performing medical interventions, causing untoward physical and psychological effects.[23]

Castration for transgender women involves removal of the penis and scrotum without the construction of female genitals. The underlying reasons for seeking castration and gender affirming surgery can go further than relief from physical dysphoria and perceived needs for compatible and socially acceptable sex-gender aligned lifestyles. The meaning of castration can vary—for example, for some hijra, it represents sociocultural restructuring through which they ensure their economic survival by their engagement with the hijra community.[23] Members of this community can earn their living through traditional hijra occupations (known as *badhai*), such as collecting money from the market places (*bazar tola*) and blessing newborn babies (*bachcha nachano*).[24] Castration can also enhance their self-esteem, power, and status within and outside of the hijra community; through castration they become "real" hijras[21,23] who can earn more than noncastrated hijras through badhai and by selling sex.

Not all transgender women go through castration or gender-affirming surgery. Instead, many adopt feminine gestures, clothing, voices, and roles. This type of sociocultural adaptation enables the individual to have the experience of being transgender without any medical or surgical intervention. Those who have undergone castration often report substantial physical side effects, such as urethral strictures, severe infections, and loss of libido.[23,25-27] Moreover, social and legal dilemmas exist. For example, some noncastrated hijra believe that medical intervention may reemphasize the dominant binary gender construction that ignores transgender as a separate gender. This is seen as a violation of their basic rights to life and survival.

1

People whose gender identity does not align with a rigid male/female dichotomy have been ostracized, leading to pervasive stigma and discrimination in all areas of life for transgender people. Normative notions often marginalize transgender people and place them in an abusive sociolegal environment, in which they are sociopolitically, religiously, and economically excluded from the mainstream, which in turn may enhance their risk-taking behaviors.[3] Pathologization of gender and sexual minorities in the Western medical model[28] has often resulted in transgender people being labeled as deviant individuals requiring medical and legal attention. As cross-cultural diversity and fluidity of gender and sexuality have received attention, it is expected that standard care and services for transgender people will become available in most countries within the framework of human rights.

Legislative Changes and Trends

Many countries do not offer legal or administrative measures enabling gender recognition for transgender people. Even in Europe, which is often seen as progressive on these matters, 8 out of 49 states fail to offer any such measures. Worryingly, among the 33 states where measures are available, 17 impose sterilization requirements on those who seek recognition, despite opposition from authoritative voices in health and human rights, who view such requirements as a form of coercive medicine. Some states are moving towards less intrusive legal arrangements for gender recognition. In Europe, 10 states (Austria, Belarus, Denmark, Germany, Ireland, Malta, Moldova, the Netherlands, Portugal, and the United Kingdom) have dispensed with requirements for any type of medical intervention.[29] Steps towards less onerous legal requirements have also taken place in parts of Canada, the United States, Australia, New Zealand, Nepal, India, and Pakistan.

Three European countries—Denmark, Malta, and Ireland—have stopped their medical requirements altogether (even a requirement for a diagnosis), following the lead of Argentina in adopting a so-called declaration model, in which transgender people are able to determine their gender through a simple administrative procedure.[30]

The Argentinian and Maltese laws are particularly progressive.[31,32] First, they extend legal gender change rights to children and young people. At least two children in Argentina, one of whom was aged 6 years, have availed themselves of this right. Second, these laws explicitly affirm the right of transgender people to appropriate health care. The Maltese law arguably goes the furthest. It contains antidiscrimination provisions offering protection on the grounds of not only gender identity but also gender expression.

There are also provisions that are of particular importance for intersex infants and young children, as they prohibit any medical procedures on the sex characteristics of a minor until that minor can provide informed consent. Several countries are also providing opportunities for transgender people to be recognized outside the gender binary. New Zealand, Australia, Nepal, Pakistan, and India have moved, or are moving, towards such changes.

Community-based organizations continue to fight for gender recognition rights and for removal of onerous requirements for approval.[33] Research on the effect of legislative changes on gender recognition is sparse. Available findings suggest that such changes can positively affect transgender people's quality of life.[34]

Terminology: Spectrum of Gender Identity and Expression

CISGENDER PERSON

A person whose gender identity matches his or her sex assigned at birth and who therefore, unlike transgender people, experiences no gender incongruence.

GENDER

The attitudes, feelings, and behaviors linked to the experience and expression of one's biological sex.

GENDER IDENTITY

The personal experience of oneself as a boy or man, girl or woman, as a mix of the two, as neither, or as a gender beyond man or woman. Some individuals (particularly in cultures which accept the idea of genders beyond man and woman) identify as members of "third genders" or use indigenous gender labels.

GENDER EXPRESSION

The expression of one's gender identity, often through appearance and mode of dress, and also sometimes through behavior and interests. Gender expression is often influenced by gender stereotypes.

GENDER STEREOTYPES

Ideas, current in the culture and times in which a person lives, about the different characteristics that men and women have and should have. Many transgender people can encounter rejection and hostility because of departure from a gender stereotype.

GENDER INCONGRUENCE

Incongruence between a person's own experience of their gender (gender identity) and the sex assigned to them at birth (birth-assigned sex).[35]

Gender incongruence can have two aspects: social incongruence, between a person's gender identity and the gender that others recognize on the basis of that person's birth-assigned sex; and physical incongruence, between a person's gender identity and their primary or secondary sex characteristics.

GENDER DYSPHORIA

Discomfort or distress connected with one's own gender incongruence (social, physical, or both).

GENDER TRANSITION

A person's adoption of characteristics that they feel match their gender identity.[35] Gender transition can involve social aspects such as changing appearance (including styles of dress and hair) and name, arranging new identity documents, or simply the use of a more suitable gendered pronoun. It can also involve a change in physical characteristics. Physical transition can facilitate social transition, enabling styles of dress, social activities, and (in many countries) changes in documentation that would not otherwise be possible. Those who engage in a physical transition are often popularly described as transsexual people.

SEX

A person's biological status (chromosomal, hormonal, gonadal, and genital) as male or female. An individual's sex at birth (birth-assigned sex) is usually determined on the basis of genital appearance.

SEXUAL ORIENTATION

Sexual orientation is about whom one is sexually attracted to and is not the same as gender identity.

TRANSGENDER PERSON

Transgender people experience a degree of gender incongruence. Some intersex people, as well as some people considered by others to be cross dressers or transvestites, experience gender incongruence and accompanying dysphoria.

TRANSGENDER MAN

A person assigned female who identifies as a man or in similar terms (e.g., as a "trans man" or "man of transgender experience").

TRANSGENDER WOMAN

A person assigned male at birth who identifies as a woman or in similar terms (e.g., as a "trans woman" or "woman of transgender experience").

Epidemiology and Population Trends

We do not know how many transgender people there are or how many experience a need for health care, which poses a problem for health-care planners. The first task for the researcher in this area is to decide whom to count and by what means. Transgender people are a very diverse group. Some live with their gender incongruence but decide not to transition. Some make a social transition only, without accessing any gender-affirming health care. Some buy hormones from nonmedical providers (or on the internet), or visit their local doctors rather than attending specialized clinics. In many parts of the world, stigma discourages transgender people from making their transgender status known to others or accessing health care of any sort. These and other considerations present challenges to the researcher attempting to ascertain the size of the transgender population.

Faced with these difficulties, researchers have tended to focus on the most easily counted subgroup: those who seek gender-affirming health care at specialist clinics. Clinic-based data are important for the planning of clinic-based services. However, such numbers grossly underestimate the size of the broader population of transgender people who cannot or do not access clinics, and tell us little about the much larger numbers who may benefit from information and counseling services.

More direct methods for estimating population sizes, in which samples from the general population are questioned about their identity, generate estimates ranging from 0.5% to 1.3% for birth-assigned males and from 0.4% to 1.2% for birth-assigned females (Table 1.1). If one of the lower estimates in the table is extrapolated to a global population of 5.1 billion people aged 15 years and older (US Census Bureau, estimates for mid-2011), we arrive at a figure of approximately 25 million transgender people worldwide. This gives some idea of the potential worldwide (and currently largely unmet) need for transgender health care.

Etiology

A growing body of scientific evidence is now available to inform debate on the extent to which biological factors (especially hormonal and genetic), rather than factors such as parenting or social environment, contribute to the development of gender identity. Putative contributing factors that are not biological are not within the scope of this section. However, gender outcomes are probably influenced by interactions between underlying biology and cultural norms, which generate social pressures on children (including those from parents) to conform to behaviors typically associated with the sex assigned at

TABLE 1.1	Population Studies Yielding Prevalence Data for Transgender People				
	Sample	Measure	PREVALENCE OF TRANSGENDER PEOPLE BY BIRTH-ASSIGNED SEX		
			Male	Female	All
Glen and Hurrell[36] United Kingdom	9950 adults	Identification as other gender or in another way	0–6%	0.4%	0.5%
Clark et al.[36a] New Zealand	7729 high school students	Identification as transgender	1.3%	1.2%	1.2%
Kuyper and Wijsen[36b] Netherlands	8064 adults	Identification on gender spectrum	1–1%	0–8%	0.9%
Van Caenegem et al.[36c] Belgium	1832 adults	Identification on gender spectrum	0.7%	0–6%	0–6%

From Winter S, Diamond J, Green J, et al. Transgender people: health at the margins of society. *The Lancet.* 2016;388:390–400.

birth. Despite these pressures, gender-variant children identify in a way that is incongruent with their birth-assigned sex,[37] which they may express in behaviors that contravene the norms of their culture. To date, research has established no clear correlations between parenting and gender incongruence.[38,39] In circumstances where infants have been born with ambiguous genitalia, neither genital surgery intended to "correct" the sex anatomy, nor parental upbringing in a social role consistent with that anatomy, guarantees that the child develops a gender identity congruent with the one to which he or she has been surgically and socially assigned. Similarly, when a male infant has been surgically assigned to female anatomy after accidental damage to the penis, it is impossible to guarantee that the child will grow up identifying as a girl. These findings indicate that early brain development seems to have an indelible effect on gender identity that is resistant to normative social pressures[40-45] and that may result from prenatal sex hormones,[46] direct genetic effects,[47] or both.

Biological influences are evident in several other research findings. Two studies have reported the presence of repeat polymorphisms in the gene coding for the androgen receptor in transgender women, suggesting that these individuals have an atypical response to testosterone.[48,49] Other research has shown that some chromosome anomalies in individuals with a male phenotype (such as XXY, XYY, and mosaicism) are associated with a raised incidence of individuals who identify as women.[50,51] There is also evidence that low androgen levels associated with medication use in pregnancy may be associated with a higher incidence of gender dysphoria in an XY fetus.[52]

Additional studies of family cooccurrence of gender dysphoria indicate that there may be a genetic link in a subset of transgender individuals.[53] Studies of twins have shown that monozygotic twins have a significantly higher likelihood of concordance for transgenderism than dizygotic twins. In one study, 33% of male monozygotic twin pairs (where at least one twin had transitioned) were concordant for transition, including two pairs of twins who were reared apart from birth. Concordance for transition was 23% among female monozygotic twins where one twin had transitioned to live as a man, and this included one pair of twins who were raised apart. By contrast, concordance for transition among male or female dizygotic twins was reported to be low.[54]

Studies of cerebral lateralization of neural pathways associated with listening ability reveal differences between male and female brains in cisgender individuals (persons who identify in a way that is consistent with their assigned sex at birth). A study of click-evoked otoacoustic emissions in untreated children and adolescents experiencing gender incongruence (24 assigned male at birth, identifying as girls), demonstrated responses that were more in agreement with those of 62 cisgender girl controls than with those of 65 cisgender boys. The findings did not support the hypothesis that increased prenatal exposure to androgens had an opposite effect, in relation to otoacoustic emissions, on gender incongruent young people assigned female at birth. However, in cases of gender incongruent birth-assigned males, the authors postulate that atypically low in utero testosterone levels may affect the crucial period of sex differentiation in the brain. Similarly, a study of dichotic listening in transgender women showed that their lateralization resembled that of cisgender women rather than that of cisgender men.[55] The cohort of transgender men and women involved in this study also showed a markedly raised prevalence of non-right-handedness compared with the cisgender population. This finding augments those of previous studies, and it is highly likely that there is an association between gender incongruence and atypical brain development.[56,57]

Other studies have also shown that sensitivity to odors may be different in transgender individuals compared with those who are cisgender. Transgender women have demonstrated certain odor sensitivity patterns that reflect their gender identity, rather than their assigned birth sex, suggesting that there may be sex-atypical physiologic responses in specific hypothalamic circuits.[58]

Not all cadaveric or in vivo studies of transgender individuals have revealed cross-sex characteristics,[59] but there are many studies that have. For example, post-mortem studies of small numbers of transgender individuals, two of which focused on the central subdivision of the bed-nucleus of the stria terminalis, and one on the uncinate nucleus, suggest neural differentiation that is discordant with genital and gonadal characteristics at birth but similar to that of cisgender individuals of the same gender identity.[60-63] A study based on scans of the white matter in the brains of transgender men who had not yet undergone hormone treatment showed that their neural patterns were masculinized and closer to those of birth-assigned males than to those of birth-assigned females.[64] Scans in untreated transgender women showed that their patterns were feminized and were substantially different than those of birth-assigned male and female controls.[65]

In summary, the aforementioned research provides compelling evidence that the neurobiology of the brain is important in predisposing an individual to incongruence between his or her gender identity and his or her assigned sex at birth. However, people experiencing gender incongruence, including those who are gender dysphoric, might have one, more than one, or none of these markers. Therefore these indicators cannot be used diagnostically and only serve to help us better understand the etiology of transgenderism.

Guidelines: Framework for Transition and Care

The World Professional Association for Transgender Health (WPATH) is an international, multidisciplinary professional association that promotes evidence-based care, education, research, advocacy, public policy, and respect in transsexual and transgender health care. The association first published its standards of care in 1979 with the goal of advancing this underserved population's access to evidence-based health care, social services, justice, and equality. The most recent version (version 7, published in 2012) maintains the aim of promoting safe and effective pathways that allow transsexual, transgender, and gender nonconforming individuals to achieve lasting personal comfort with their gendered selves, maximize their overall health, and promote psychological well-being and self-fulfillment. The standards of care document is intentionally worded to allow flexibility, in order to meet diverse health-care needs, and the core principles can be applied to a wide range of settings.

The 7th version of the standards of care contains several improvements. First, it includes the concept that gender nonconformity is not, in and of itself, pathologic. However, the guidelines acknowledge that those who experience distress related to gender dysphoria and who want to make a physical transition are entitled to and should have access to medically necessary treatment.

Second, the guidelines now clarify that, although psychotherapy is not an absolute requirement for individuals to access medical interventions, an assessment and referral by a healthcare professional with training in transgender health is essential. There is an emphasis on the importance of the role of the mental health professional in helping to improve overall health and fulfillment. Mental health professionals are able to address the negative effects of stigma and prejudice experienced by many transgender individuals, they help their clients to find their most comfortable and fulfilling gender expression, and, if applicable, they can assist with gender role changes and mitigate the challenges that are associated with coming out.

Third, the most recent version of the standards of care provides a very clear set of guidelines for patients wishing to start hormone therapy or who desire to undergo breast or chest surgery. Patients must present with persistent, well-documented gender dysphoria; must demonstrate the capacity to make a fully informed decision and to consent for treatment; and must be the legal age of adulthood in the country of treatment (Table 1.2). If substantial medical or mental health concerns are present, documentation must show that these conditions are well managed. Although not an explicit criterion, the guidelines recommend that individuals undergoing feminizing transition undergo feminizing hormone therapy for a minimum of 12 months before breast construction surgery. This approach maximizes breast growth, which allows for better surgical (aesthetic) results, and also confirms the steadiness of the desire to transition. To be qualified to write a recommendation for hormone therapy or breast or chest surgery, a healthcare professional should have appropriate training and professional licensure in behavioral health and have demonstrated competency in the assessment of gender dysphoria. This experience is particularly important when the professional is part of a multidisciplinary specialist team that provides access to feminizing or masculinizing hormone therapy.

Fourth, in addition to the criteria set for hormone therapy, the standards of care recommend 12 months of continuous living in a gender role that is congruent with the person's gender identity for genital surgery, which includes metoidioplasty or phalloplasty in female-towards-male transition, and vaginoplasty in male-towards-female transition (Table 1.3). Twelve

months of hormone therapy is recommended for hysterectomy or ovariectomy in female-towards-male transitions or orchiectomy in male-towards-female transitions. A letter of recommendation from a qualified mental health professional is required for hormone therapy referral or breast surgery, and two letters from two independent qualified mental health professionals are required for genital surgery.

Fifth, the guidelines state that any adolescent requesting puberty-suppressing hormones should demonstrate a long-lasting and intense pattern of gender nonconformity or gender dysphoria (whether suppressed or expressed), with gender dysphoria emerging or worsening with the onset of puberty (at least Tanner stage 2). As in adults, any coexisting psychological, medical, or social problems that could interfere with treatment (e.g., factors that might compromise treatment adherence) should be successfully managed before hormone therapy is started. In addition, the document states that adolescents may be eligible to begin feminizing or masculinizing hormone therapy, preferably with parental consent. Intervention usually starts with the use of Gonadotropin-releasing hormone (GnRH) agonists or antagonists, which block the development of secondary sexual characteristics of the natal sex. If these treatments are stopped, secondary sex characteristics will develop along the lines of the individual's sex assigned at birth.

In adolescents, cross-sex hormones are added later in the treatment pathway; in many countries this occurs when the legal age of independent medical decision making has been reached. The adolescent must provide written assent to treatment, in addition to the informed consent obtained from parents or legal guardians. In many countries, 16 year olds are legal adults for the purpose of medical decision making and do not require parental consent. Ideally, treatment decisions should be made in collaboration between the adolescent, the family, and the treatment team. Although chest surgery can be performed earlier, genital surgery should not be undertaken until the patient has reached the legal age of adulthood in the

TABLE 1.2 Criteria for Hormones and Upper Body Surgery, WPATH Standards of Care (Version 7)			
Criteria for Adults: 1 Letter	Hormone Therapy	Chest Surgery	Breast Augmentation*
Persistent, well-documented gender dysphoria	✓	✓	✓
Capacity to make a fully informed decision and to consent for treatment	✓	✓	✓
Age of majority in a given country	✓	✓	✓
If significant medical or mental concerns are present, they must be reasonably well controlled	✓	✓	✓

*means the criteria one should meet in order to do the procedure.
WPATH, World Professional Association for Transgender Health.
From Wylie K, Knudson G, Khan SI, et al. Serving transgender people: clinical care considerations and service delivery models in transgender health. *The Lancet.* 2016;388:401–411.

TABLE 1.3 Criteria for Lower Body Surgery, WPATH Standards of Care (Version 7)		
Criteria for Adults: 2 Letters	Gonadectomy	Genital Surgery*
Persistent, well-documented gender dysphoria	✓	✓
Capacity to make a fully informed decision and to consent for treatment	✓	✓
Age of majority in a given country	✓	✓
If significant medical or mental concerns are present, they must be well controlled	✓	✓
12 continuous months of hormone therapy as appropriate to the patient's gender goals (unless the patient has a medical contraindication or is otherwise unable or unwilling to take hormones)	✓	✓
12 continuous months of living in a gender role that is congruent with their gender identity		✓

*means the criteria one should meet in order to do the procedure.
WPATH, World Professional Association for Transgender Health.
From Wylie K, Knudson G, Khan SI, et al. Serving transgender people: clinical care considerations and service delivery models in transgender health. *The Lancet.* 2016;388:401–411.

country of treatment and has lived continuously for at least 12 months in the gender role that is congruent with their gender identity.

The WPATH standards of care provide clear guidelines for the health care and transition care of patients. They also represent an advocacy platform for the advancement of public policies and legal reforms that promote tolerance and equity for gender and sexual diversity, to eliminate prejudice, discrimination, and stigma. There are also many country-specific guidelines that exist (e.g., in the United Kingdom[66]), and these are informed by the WPATH standards of care.

REFERENCES

1. Connell RW. *Gender.* Cambridge: Polity; 2002.
2. Wirth JH, Bodenhausen GV. The role of gender in mental-illness stigma: a national experiment. *Psychol Sci.* 2009;20:169–173.
3. Khan SI, Hussain MI, Parveen S, et al. Living on the extreme margin: social exclusion of the transgender population (hijra) in Bangladesh. *J Health Popul Nutr.* 2009;27:441–451.
4. Hines S. *Transforming Gender: Transgender Practices of Identity, Intimacy and Care.* Bristol: The Policy Press, University of Bristol; 2007.
5. Rice ME, Harris GT. Is androgen deprivation therapy effective in the treatment of sex off enders? *Psychol Public Policy Law.* 2011;17:315–332.
6. Sam H. *Transgender Representations.* Singapore: National University of Singapore; 2010.
7. Chokrungvaranont P, Selvaggi G, Jindarak S, et al. The development of sex reassignment surgery in Thailand: a social perspective. *Scientific World J.* 2014;2014(2):182981.
8. Doussantousse S, Sakounnavong B, Patterson I. An expanding sexual economy along National Route 3 in Luang Namtha Province, Lao PDR. *Cult Health Sex.* 2011;13(suppl 2):S279–S291.
9. *Pew Research Center.* The global divide on homosexuality. Greater acceptance in more secular and affluent countries. http://www.pewglobal.org/2013/06/04/the-global-divide-on-homosexuality/; Accessed 14.12.18.
10. Melayu B. World Report 2015: Malaysia. In: *Human Rights Watch*: 2015.
11. Offord B, Cantrell L. Homosexual rights as human rights in Indonesia and Australia. *J Homosex.* 2001;40:233–252.
12. Laurent E. Sexuality and human rights: an Asian perspective. *J Homosex.* 2005;48:163–225.
13. Nandi J. Germany got it right by offering a third gender option on birth certificates. In: *Guardian (London)*: 2013.
14. Karim M. *Hijras Now a Separate Gender.* Dhaka: Dhaka Tribune; 2013.
15. Mahapatra D. *Supreme Court Recognizes Transgenders as 'Third Gender'.* New Delhi: Times of India; 2014.
16. Chin J. Nepal issues its first third-gender passport to recognize LGBT citizens. *Huffington Post Canada.* 2015;.
17. Vidal-Ortiz S. Transgender and transsexual studies: sociology's influence and future steps. *Soc Compass.* 2008;2:433–450.
18. Guadamuz TE, Wimonsate W, Varangrat A, et al. HIV prevalence, risk behavior, hormone use and surgical history among transgender persons in Thailand. *AIDS Behav.* 2011;15:650–658.
19. Winter S, Doussantousse S. Transpeople, hormones, and health risks in southeast Asia: a Lao study. *Int J Sex Health.* 2009;21:35–48.
20. Master V, Santucci R. An American hijra: a report of a case of genital self-mutilation to become India's "third sex". *Urology.* 2003;62:1121.
21. Nanda S. *Neither Man nor Woman.* Belmont, TN: Wadsmorth Publishing; 1990.
22. Nanda S. The hijras of India: cultural and individual dimensions of an institutionalized third gender role. *J Homosex.* 1985;11:35–54.
23. Shreshtha S. *Exploring the Consequences of Castration in the Life of Hijra in Bangladesh.* Dhaka: BRAC University; 2011.
24. Khan SI, Hussain MI, Gourab G, et al. Not to stigmatize but to humanize sexual lives of the transgender (hijra) in Bangladesh: condom chat in the AIDS era. *J LGBT Health Res.* 2008;4:127–141.
25. Brett MA, Roberts LF, Johnson TW, Wassersug RJ. Eunuchs in contemporary society: expectations, consequences, and adjustments to castration (part II). *J Sex Med.* 2007;4:946–955.
26. Masumori N. Status of sex reassignment surgery for gender identity disorder in Japan. *Int J Urol.* 2012;19:402–414.
27. Wassersug RJ, Johnson TW. Modern-day eunuchs: motivations for and consequences of contemporary castration. *Perspect Biol Med.* 2007;50:544–556.
28. Monro S. Transmuting gender binaries: the theoretical challenge. *Sociol Res Online.* 2007;12. https://doi.org/10.5153/sro.1514.
29. *ILGA-EUROPE.* Rainbow map (index). https://www.ilga-europe.org/resources/rainbow-europe/rainbow-europe-2018; Accessed 14.12.18.
30. *Transgender Europe.* Trans rights Europe 2016 map and index 2016. http://tgeu.org/trans-rights_europe_map_2016; Accessed 23.05.16.
31. *Government of Malta.* Gender identity, gender expression and sex characteristics act. http://justiceservices.gov.mt/DownloadDocument.aspx?app=lom&itemid=12312&l=1; 2015 Accessed 18.11.15.
32. *Global Action for Trans* Equality.* English translation of Argentina's gender identity law as approved by the Senate of Argentina on May 8, 2012. http://globaltransaction.files.wordpress.com/2012/05/argentina-gender-identity-law.pdf; 2013 Accessed 23.02.14.
33. Kohler R, Recher A, Ehrt J. *Legal Gender Recognition in Europe Toolkit.* Berlin: Transgender Europe; 2013.
34. Aristegui I, Romero M, Zalazar V, et al. Transgender people perceptions of the impact of the gender identity law in Argentina. In: *20th International AIDS Conference*; 2014. Melbourne, http://pag.aids2014.org/Abstracts.aspx?SID=1112&AID=7341 2014. Accessed 23.05.16.
35. World Professional Association for Transgender Health. *Standards of Care for the Health of Transsexual, Transgender, and Gender Nonconforming People.* 7th ed. Minneapolis, MN: WPATH; 2012.
36. Glen F, Hurrell K. *Technical Note: Measuring Gender Identity.* Manchester: Equality and Human Rights Commission; 2012.
36a. Clark T, Lucassen M, Bullen M, et al. The health and well-being of transgender high school students: results from the New Zealand adolescent health survey (Youth'12). *J Adolesc Health.* 2014;55:93–99.
36b. Kuyper L, Wijsen C. Gender identities and gender dysphoria in the Netherlands. *Arch Sex Behav.* 2014;43:377–385.
36c. Van Caenegem E, Wierckx K, Elaut E, et al. Prevalence of gender nonconformity in Flanders, Belgium. *Arch Sex Behav.* 2015;44:1281–1287.
37. Diamond M. Transsexuality among twins. *Int J Transgend.* 2013;14:24–38.
38. Stevens M, Golombok S, Beveridge M. Does father absence influence children's gender development? Findings from a general population study of pre-school children. *Parent Sci Pract.* 2002;2:47–60.
39. Zucker KJ, Bradley SJ. *Gender Identity Disorder and Psychosexual Problems in Children and Adolescents.* New York, NY: Guilford Press; 1995.
40. Diamond M, Sigmundson HK. Sex reassignment at birth. Long term review and clinical implications. *Arch Pediatr Adolesc Med.* 1997;151:298–304.
41. Kipnis K, Diamond M. Pediatric ethics and the surgical assignment of sex. *J Clin Ethics.* 1998;9:398–410.
42. Ochoa B. Trauma of the external genitalia in children: amputation of the penis and emasculation. *J Urol.* 1996;160:1116–1119.
43. Bradley SJ, Oliver GD, Chernick AB, Zucker KJ. Experiment of nurture: ablatio penis at 2 months, sex reassignment at 7 months, and a psychosexual follow-up in young adulthood. *Paediatrics.* 1998;102:e9.
44. Hines M. *Brain Gender.* New York, NY: Oxford University Press; 2004.
45. Dessens AB, Froukje ME, Slijper FME, Stenver LS, Drop SLS. Gender dysphoria and gender change in chromosomal females with congenital adrenal hyperplasia. *Arch Sex Behav.* 2005;34:389397.
46. Bao A-M, Swaab DF. Sexual differentiation of the human brain: relation to gender identity, sexual orientation and neuropsychiatric disorders. *Front Neuroendocrinol.* 2011;32:214–226.
47. Dewing P, Shi T, Horvath S, Vilain E. Sexually dimorphic gene expression in mouse brain precedes gonadal differentiation. *Mol Brain Res.* 2003;118:82–90.
48. Hare L, Bernard P, Sanchez FJ, et al. Androgen receptor repeat length polymorphism associated with male to female transsexualism. *Biol Psychiatry.* 2008;65:93–96.
49. Henningsson S, Westberg L, Nilsson S, et al. Sex steroid related genes and male to female transsexualism. *Psychoneuroendocrinology.* 2005;30:657–664.
50. Snaith RP, Penhale S, Horsfield P. Male-to-female transsexual with XYY karyotype. *Lancet.* 1991;337:557–558.

51. Wylie KR, Steward D. A consecutive series of 52 transsexual people presenting for assessment and chromosomal analysis at a gender identity clinic. *International Journal of Transgenderism*. 2008;10:147–148.

52. Dessens AB, Cohen-Kettenis PT, Mellenbergh GJ, van der Poll NE, Koppe JG, Boer K. Prenatal exposure to anticonvulsants and psychosexual development. *Arch Sex Behav*. 1999;28:31–44.

53. Green R. Family co-occurrence of gender dysphoria: ten sibling or parent-child pairs. *Arch Sex Behav*. 2000;29:499–507.

54. Burke S, Menks W, Cohen-Kettenis P, et al. Click-evoked otoacoustic emissions in children and adolescents with gender identity disorder. *Arch Sex Behav*. 2014;43:1515–1523.

55. Govier E, Diamond M, Wolowiec T, Slade C. Dichotic listening, handedness, brain organisation and transsexuality. *Int J Transgender*. 2010;12:144–154.

56. Green R, Young R. Hand preference, sexual preference, and transsexualism. *Arch Sex Behav*. 2001;30:565–574.

57. Zucker KJ, Beaulieu N, Bradley SJ, et al. Handedness in boys with gender identity disorder. *J Clin Child Psychol Psychiatr*. 2001;42:767–776.

58. Burglund H, Lindstrom P, Dhejne-Helmy C, Savic I. Male-to-female transsexuals show sex-atypical hypothalamus activation when smelling odorous steroids. *Cereb Cortex*. 2008;18:1900–1908.

59. Savic I, Arver S. Sex dimorphism of the brain in male-to-female transsexuals. *Cereb Cortex*. 2011;21:2525–2533.

60. Luders E, Sánchez FJ, Gaser CW, et al. Regional gray matter variation in male-to-female transsexualism. *Neuroimage*. 2009;46:904–907.

61. Zhou J-N, Swaab DF, Gooren LJ, Hofman MA. A sex difference in the human brain and its relation to transsexuality. *Nature*. 1995;378:68–70.

62. Kruijver FPM, Zhou J-N, Pool CW, et al. Male to female transsexuals have female neuron numbers in a limbic nucleus. *J Endocrinol Metabol*. 2000;85:2034–2041.

63. Garcia-Falgueras A, Swaab DF. A sex difference in the hypothalamic uncinate nucleus: relationship to gender identity. *Brain*. 2008;131:3132–3146.

64. Rametti G, Carrillo B, Gómez-Gil E, et al. White matter microstructure in female to male transsexuals before cross-sex hormonal treatment. A diffusion tensor imaging study. *J Psychiatr Res*. 2011;45:199–204.

65. Rametti G, Carrillo B, Gómez-Gil E, et al. The microstructure of white matter in male to female transsexuals before cross-sex hormonal treatment. A DTI study. *J Psychiatr Res*. 2011;45:949–954.

66. Wylie K, Barrett J, Besser M, et al. Good practice guidelines for the assessment and treatment of adults with gender dysphoria. *Sex Relatsh Ther*. 2014;29:154–214.

Mental Health Care for the Adult Transgender Patient

DAN H. KARASIC

Introduction

Transgender identity is not a mental illness; however, mental health assessment and care is an integral part of transgender care. Transgender people may present with gender dysphoria, for help in exploring their gender identity, or for mental health conditions like depression, anxiety, or substance abuse that may be related to societal prejudice and trauma, which are commonly experienced by trans people.[1] Misunderstanding or failure to recognize an individual's affirmed gender may worsen their mental health symptoms while acknowledgement of their name and/or gender may help to reduce depression and suicidal thinking.[2]

The role of the mental health provider is to provide a safe and supportive space, incorporating the principles of cultural humility in the provision of care to patients.[3] In addition to providing mental health care, providers have a key role in assessing clients/patients for transition-specific medical and surgical care. This role is described in detail by the World Professional Association for Transgender Health (WPATH) in their standards of care (SOC), currently in its seventh version.[4]

Evolution of the DSM and Diagnostic Criteria in DSM 5

A diagnosis of *Transsexualism* entered the *Diagnostic and Statistical Manual of Mental Disorders* (DSM) with the publication of DSM III in 1980.[5] The criteria for diagnosis included discomfort with one's assigned sex, dressing as the other sex, and a desire to change primary and secondary sex characteristics. In DSM III-R, published in 1987, *Transsexualism* was placed in the category of Disorders Usually First Evident in Infancy, Childhood, or Adolescence. *Gender Identity Disorder (GID) of Childhood* was a diagnosis given to prepubertal children in the DSM III and III-R.[6] The DSM III-R also included a diagnosis called *Gender Identity Disorder (GID) of Adolescence or Adulthood, Nontranssexual Type*.

In the DSM IV, published in 1994, diagnoses of *Transsexualism* and *GID of Children* were both replaced with *GID* alone, with criteria for adolescents and adults and a separate set of criteria for children, in the *Sexual and Gender Identity Disorders* chapter.[7] *GID in Adolescents and Adults* in the DSM IV and DSM IV-TR (2000) is characterized by "a strong and persistent cross-gender identification" and a persistent discomfort with one's sex or gender role, a desire for medical or surgical treatment, and a belief that one was "born the wrong sex."[8] *GID in Adolescents and Adults* was criticized for a number of reasons. First, the diagnosis was binary, with references made to a "cross-gender identity" and "opposite sex." Second, a belief that one was born the wrong sex was considered inaccurate criteria because this type of belief could persist posttransition. Third, using this diagnosis, a desire for treatment was considered a symptom of a disorder,

rather than a healthy response to distress. And last, the name of the diagnosis itself implied that transgender identity was a mental disorder.[9,10] Furthermore, the chapter on *Sexual and Gender Identity Disorders* included a section on paraphilias, which included transvestic fetishism and other paraphilias, some of which involved criminal behavior, such as pedophilia.

The *GID in Children* diagnosis in the DSM IV and DSM IV-TR was also criticized. *GID in Children* criteria included gender nonconforming behaviors. Only one criterion was related to cross-gender identity, and it was not required to make the diagnosis. As a result, persistent gender nonconformity in youth without transgender identity could be assigned the diagnosis. One of the biggest criticisms of persistence and desistance of gender dysphoria from prepubertal childhood into adulthood is that several studies examining this used the *GID in Children* diagnosis, which could be made with gender nonconforming behavior alone, without transgender identity.[11]

The most recent version of the DSM is the DSM 5, which was published in 2013, and replaced *GID* with a diagnosis of *Gender Dysphoria (GD)*. In addition, *GD* was removed from the chapter that included the paraphilias. The most significant changes from the *GID* diagnosis to *GD* include the following: (1) As indicated by the terminology change, *GD* is the distress related to the difference between one's assigned gender and one's experienced gender, rather than the identity that is associated with being transgender. An individual has the diagnosis as long as there is clinically significant distress or social/occupational impairment related to the incongruence between their identity and how they were born. The diagnosis does include a posttransition specifier, which allows for ongoing treatment, for example, with hormones. (2) Unlike *GID*, which describes a binary trans identity and transition, *GD* includes nonbinary people. Identity and transition do not have to be related to the "opposite" sex, but rather can be related to any identity along the gender spectrum, including identifying as nonbinary or agender (Table 2.1).[12]

The World Health Organization released the International Classification of Diseases, 11th Revision (ICD 11) in 2018. ICD 11 replaces *transsexualism* from the ICD 10 with *Gender Incongruence*.[13] Like *GD*, *Gender Incongruence* includes nonbinary gender identities and reduces the length of duration of symptoms to several months to formally make the diagnosis. *Gender Incongruence* is not distressed-based like *GD* and belongs in a *Conditions Related to Sexual Health* chapter, apart from the mental disorders, so as to not psychopathologize trans identity (Table 2.2).

WPATH Requirements for Mental Health Professionals

The WPATH has been publishing consensus guidelines for care since 1979. WPATH released the SOC version 7 (SOC 7) in

TABLE 2.1	DSM 5 Criteria for Gender Dysphoria in Adolescents and Adults

A. A marked incongruence between one's experienced/expressed gender and assigned gender, of at least 6 months duration, manifested by at least two of the following:
  1. A marked incongruence between one's experienced/expressed gender and primary or secondary sex characteristics.
  2. A strong desire to be rid of primary or secondary sex characteristics.
  3. A strong desire for the primary or secondary sex characteristics of the other gender.
  4. A strong desire to be the other gender (or some alternative gender).
  5. A strong desire to be treated as the other gender (or some alternative gender).
  6. A strong conviction that one has the typical feelings and reactions of the other gender (or some alternative gender).
B. The condition is associated with clinically significant distress or impairment in social, occupational, or other important areas of functioning.

Specifiers:
With a disorder of sex development
Posttransition

DSM, Diagnostic and Statistical Manual of Mental Disorders.

TABLE 2.2	ICD 11 Criteria for Gender Incongruence of Adolescence and Adulthood

Characterized by a marked and persistent incongruence between an individual's experienced gender and the assigned sex, as manifested by at least two of the following:
1. A strong dislike or discomfort with the one's primary or secondary sex characteristics (in adolescents, anticipated secondary sex characteristics) due to their incongruity with the experienced gender.
2. A strong desire to be rid of some or all of one's primary and/or secondary sex characteristics (in adolescents, anticipated secondary sex characteristics) due to their incongruity with the experienced gender.
3. A strong desire to have the primary and/or secondary sex characteristics of the experienced gender.

The individual experiences a strong desire to be treated (to live and be accepted) as a person of the experienced gender.
The experienced gender incongruence must have been continuously present for at least several months.
The diagnosis cannot be assigned prior to the onset of puberty.
Gender variant behavior and preferences alone are not a basis for assigning the diagnosis.

2011, and the SOC 8 will soon be published. The WPATH SOC is an easily accessible document, and it is available in many languages. The SOC are guidelines that outline the role of the licensed and qualified mental health professional who performs mental health assessments for transgender patients seeking medical and surgical transition. Per the SOC, these qualified mental health professionals can have either a master's or doctoral degree. Assessments may be done with clients or patients in therapy, or people may seek assessments only. Importantly, psychotherapy is not required for these assessments.[4]

The assessment for hormones under the SOC may be done by a mental health professional or, alternatively, a knowledgeable primary care provider or endocrinologist. Criteria for adults to initiate hormone therapy include persistent gender dysphoria, the capacity to give informed consent, and "reasonably well-controlled" mental illness, if present. Individuals who are exploring gender identity or who are addressing their gender dysphoria for the first time may present with significant distress that may be relieved with social transition and the initiation of hormones. Therefore it is important for mental health providers to recognize when this distress should not delay referral for hormone therapy. Conversely, patients with concurrent psychiatric conditions like bipolar disorder or schizophrenia may benefit from stabilization prior to transitioning. The risks and benefits of starting medical transition versus delaying initiation of medical care must be weighed under these circumstances. The ability of the person to give informed consent should be unimpaired, and the benefits of initiation of hormones should outweigh the risks. In clinical practice, stabilization of mental illness and substance abuse often happens concurrently with hormonal transition.[3]

For chest surgery, the SOC require one letter of recommendation and support from a mental health professional. Similar to initiation of hormones, the adult patient must have persistent gender dysphoria and the ability to give informed consent, and concurrent mental illness must be relatively well controlled. For some, chest surgery comes as an early step in transition and may occur before social transition or treatment with hormones. For example, a transmasculine person or trans man may wish to have chest surgery before social transition, because breast binding is uncomfortable and may not be sufficient for the individual to feel comfortable presenting publicly as male. Significant chest dysphoria may occur in individuals assigned female at birth who do not want to start testosterone; these individuals may identify as nonbinary. For trans women, hormone treatment for 1 year is recommended but not required for feminizing mammoplasty. Significant breast tissue development may occur on feminizing hormones, so for some people, surgical augmentation may not be necessary.

For genital surgery, two independent assessments and letters from mental health professionals are required. For adults, persistent gender dysphoria and the ability to give informed consent are required. The person must be on hormones for the 1 year prior to surgery, unless it is clinically not indicated. Social transition to the gender with which the individual identifies is required for 1 year prior to surgery for vaginoplasty, metoidioplasty, and phalloplasty but not for orchiectomy or hysterectomy and/or oophorectomy.[4]

As previously mentioned, the SOC recommend that mental illness must be "reasonably well-controlled" prior to chest or breast surgery and "well-controlled" prior to genital surgery. Note the wording is stronger for genital surgical guidelines than it is for medical transition and chest/breast surgery. Mental illness and substance abuse may impair the individual's ability to give informed consent for surgery. Genital surgery in particular is associated with a significant risk of complications, and these should be well-understood before surgery is performed. Mental illness and substance abuse may impair the patient's ability to keep appointments and follow perioperative instructions. Important postoperative issues, such as regular dilation after vaginoplasty, or being observant for complications may be compromised. Moreover, substance abuse may affect anesthesia or lead to postoperative withdrawal, which can have deleterious consequences. Lastly, tobacco smoking and other nicotine use impairs healing, and cessation needs to be addressed before surgery.

Prevalence and Management of Co-Occurring Mental Health Conditions

Data on the prevalence of co-occurring mental health conditions in trans people suffer from selection bias—many assessments of co-occurring conditions were performed in clinical settings, many of which had gender clinics. However, across studies, the prevalence of both depressive and anxiety disorders is high in this patient population, whereas rates of bipolar disorder and schizophrenia are close to the general population.[14] In one study, dissociative disorders were present in 29.6% of 118 trans patients assessed at a gender clinic.[15] A large web survey showed that 41% of trans people responding had experienced suicidality. Suicidal ideation is particularly common in trans youth.[16] Mental health was substantially improved post transition treatment. In one study of 62 gender clinic patients, 29% made suicide attempts prior to gender confirming surgery, versus 5% afterwards.[17] Interestingly, one study of Swedish mortality records found high rates of suicide in post–gender confirmation surgery patients in the early years of the study, but the difference from the control group was not significant in those receiving surgery in the later years of the study, from 1989 to 2010.[18]

In addition to the distress that is associated with gender dysphoria, many trans people also suffer from trauma and minority stress, often as a result of rejection by family and discrimination in schools and workplaces, and they are unfortunately often the victims of harassment and violence.[19]

Transition often brings great relief of gender dysphoria, but it can also bring new stressors. Trans people may face rejection from those they have counted on for support—partners, family, and friends. Some may face discrimination in the workplace. There may be a period in early transition in which the individual is recognizable to others as trans or gender nonconforming, and they may be sensitive to being identified as such in public.

The clinician should treat co-occurring mental illness, in addition to providing support and guidance in transition. Major depressive disorder, posttraumatic stress disorder, and panic disorder with agoraphobia may respond to medications, such as serotonin reuptake inhibitors, as well as to cognitive behavior therapy and other psychotherapies. Psychotherapy can be a safe and a supportive place to explore options for addressing gender dysphoria, as well as a way to cope with past trauma or with suicidal thoughts. Bipolar disorder and schizophrenia in transgender patients are treated similarly to other patients. Psychosis—hallucinations and delusions—can impair a patient's ability to give informed consent and should be addressed as symptoms are recognized. Some disorders diagnosed in childhood—autism spectrum disorder and attention-deficit/hyperactivity disorder—may remain clinical issues into adulthood.[20] Dissociative disorders should be diagnosed when present. Symptoms may emerge when coping with trauma and other stressors, and rarely, such as with dissociative identity disorder, may intersect with a person's sense of gender identity.[1]

Substance use disorders must also be addressed when present. Some patients may suffer from substance abuse as a means of avoidance coping when trying to suppress gender dysphoria prior to transition. Substance use disorders significantly impact quality of life in people regardless of whether they are cis or trans. In trans people, substance use can interfere with following through on transition care. For those seeking surgery, substance use disorders should be addressed, including tobacco use cessation prior to surgery.

Role of the Mental Health Professional Before, During, and After Transition

Much of the literature on trans care comes from gender clinics and other care providers focusing specifically on transition. Although more youth are transitioning early, trans people continue to present across the life span, seeking transition care. Adults who present for care may recall having an affinity toward another gender from early in their childhood and may recall increasing discomfort with their bodies at puberty. Often, patients will describe not being able to act on their feelings in childhood, even if their sense of gender identity was clear. Some people recognize a sense of difference but do not identify this as being transgender until later into adulthood. People may start careers, marry, and have children, and these may become additional barriers to transition because individuals may fear giving up the life they have for something unknown.[3] If the person has made the decision to transition, a therapist can help them to navigate the process of coming out to family, friends, and the workplace. Issues such as security of housing, finances, and personal safety may be present, depending on the circumstance.

The therapist can help the client to navigate medical and surgical systems, while providing psychoeducation and support.[21] For this, it is important that the mental health professional be knowledgeable on the process of transition, including understanding the benefits and risks for their clients. Exploration of gender identity should be nonjudgmental, and the mental health therapist should not impose their narrative on the client.[3] The mental health professional should ask about gender identity in an open-ended way, without a binary assumption or an assumption that any given transition steps need to be taken. Instead, the mental health professional should follow the client's lead about their identity and the steps they foresee in addressing it.[3] The mental health professional can provide information on the transition process with referrals for medical and surgical care as appropriate, including the assessments and letters needed by other clinicians per the WPATH SOC, or as necessary for insurance coverage. The mental health professional can provide support through the coming out process. Referrals for peer support may be helpful.

A client in therapy may at some point ask for a mental health assessment letter per the SOC or may contact the mental health professional for an evaluation only. Often the evaluation for initiation of hormones may be done by the medical provider, but the prescribing medical provider may request that a mental health professional do the evaluation. For surgery, the evaluations and letters must come from one or two mental health professionals, as described earlier.

The contents of the mental health assessment letter for surgery should include the following:

1. Date and address to surgeon
2. Name and date of birth of patient
3. Who the mental health assessor is and the assessor's relationship with the patient; for example, "I am a licensed clinical social worker and saw AB weekly from July to December, 2018, for psychotherapy and for an assessment for genital surgery
4. The history of the patient's gender dysphoria, what treatment (e.g., psychotherapy, hormones, other surgeries) the patient has already undergone, and their response to prior treatment
5. The patient's social transition, with pertinent details; for example, when the patient started living full time in their

current gender role, relationships and functioning in current gender role, legal name/gender change

6. For genital surgery, specify length of time on hormones and in current gender role, meeting SOC 7 1-year requirement
7. History of mental illness and substance abuse
8. Current medical or mental health conditions, current medications, and level of stability of these conditions
9. Capacity for informed consent, and patient's understanding of the risks and benefits of the planned surgery
10. Fertility discussion, when appropriate
11. Psychosocial stability: housing, support, plan for postoperative period
12. Diagnosis: *Gender Dysphoria (GD)*, co-occurring conditions if present
13. A statement that the patient meets SOC 7 criteria for the surgery
14. A statement that the requested surgery is a medically necessary treatment for GD (this may be helpful for insurance coverage because insurance may cover medically necessary but not cosmetic treatments)
15. A request that the surgeon contact the mental health professional if further information is needed

For genital surgery, a second assessment is usually done after reviewing the first assessment and discussing the case with the primary mental health professional who has written the first letter. This is especially the case if that person knows the client better, for example, if the person was in therapy with the first letter-writer. Otherwise, the second assessment is an independent assessment of the patient, including history, co-occurring conditions, ability to provide informed consent and thorough understanding of the risks and benefits of the planned surgery, current psychosocial stability, and aftercare plan and diagnosis. The second letter should also include the 15 points listed previously.[22]

Some letters are not required by the SOC but may be required by the patient's insurance company. For example, if insurance covers facial feminization surgery when medically necessary, a letter may be required to obtain coverage for services. These letters follow the same format and should emphasize specifically why the surgery is a medically necessary treatment for GD (e.g. how the surgery will help to relieve distress and improve functioning).

During the time of transition surgeries and afterwards, the mental health professional should remain available to provide care for their client.[21] The mental health professional can assist the client in planning for surgeries, including the client enlisting supports, usually family and friends, who might assist with practical support in the perioperative period. The process might be quite stressful. Ideally, the patient has a realistic understanding of the risks and benefits of surgery. Although most have relief of gender dysphoria with medical and surgical treatment, there may be unrealistic expectations about the effects of surgery on their life or existing issues unrelated to gender dysphoria may remain, such as the effects of trauma earlier in life that may still be present. Interpersonal issues, social isolation, maladaptive coping, or substance abuse that are present before transition may also remain afterwards. For some trans people as they age, ruptured relationships with parents, siblings, partners, and children may contribute to social isolation. The mental health professional can assist their client as they age, in building new social supports and relationships and with coping with the stressors of aging.[3]

REFERENCES

1. Byne W, Karasic DH, Coleman E, et al. Gender dysphoria in adults: an overview and primer for psychiatrists. *Transgend Health*. 2018;3(1):57–70.
2. Russell ST, Pollitt AM, Li G, Grossman AH. Chosen name use is linked to reduced depressive symptoms, suicidal ideation, and suicidal behavior among transgender youth. *J Adolesc Health*. 2018; [Epub ahead of print]. https://doi.org/10.1016/j.jadohealth.2018.02.003.
3. Karasic DH. Transgender and gender nonconforming patients. In: Lim RF, ed. *Clinical Manual of Cultural Psychiatry*. 2nd ed. Arlington, VA: American Psychiatric Publishing; 2015: 397–410.
4. Coleman E, Bockting W, Botzer M, et al. Standards of care for the health of transsexual, transgender, and gender—nonconforming people, version 7. *Int J Transgend*. 2012;13(4):165–232.
5. American Psychiatric Association. *Diagnostic and Statistical Manual of Mental Disorders III*. Washington, DC: American Psychiatric Association; 1980.
6. American Psychiatric Association. *Diagnostic and Statistical Manual of Mental Disorders*. 3rd ed (rev. ed) Washington, DC: American Psychiatric Association; 1987.
7. American Psychiatric Association. *Diagnostic and Statistical Manual of Mental Disorders IV*. Washington, DC: American Psychiatric Association; 1994.
8. American Psychiatric Association. *Diagnostic and Statistical Manual of Mental Disorders IV*.

Washington, DC: American Psychiatric Association; 2000.
9. Karasic D, Drescher J. Introduction. In: Karasic D, Drescher J, eds. *Sexual and Gender Diagnoses of the Diagnostic and Statistical Manual (DSM)*. New York, NY: Routledge; 2005:1–5.
10. Winters K. Gender dissonance: diagnostic reform of gender identity disorder for adults. In: Karasic D, Drescher J, eds. *Sexual and Gender Diagnoses of the Diagnostic and Statistical Manual (DSM)*. New York, NY: Routledge; 2005: 71–90.
11. Hill DB, Rozanski C, Carfagnini J, Willoughby B. Gender identity disorders in childhood and adolescence: a critical inquiry. In: Karasic D, Drescher J, eds. *Sexual and Gender Diagnoses of the Diagnostic and Statistical Manual (DSM)*. New York, NY: Routledge; 2005:7–34.
12. American Psychiatric Association. *Diagnostic and Statistical Manual of Mental Disorders 5*. Washington, DC: American Psychiatric Publishing; 2013.
13. *ICD 11*. World Health Organization. https://icd.who.int/ Accessed 29.06.18.
14. Dhejne C, Van Vlerken R, Heylens G, Arcelus J. Mental health and gender dysphoria: a review of the literature. *Int Rev Psychiatry*. 2016;28(1):44–57.
15. Colizzi M, Costa R, Todarello O. Dissociative symptoms in individuals with gender dysphoria: is the elevated prevalence real? *Psychiatry Res*. 2015;226(1):173–180.

16. Veale JF, Watson RJ, Saewyc EM. Mental health disparities among Canadian transgender youth. *J Adolesc Health*. 2017;60(1):44–49.
17. De Cuypere G, Elaut E, Heylens G, et al. Long-term followup: psychosocial outcome of Belgian transsexuals after sex reassignment surgery. *Sexologies*. 2006;15(2):126–133.
18. Dhejne C, Lichtenstein P, Boman M, et al. Long-term follow-up of transsexual persons undergoing sex reassignment surgery: cohort study in Sweden. *PLoS One*. 2011;6(2). e16885. https://doi.org/10.1371/journal.pone.0016885.
19. Grant JM, Mottet L, Tanis JE, et al. *Injustice at Every Turn: A Report of the National Transgender Discrimination Survey*. Washington, DC: National Center for Transgender Equality and National Gay and Lesbian Task Force; 2011.
20. Strang JF, Kenworthy L, Dominska A, et al. Increased gender variance in autism spectrum disorders and attention deficit hyperactivity disorder. *Arch Sex Behav*. 2014;43:1525–1533.
21. Karasic DH, Fraser L. Multidisciplinary care and the standards of care for transgender and gender nonconforming individuals. *Clin Plastic Surg*. 2018;45(3):295–299.
22. Karasic D. Mental health assessments of transgender adults. Webinar, February 17, 2015. The National LGBT Health Education Center. https://www.lgbthealtheducation.org/webinar/mental-health-assessment-trans-adults/ Accessed 29.06.18.

3

Mental Health Care for the Child and Adolescent Transgender Patient

DAVID CALL | JAMES MURPHY

Introduction

The Lesbian, Gay, Bisexual, and Transgender (LGBT) community has built tremendous momentum in raising awareness of its presence in our communities, and in the past several decades we have seen the positive impacts that LGBT and ally groups have made on society. However, despite these great strides, the community is still significantly marred by stigma, hate, and isolation and is often susceptible to the immense burden of grouping a diverse population under one common flag. In the past decade, the transgender community has made some of the most significant strides in bringing about awareness and acceptance of individuals who may not identify with their assigned birth genders or with society's binary construct of gender. Increasing evidence has shown that children and youth who struggle with gender identity benefit from compassionate and informed care. With appropriate management, health care providers can help to safely affirm and assist children and youth who identify as transgender in navigating their individual journeys while minimizing physical and mental health risks.

When treating children and adolescents whose gender identity differs from their assigned sex at birth, correct use of terminology is important. Box 3.1 defines some of the more common terms currently used in the field. However, it important to note that language related to gender identity may vary and may not have the same meaning to all individuals. Some individuals may find certain terms outdated or even offensive, whereas others may still prefer the use of them to describe their experience. It is therefore important for clinicians to preemptively ask patients and their families which terms they prefer, especially with regard to identity and use of pronouns.

Trends in Gender Nonconforming Behavior and Gender Variance

Transgender youth make up a unique and vulnerable population that requires comprehensive treatment approaches and considerations. There is currently more literature studying and describing the adult lesbian, gay, and bisexual population, with limited data on youth populations. This is especially true with regard to research related to transgender youth and their health outcomes. Given that the percentage of individuals who identify as LGBT in the community is small, studies also tend to have small population sizes and/or are case studies. In 2016 the Williams Institute published a study looking at data from the Centers for Disease Control and Prevention (CDC) Behavioral Risk Factor Surveillance System and estimated that 0.6% of adults in the United States identify as transgender.[1] An earlier study based on a smaller data set at the state level had estimated that the prevalence of transgenderism within the United States was 0.3%.[2] In addition to increasing efforts in gathering data on the transgender community, it is also possible that increased acceptance and visibility of transgender individuals in society may also be contributing to more transgender individuals identifying themselves as such on survey data. To estimate prevalence in youth populations, it is even more difficult because the data are limited to even smaller data sets. We must also consider the likelihood that transgender youth are less willing to identify themselves in surveys as a result of fear related to confidentiality issues or because many youth are still exploring their gender identity and may not be sure how to answer the survey question related to gender and identity.

As mentioned, studies looking specifically at prevalence rates in youth populations remain limited. One study done in New Zealand surveyed 8500 youth and found that 1.2% of respondents identified as transgender. Interestingly, the study also had options for students to indicate if they were not sure of their gender (2.5%) or if they did not understand the question (1.7%).[3] In their 2016 review, Connolly et al. looked at the existing data on transgender youth. They found variance in the reported prevalence of youth who identify as transgender, between 0.17% and 1.3%. It is important to note that these studies relied on a binary system of describing gender (male or female) and were not inclusive of other gender-fluid identities.[4] Previous studies, such as the one published in 2009 by Almeida et al., found that in a sample of more than 1000 students in Boston, 1.6% identified as transgender.[5] Gender clinics specializing in gender nonconforming and transgender youth have also seen a significant increase in referrals in recent years,[6–9] and the number of total gender clinics has also grown.[10]

In 2015, the US Transgender Survey aimed to better understand the experience of the transgender community by surveying 27,000 transgender adult respondents in the United States. Although the survey focused on adults, it asked a number of questions regarding the individual's childhood experiences. In this portion of the survey, 54% of respondents recalled being verbally harassed in their K-12 experience, 24% were physically attacked, and 13% were sexually assaulted because of their gender identity. Of the respondents who disclosed their gender identity to their families, 10% experienced violence from one or more family members and 8% were kicked out of the home. Mental health concerns were also brought to light in this survey, because 39% of respondents reported experiencing serious psychological distress in the past month, 40% reported a suicide attempt in their lifetime, and 7% reported a suicide attempt in the past year.[11]

The most current version of the Diagnostic and Statistical Manual of Mental Disorders, the DSM 5, describes the diagnosis of *Gender Dysphoria* as "the distress that may accompany the incongruence between one's experienced or expressed gender and one's assigned gender."[12] This more recent diagnosis marked a change from the previous version of the DSM-IV,

BOX 3.1 TERMINOLOGY

Sex	Birth classification, generally as male and female, based on gender-specific anatomy (internal and external reproductive organs), chromosomal classification.
Intersex	Used to describe an individual with ambiguous gender-specific anatomy and/or chromosomal makeup.
Gender	Social and psychological constructs and expectations held for individuals based on their assigned sex.
Gender Identity	The internalized sense of gender, this may correlate with assigned sex (cisgender), conflict with assigned sex (transgender), or be represented in varying degrees (see below).
Gender Expression	External expression of gender identity; clothing, hair, and behavior (including voice, body morphology), as well as the use of preferred names and pronouns.
Sexual Orientation	A person's physical, romantic, emotional, and sexual attraction to another person. A person can be lesbian, gay, straight, bisexual, or queer based on their gender identity.
Transgender	A person whose gender identity and expression differ from their assigned sex at birth.
Cisgender	A person's whose gender identity and expression match their assigned sex at birth.
Gender Nonconforming	Term often used to describe when aspects of one's gender expression does not conform to the social expectations of femininity or masculinity. Gender nonconforming individuals can identify as transgender or cisgender.
Nonbinary Identities (can include various terms including "nonbinary," "genderqueer," "neutrois")	A person whose gender identity does not meet conventional expectations of gender in a binary form (e.g., male vs. female). Gender identity can be fluid, identifying with aspects of either gender, or neither.
Transitioning	Refers to the process by which a person begins to alter their sex and begin expressing their gender identity. This is a complex process that involves social transitioning (living socially as their identified gender), may include medical interventions such as pubertal suppression, cross-sex hormone therapy (see below), or gender-confirming surgery (see below).
Cross-Sex Hormone Therapy (also referred to as Gender Affirming Hormone Therapy)	The use of feminizing hormones on a biologic male, or the use of masculinizing hormones on a biologic female.
Gender-Confirming Surgery (also referred to as Gender Affirming Surgery)	A series of surgical procedures performed with a goal of adopting a person's preferred sexual anatomy. This may include masculinizing or feminizing cosmetic procedures as well.

From Gay & Lesbian Alliance Against Defamation. Media Reference Guide—Transgender. Retrieved from https://www.glaad.org/reference/transgender and American Psychiatric Association. *Diagnostic and Statistical Manual of Mental Disorders.* 5th ed. Arlington, VA: American Psychiatric Association; 2013.

which diagnosed transgender individuals with *Gender Identity Disorder* (GID).[13] By changing the terminology and omitting "disorder" from the diagnosis, there was a shift in the paradigm with regard to what it means to be transgender. There is now less of an emphasis on an individual being disordered, and there is more of a focus on the distress that some individuals may experience as a result of being transgender. An important take away point from this change in nomenclature is that the term *Gender Dysphoria* does not simply refer to behavior that is nonconforming with stereotypical gender roles, but rather, it describes an individual's distress or impairment as a result of the incongruence between their experienced and assigned gender. The main purpose for changing the terminology was to refine the diagnosis and to help avoid stigma against patients.[14] In the past, it has been easy to misinterpret the former diagnosis of GID to mean that transgender individuals are inherently mentally ill or that their identity can be changed through treatment as in any other disorder.

In the DSM 5 criteria for *Gender Dysphoria* a distinction is made between *Gender Dysphoria in Childhood* and *Gender Dysphoria in Adolescents and Adults* (Box 3.2). In the criteria for *Gender Dysphoria in Childhood*, there must be a desire or insistence that the individual is of the other or an alternative gender. Some children present voicing a strong insistence that they are the other gender, and they may exhibit their distress as a result of this in the form of behavioral problems or temper tantrums when those around them treat them as their assigned gender. On the other hand, some children exhibit interests that might challenge our society's expectations for their assigned gender (e.g., a natal boy who likes to play dress up in princess gowns, or a natal girl who may refuse to wear a dress or play with dolls) but continue to insist that their gender identity is in line with their assigned gender.

In addition to the desire to be the other or some alternative gender, to meet criteria for *Gender Dysphoria* in childhood, a child must have six out of eight criteria that include various preferences in types of play and activities, clothing, roles in pretend play, and gender of their playmates. Two of the eight criteria refer to either a dislike of their sexual anatomy or a desire for the primary/secondary sex characteristics of their experienced gender.

The requirements for diagnosis in adolescents differ slightly from the diagnosis of children. To make the diagnosis in adolescence, two out of the following six criteria must be met: a marked incongruence between one's experienced gender and assigned gender; a strong desire to be rid of their primary/secondary sex characteristics because of the incongruence; a strong desire for the primary/secondary sex characteristics of the other gender; a strong desire to be a different gender from their assigned gender; a strong desire to be treated as the other gender; or a strong conviction that one has the feelings and reactions of the other gender.

The aforementioned criteria must be present for at least 6 months for *Gender Dysphoria* to be formally diagnosed in either childhood or in adolescence, and they must be associated with marked distress or impairment in functioning. It is possible

BOX 3.2 DSM 5 CRITERIA FOR DIAGNOSIS OF GENDER DYSPHORIA IN CHILDREN

A. A marked incongruence between one's experienced/expressed gender and assigned gender, of at least 6 months' duration, as manifested by at least six of the following (one of which must be Criterion A1):
 1. A strong desire to be of the other gender or an insistence that one is the other gender (or some alternative gender different from one's assigned gender).
 2. In boys (assigned gender), a strong preference for cross-dressing or simulating female attire; or in girls (assigned gender), a strong preference for wearing only typical masculine clothing and a strong resistance to the wearing of typical feminine clothing.
 3. A strong preference for cross-gender roles in make-believe play or fantasy play.
 4. A strong preference for the toys, games, or activities stereotypically used or engaged in by the other gender.
 5. A strong preference for playmates of the other gender.
 6. In boys (assigned gender), a strong rejection of typically masculine toys, games, and activities and a strong avoidance of rough-and-tumble play; or in girls (assigned gender), a strong rejection of typically feminine toys, games, and activities.
 7. A strong dislike of one's sexual anatomy.
 8. A strong desire for the primary and/or secondary sex characteristics that match one's experienced gender.
B. The condition is associated with clinically significant distress or impairment in social, school, or other important areas of functioning.

From Diagnostic and Statistical Manual of Mental Disorders (DSM 5), Fifth edition. American Psychiatric Association. 2013

for a child or adolescent to identify as another gender, and some patients may even consider themselves transgender without there being associated distress or impairment. These individuals do not meet criteria for *Gender Dysphoria*, but it is important to acknowledge that this does not mean that the individual's gender identity is any less valid, nor does it mean that they may not need mental health care services. Many gender-nonconforming youth who do not have gender dysphoria may still be subject to stressors such as teasing or bullying around their gender expressions that can lead to the development of problems such as school avoidance, anxiety, and/or depression.

EPIDEMIOLOGY

As previously mentioned, understanding the true prevalence of transgenderism and gender dysphoria has been challenging because there is limited research in this area. Most of the data that exist have been subject to both selection and recall bias as a result of how samples are chosen and the need to rely on self-reporting. Individuals may not be comfortable identifying themselves as a gender minority, which leads to an underestimation of the prevalence of this patient population. Early estimates in children and adolescence have been based more on behavior, making them more difficult to interpret because exhibiting behavior that is more typical of the other gender does not equate to having a transgender identity or meeting criteria for *Gender Dysphoria*. Some of these earlier estimates used the Child Behavior Checklist (CBCL), which contains questions for parents to indicate whether their child behaves like the opposite sex or wishes to be of the opposite sex. Zucker et al. found that using the CBCL, when asked, mothers reported the following: their child behaves like the opposites sex (for natal boys 3.8% sometimes, 1% often; for natal girls 8.3% sometimes, 2.3% often) and their child wishes

to be the opposite sex (for natal boys 1% sometimes, 0% often; for natal girls 2.5% sometimes, 1% often).[15] A large Dutch twin study also looked at parental endorsement of cross-gender behavior and identification and found similar results (for natal boys at 7 years old 3.4% behaving like the other gender and 1% wishing to be the opposite sex, at 10 years old 2.4% behaving like the opposite sex and 1% wishing to be the opposite sex; for natal girls at 7 years old 5.2% behaving like the opposite sex and 1.7% identifying as the opposite sex, and at 10 years old 3.4% behaving like the opposite sex and 0.9% identifying as the opposite sex).[16] Again, we would like to emphasize that it is hard to interpret these data because cross-gender behavior is not necessarily a surrogate for *Gender Dysphoria*.

SOCIAL TRANSITIONS IN PREPUBERTAL YOUTH

Social transition can refer to various decisions and choices one can make to show themselves as the gender they identify as. This can include changing one's name to one that is more stereotypically associated with their experienced gender, changing the use of pronouns or changing the way they express their gender in a way that fits their experienced gender. One who is or has socially transitioned may make some of the aforementioned choices in some or in all settings. As visibility has increased around transgender identities, there has been a growing number of families that present to gender clinics and specialists looking for guidance in making some of these decisions at an early age.

There is controversy surrounding the best approach for working with children with gender dysphoria. As such, there are a number of different treatment approaches that specialists have taken in caring for young patients. Families sometimes present very anxious about their child's behaviors when they are outside of the social norms for what is expected of the child's assigned birth gender. A very frequent concern and question that many parents have is if it is too early in development for their child to truly know their gender identity. Current psychological theories do point to children having an early awareness of their gender identity and having an ability to label themselves as being a boy or girl as young as 2 or 3 years of age.[17] However, parents often raise concerns that their child may change their mind and they worry about the damage that could be done if a "wrong" decision is made with regard to their child's transition.

There have been a number of studies that have looked at the development of youth that exhibit gender nonconforming behaviors at an early age. Overall, these studies show that a significant percentage of these youth "desist" in their presentations and ultimately identify as their assigned gender at birth. Studies show variable rates of persistence in children identifying as the other gender, ranging from 2% to 39%.[18–26] Of note, very few studies use the most up-to-date DSM 5 definition of *Gender Dysphoria*. More recent research has looked into the differences that exist between the groups of children that "persist" and those that do not. In a prospective study of 77 children referred for *Gender Dysphoria*, Wallien and Cohen-Kettenis showed that those children who persisted had a much higher incidence of being assigned a formal diagnosis of GID (as defined by DSM-IV at the time of the study), more gender variant behavior, and a higher intensity of dysphoria in childhood. Steensma et al. followed 127 adolescents and found that "persisters" tended to be more explicit in their belief that they were the other sex and had higher intensity of gender dysphoria in childhood, more gender variant behavior, and more dissatisfaction with their bodies compared with children that did not remain persistent.[27]

The aforementioned findings have led many parents and providers to adopt the now commonly used phrase of looking for an "insistent, consistent, and persistent" pattern to help determine which children may be more likely to persist in their presentation through adolescence and adulthood. This concept has been further validated by researchers such as de Vries et al., who showed that in a cohort of 55 adolescents belonging to a Dutch gender clinic, all of the patients were children who continued to identify as transgender in young adulthood.[28] Interestingly, review of persistence and desistance studies reveals that the rates of persistence have increased to a range of 12% to 39% compared with studies published before the year 2000 which showed lower persistence rates of 2% to 9%. Some have theorized that this may be a result of changes in our societies with more individuals identifying as transgender because of less stigma and social pressures.[29]

Role of the Mental Health Professional in the Assessment and Treatment of Adolescents with Gender Nonconforming Behavior

ASSESSMENT OF CO-OCCURRING PSYCHIATRIC CONDITIONS

With suicide currently as the second leading cause of death in US youth, it is important to remember that sexual and gender minority youth are at a particularly higher risk for suicidal ideation, self-injurious behavior, and suicide attempts. Mental health can be a stigmatized subject, and transgender youth may have difficulty fully disclosing their concerns with providers. Major contributors to this are social factors such as a higher risk of bullying and victimization as a result of disclosure. Seventy-five percent of sexual and gender minority youth experience bullying and are afraid or may not feel supported if they disclose this at home or in their school community. Bullying and victimization at school and home put transgender youth at a particularly high risk for running away behavior, which contributes to their overrepresentation in the homeless youth population.[30] Without a stable environment in which to develop, these youth are at risk for comorbid depression, anxiety, substance use (sexual minorities have the greatest risk of reporting lifetime substance use problems, especially sexual minority women of color),[31] use of illegally obtained street-hormones, engaging in prostitution and "survival sex," and associated physical health concerns such as communicable diseases.

A number of studies have looked at the presence of mental health comorbidities in youth with gender dysphoria. In one study, 44% of youth followed in a multidisciplinary gender clinic had a significant psychiatric history, 58% had been diagnosed with depression, 16% with generalized anxiety, 21% had a history of self-mutilation, and 9% had at least one previous suicide attempt.[32] A Dutch study found that out of 120 children referred to a gender clinic, 52% had a mental health diagnosis other than GID (the term used at the time) and a higher incidence of internalizing disorders (e.g., anxiety and mood disorders) compared with externalizing disorders (e.g., disruptive behavioral disorders): 37% versus 23%.[33] Similarly, a study performed in

the Gender Identity Development Service (GIDS) in London examined adolescents with gender dysphoric features and also found higher rates of internalizing symptoms compared with externalizing symptoms.[34]

Reisner et al. showed that transgender youth have significantly more comorbid psychiatric conditions when compared with cisgender controls.[35] In their study, youth who identified as transgender were more likely to be diagnosed with a depressive disorder (50.6% vs. 20.6%) or anxiety (26.7% vs. 10%), to have presence of suicidal ideation (17.2% vs. 6.1%), presence of self-injurious behavior (16.7% vs. 4.4%), a history of inpatient psychiatric treatment (22.8% vs. 11.1%), or to report being in an outpatient psychiatric treatment at the time of the study (45.6% vs. 16.1%). In this study, there were no significant differences in the aforementioned mental health conditions between transgender males and females.

A number of studies have also been done looking at suicidality. One study interviewed a sample of youth and young adults who identified as transgender and found that 45% seriously thought of suicide, with even higher rates reported by those that identified as having experienced verbal or physical abuse by parents, and 26% reported a history of a suicide attempt.[36]

A retrospective analysis by the GIDS in London also showed that youth with gender dysphoric features often have high rates of bullying (47%), low mood or depression (42%), and self-harm behavior (39%).[37] Their study also compared youth aged 5 to 11 years and youth aged 12 to 18 years and showed that puberty was a time of increased distress with even higher rates of depression, self-harm, and suicidal thoughts in the younger age group. In a study published by Olson et al., 20% ($n = 96$) of youth aged 12 to 24 years of age seeking care in a transgender youth clinic had Beck Depression Inventory rating scale scores in the moderate to extreme range, 51% had a history of suicidal thoughts, and 30% had a history of a suicide attempt.[38]

Similarly, in a comprehensive review by Connolly et al., the authors found that transgender youth were more likely to be depressed than their cisgender peers, with up to 50.6% of youth diagnosed with depression. They also showed that transgender youth were at a higher risk for attempted suicide and suicidal ideation, with rates reported in some studies as high as 19.8% and 56%, respectively.[4] In their 2016 study looking at the prevalence of suicidal thoughts and behaviors in children (aged 3 to 12 years) seen in a gender identity clinic, Aitken et al. noted that children referred to gender clinics had more behavior problems and had poorer peer relations than a nonreferred group of children. The referred group was also more likely to talk about killing themselves (22.7%), more likey to be deliberately harming themselves and attempting suicide (18.6%). There appeared to be an age relationship: as children got older, the gender-referred group was 15 times more likely to talk about suicide.

It is no surprise that social supports and perception of safety play a significant role in the well-being of transgender youth, and assessment of this is important when conducting a mental health evaluation. LGBT youth who report low levels of support from their families, communities, or social relationships are more likely to report depressive symptoms and suicidality.[39] In their 2014 study of LGBT youth in Boston, Duncan and Hatzenbuehler found a correlation between suicidal ideation and suicide attempts in LGBT youth who lived in neighborhoods that had high rates of LGBT-related hate crimes.[40]

Lastly, Connolly et al. also reported a higher prevalence of eating disorders among transgender adolescents, with overall rates as high as 15.8%. The authors revealed that 13.5% of youth reported using diet pills and 15.1% described purging behaviors.[4]

EXPLORATION OF GENDER IDENTITY/EXPRESSION

At the time of assessment, a diagnosis of *Gender Dysphoria* may or may not be made depending on whether the child or adolescent meets criteria for the diagnosis. Regardless of the formal diagnosis that is made, the mental health provider's role is also to help children and adolescents further explore and discern their gender identity and gender expression. Some youth may not show much desire to "explore," because they may express certainty about their gender identity. Conversely, other children and adolescents present to the mental health provider with difficulty in articulating their internal sense of their gender identity. This is often the case for those individuals who may not identify in the binary (male vs. female) sense of gender. Some children present identifying neither as male nor female and, when asked, may find difficulty in labeling their gender identity. Adolescents who feel certain with their gender identity may still desire counseling regarding ways to express their gender. Great care must be taken in eliciting conversations about gender identity. Some youth may choose to not to disclose their gender identity or express their gender the way they truly wish to out of fear of bullying or harassment. In other cases, it may be the parents who wish to limit certain expressions out of safety fears for their child.

There is a lot of controversy surrounding models of care for prepubertal youth who have gender variant behaviors. Past approaches have included efforts to help youth be more comfortable with their assigned gender at birth through different interventions, such as promoting interactions with same-sex peers, relationships with the same-sex parent, and encouraging more typical behaviors of the assigned sex at birth. The rationale behind these approaches are to help hasten desistence, which is based on previous literature that suggests that many prepubertal youth who have gender nonconforming behaviors desist through development and eventually stop identifying as the opposite gender thereby minimizing the potential risks of being rejected by peers and family and developing symptoms of anxiety or depression.[41] It is important to note that these approaches lack strong evidence and have not been studied in randomized controlled trials designed to show efficacy.[42] As noted earlier, the literature that exists on rates of persistence and desistance has a number of limitations. The biggest concern related to this approach is the potential risk of harm that could occur in the individual who does not desist, but rather persists. The approach sends a message of lack of acceptance or tolerance, and this type of rejection may be at the core of some of the disparities in mental health seen in transgender youth.

Other approaches have taken a "watchful waiting" stance, where risks of transitioning are taken into consideration given potential negative reactions or responses from others. In this approach, parents may have their child wait before undergoing a social transition until further development into puberty, while still trying to balance an accepting approach.[6] Some approaches try to balance this by encouraging acceptance and tolerance of any behaviors or interests that are considered gender nonconforming, but potentially limiting expression or deferring timing of social transitions when accounting for potential risks.[43]

Finally, the affirmative model focuses on building resilience and positive self-esteem, and youth desiring a social transition are affirmed and supported in their attempts to transition.[44] More recent research has looked at prepubertal transgender youth who have undergone social transition. Compared with cisgender controls, affirmed transgender youth seem to have no significant differences in depressive symptoms and only mild elevation in anxiety ratings that are not considered clinically concerning.[45]

Controversy remains among multiple professional societies[42,46,47] regarding the acceptability of allowing a child to transition to their self-affirmed gender. However, what is agreed upon is that decisions around social transitions must be tailored to various factors, including the temperament of the child, the level of social supports, acceptance and understanding of those around the child, and of course, the child's desires. Some children desire a social transition early and want to disclose their identity as transgender to many of their peers and those around, whereas other children may want to defer transitioning due to anxieties or fears of being stigmatized, harassed, or bullied and may express their gender identity only in limited settings.

SUPPORT FOR BOTH THE CHILD/ADOLESCENT AND PARENTS

Families may bring their child to the mental health professional for a variety of reasons. Many families are concerned about whether their child truly is transgender and wonder if this may be "just a phase." Other families may be convinced that their child is transgender and may have worries and anxieties around how to help their child face potential obstacles and barriers, such as teasing and bullying, or the fear of their child being assaulted or discriminated against. Still other families may present hoping that the mental health professional can in some way change the development of the child such that he or she no longer has cross-gender expressions or identification. Mental health professionals need to be prepared for the variety of presentations from families and how to best address their concerns, while maintaining what is in the best interest of the child.

In working with parents of gender nonconforming and transgender youth, it is important to realize that without working and addressing the parents' concerns and questions, one may inadvertently push the family away from coming in to get the help that may be needed for the child. Eliciting parent expectations and concerns is key early on in therapeutic work to help shape and determine how the provider may proceed in working with both the child and the family. Coolhart and Shipman describe a model for working with families therapeutically where the tasks in therapy are divided into two stages: the first being assessing and increasing family "attunement" (their level of understanding and peace with the child's gender identity and expression) and the second being helping explore and support options for gender expression or transition.[48] Parents who may feel that their concerns or viewpoints are not being heard or taken into consideration may result in the parents preventing their child from getting the help or support that they need.

Furthermore, it should be noted that just because the child may be gender nonconforming or identify as transgender, it may not be necessary for the child to receive mental health treatment.

It is important to recognize that the "diagnosis" that is often being evaluated for is *Gender Dysphoria* focusing on the distress and impairment that can often occur in a transgender individual's life. The clinician is not diagnosing the child's gender identity, although parents may be looking for the clinician to provide them with reassurance that their child is or is not transgender. Psychotherapy is no longer an absolute requirement for access to interventions for transitioning, such as hormone therapy or surgery as outlined in the World Professional Association for Transgender Health (WPATH) standards of care.[49] Depending on the individual child and the family, there will be different needs, and the flexibility of the mental health care provider is important in working with these families. The WPATH standards of care outline some potential roles that mental health care providers may play in working with gender nonconforming and transgender youth. These potential roles include (Box 3.3): directly addressing gender dysphoria, providing family counseling, helping youth explore their gender identity, assessing and treating any coexisting mental health concerns, referring for physical interventions (puberty suppression and gender-affirming hormones), educating and advocating for the child and their family, and providing or referring youth and their families to peer support resources.[49]

Parents themselves may experience a range of emotions and responses to their child's gender expression or identity, and the mental health provider can play a significant role in normalizing and validating the experience that many parents go through. Some parents experience grief and loss over their child's disclosure of having a non-conforming gender identity. Other parents have significant worry and anxiety about what the future may bring for their child, particularly about their safety and being accepted in society for who they are. The mental health provider can help to promote a safe space not just for the child but also for the parent to express their feelings.[50] As mentioned previously, the role of parent support groups either in the community, through organized gender programs, or through online groups can be helpful as an adjunctive source of support outside of the mental health provider's office. The ability to meet other parents who are experiencing similar feelings of loss and grief, struggling with adjusting their parenting styles, and promoting acceptance can be very powerful in helping parents problem solve issues that may come up in settings such as the family, school, and with friends.[50,51]

SUPPORT AND CONSIDERATION FOR MEDICAL INTERVENTIONS

Following the WPATH standards of care and the Endocrine Society guidelines, medical interventions, such as gender-affirming hormones, are not recommended before puberty.[49,52] For many gender-dysphoric youth, the transition into puberty can cause significant stress as there is development of secondary sex characteristics that are incongruent with their gender identity. The Dutch program pioneered the use of Gonadotropin-Releasing Hormone (GnRH) agonists to suppress estrogen or testosterone production once puberty has commenced in those youth with worsening gender dysphoria.[6,53,54] Aims of puberty suppression include helping to relieve worsening dysphoria by arresting the changes that occur at the onset of puberty but also allowing there to be more time to further explore the adolescent's desire to potentially undergo further transition with partially and completely irreversible interventions such as cross sex hormones and surgery.[6] Adolescents are often relieved that the irreversible changes that develop with puberty, such as deepening of the voice in natal males or breast development in natal females, are thwarted, thereby reducing their gender dysphoria. Pubertal suppression may also have future benefits, including potentially eliminating the need for other interventions such as the need for mastectomy in natal females or time spent in voice therapy for natal males.

Current guidelines from the Endocrine Society[52] recommend that puberty suppression be started in young individuals who have reached Tanner stage 2 or 3 of development if they have worsening gender dysphoria as a result of changes related to puberty. Criteria for starting puberty suppression include the recognition that there has been a long-lasting pattern of gender dysphoria or gender nonconformity, gender dysphoria emerged or worsened with pubertal onset, coexisting psychological, social, and medical problems that could interfere with treatment are addressed, and the adolescent, along with their guardians, has given informed consent for treatment[49] As such, close collaboration between the mental health professional and the medical professional managing puberty suppression is vital. As mentioned earlier, initiating treatment at the time of puberty appears to be critical because gender dysphoria and internalizing symptoms can worsen, so the timing of intervention is important. A prospective analysis from the Dutch program found that adolescents started on GnRH agonists who had worsening gender dysphoria with puberty had significant improvement in functioning and depressive symptoms.[55,56]

The role of the mental health provider is multifaceted during this time period. Following current guidelines such as the WPATH standards of care, mental health providers do not solely assess and make the diagnosis of *Gender Dysphoria* and refer to providers for puberty suppression. Mental health providers also have an important role in helping families understand their child's gender identity and the impact gender dysphoria is playing on their child's health. They can provide guidance to parents in helping them support their child and show acceptance, as opposed to rejecting behaviors that can lead to the development of shame or negative attitude in the child. Not all mental health providers have extensive experience in understanding the medical interventions used in the treatment of gender dysphoria, which points to the important role that close collaboration has, which is best achieved with a multidisciplinary approach. Some adolescents also benefit from hearing information regarding medical treatment from multiple providers on several occasions to help ensure that they are taking into account all of the potential risks and benefits associated with treatment before starting. For instance, although puberty suppression has been viewed as a reversible intervention,[52] there are some concerns around the potential decrease in bone mineral density that is associated with this type of treatment.[54,57] Mental health providers also should engage in discussions with the adolescent about their expectations associatd with medical therapy. It is not uncommon for some patients to misconstrue information that they may have heard online or from others, which can lead to having unrealistic goals.

The mental health provider can also further explore gender identity and expression with the adolescent once treatment has started. Discussing multiple possibilities and ways to self-identify is important because the adolescent may not even be familiar with the different identities that exist and as a result may not be able to articulate or clearly express their gender identity. During this time, it is also important to provide reassurance to the adolescent that the spectrum of transition varies among individuals and that social, medical, and surgical transition is not absolute for everyone. This is especially important in the case of the nonbinary individual who may not desire complete transition.[50] Puberty suppression can help to provide the time needed for the mental health professional to continue to work with both the adolescent and family in considering what future decisions they may want to take as they continue to develop and transition. The mental health provider can also be helpful in working with the adolescent and family in determining whether or not to go forward with other decisions, such as deciding whether or not they want to disclose their gender identity to others and decisions surrounding social transition in some or all settings, such as in school or in extracurricular activities such as sports teams. When the adolescent does make the decision to socially transition, providers can also be helpful in being an advocate for patients and their families in interacting and providing education to those involved in the adolescent's life, such as school officials and teachers.

Given that puberty suppression only pauses pubertal development, it is important to note that sometimes adolescents will continue to have some degree of gender dysphoria. As adolescents age, they may find themselves distressed or self-conscious that some of their peers are going through pubertal changes while they are not. This is another area where mental health providers can be helpful in guiding adolescents and families in other ways to manage gender dysphoria both through individual and family therapy but also support groups. Both support groups for parents and children have been found to be helpful in providing opportunities for children to socialize and meet peers who may be experiencing similar and related problems. Parent groups can also be helpful during this process so that parents can receive education and learn ways to best support their child and to provide a space where they can receive validation for some of the complex feelings they may be experiencing around their child's transition.[50]

Clinical Vignette #1

J is a 13-year-old assigned female at birth who presented with his parents for further assessment of gender dysphoria, as J came out to his parents approximately 1 year ago as identifying as male. J has been reporting feeling distressed about his body changing in ways that are not in line with his identity and the resulting frequent misgendering he experiences despite his attempts to express his gender as male. J feels that despite also telling others that he is male and requesting use of male pronouns, individuals continue to refer to him as female and he feels that much of this has to do with the pitch of his voice, his body not fitting into boy's clothing properly, and the noticeable development in his chest. He also feels distressed when having to take a shower and tries to cover up the mirrors in

his bathroom so that he does not have to see his body. His parents come to the evaluation anxious in wanting to support their child but also note that prior to coming out as a transgender boy 1 year ago, they had heard J talk about possibly identifying as a "lesbian" and then as being "nonbinary." J's parents had brought him to a therapist, who primarily spoke to J and only met with his parents briefly. They became more concerned after the initial visit when the therapist recommended that the parents should bring J to a specialist to begin hormone therapy. When the parents had questions, they felt the therapist would not talk to them in detail, and so the parents present hoping to get more education and understanding of what is going on with their child.

This vignette illustrates how well-meaning mental health providers may inadvertently push away families, where parents are also looking for guidance and support. This can be difficult when the individual provider is also trying to build rapport with the adolescent and not wanting to break trust. Sometimes, it can be helpful to collaborate with additional providers, such as a family therapist, who is also experienced in working with gender dysphoria or collaborating with a multidisciplinary gender program. Many programs allow for individual mental health providers to continue to work with the child, and the program's providers can serve in a consultative role.[6,50,58]

Once puberty suppression has been started during early puberty and after further work with the adolescent and family is underway, another decision point is whether or not to pursue interventions that are only partially irreversible, including gender-affirming cross-sex hormones. This option is also available to adolescents who may not have decided to pursue puberty suppression or may have presented for assistance in later stages of puberty when most of the secondary sex characteristics have already developed. Currently the WPATH standards of care recommend that patients be 16 years of age or older to start cross-sex hormone therapy with either testosterone or estrogen.[49] However, more recent Endocrine Society guidelines have noted that in case-by-case situations, younger patients may also have the capacity to understand the risks/benefits/limitations that are associated with hormone therapy and the potential irreversibility of some of the changes treatment can cause. The guidelines also note that with some youth receiving puberty suppression at younger ages when they reach Tanner stage 2 or 3, consideration to bone health with prolonged puberty suppression must be given, and earlier initiation of affirming hormones may prevent irreversible changes to bone density.[52]

If the adolescent is presenting for the first time at 16 or at a more fully developed stage of puberty and wanting hormone therapy immediately, mental health providers should ensure that both the adolescent and guardians (if the patient is not the age of majority) understand the risks, benefits, and limitations of hormone therapy. Current guidelines do not have a minimum time or number of sessions with a mental health professional before starting hormone therapy, because this will vary based on the individual. Depending on various factors, such as the level of acceptance of parents, level of social support to aid in transition, the adolescent's understanding of medical transition, this part of treatment can vary.

Clinical Vignette #2

G, who was assigned female at birth, presents to the Gender Development Clinic at age 17 with his parents, stating that he had identified as male since middle school when he noted significant distress with changes in puberty (such as development of his chest and changes in his body shape having a more "feminine appearance"). G states that, on reflection, he feels that he has always had a sense even before puberty of having a male gender identity but notes that he did not know that the term "transgender" existed and that it was even possible that he could have a gender identity different from that assigned at birth. G also suffers from significant generalized and social anxiety that has led to significant impairment and school avoidance. In subsequent sessions, when discussing his desire for transition, he defers on wanting to pursue testosterone therapy after learning that this could have possible impacts on his fertility status. Due to his anxiety he is very guarded on wanting to discuss this issue further. G's anxiety is managed by helping him connect with a therapist he feels more comfortable with, who "understands" gender diversity better than previous therapists who avoided talking about gender with him. He also benefits from the addition of an Selective Serotonin Reuptake Inhibitor (SSRI) to control his anxiety and ultimately is able to return to school, graduate, and gain part-time employment after socially transitioning over the course of 2 years. With the improvements in his anxiety, he is more amenable to talking about medical interventions and, in fact, brings it up after he has read a post on a social media platform indicating that testosterone has no impact on fertility. G is disappointed to learn that there is still unclear knowledge about the long-term effects of cross-sex hormones on fertility and that providers cannot guarantee that his fertility will be preserved without doing oocyte preservation. However, he states that he feels "ready" to talk more with providers about his concerns on fertility and learn about fertility preservation and eventually pursue both preservation and testosterone therapy.

This vignette shows how age is not the only factor that goes into readiness for hormones, and despite being an intelligent young man who was older than the age of 16, hormone therapy was deferred until he was able to more readily explore his desires around medical transition as it related to his hopes and attitudes about fertility. Once his mental health providers were better able to provide supportive care for his gender dysphoria and stabilize his anxiety, he was better equipped to make a decision about medical transition.

PSYCHOEDUCATION FOR THE CHILD/ADOLESCENT AND FAMILY

In addition to psychoeducation on the risks, benefits, and limitations of medical interventions, the mental health provider can also provide psychoeducation on other topics that are relevant to the child and family. This includes discussing the risks and benefits related to social transition, particularly in younger prepubertal patients. There are often many complex decisions that families and youth face, and the mental health provider can be a source of education and help in understanding what might be in the best interest of the child.

One of the roles the provider can play, particularly at the beginning, is understanding the viewpoints and background of the family to help guide further discussions. As societal views have changed, some parents may also present with feelings and opinions that are caught in between a generation of rejection and one of tolerance. For these families, it may be important to bolster peer/parent support, so that parents do not feel alone trying to counter advice from older generations while supporting their children. For many parents, initial visits can also be constructive in helping to educate them about the

diversity of gender identities and expressions. Common misconceptions include confusing gender identity with sexual orientation (e.g., "Why can't my child just be gay?"), confusing gender identity with gender expression (e.g., "I don't understand, they say they are a boy, but they still wear makeup?"), underestimating the complexity and multifaced factors that go into gender (e.g., wrongfully assuming that it was something the parent did to cause their child to be transgender), or that it is always a "phase." Parents can benefit from having a space to express their views and express their emotions around having a child that may be gender nonconforming or transgender. Providers who can validate the experience that parents are going through by acknowledging the discomfort that they may be experiencing can be helpful in allowing parents to better understand the experience of their child.[50]

Diagnosis of Gender Dysphoria in the Adolescent

When it comes to making the DSM 5 diagnosis of *Gender Dysphoria* in childhood or in adolescence, the "gold standard" is a clinical interview using the DSM criteria (see Box 3.2). However, there are also tools that clinicians can use to aid in making the diagnosis or assessing the level of or presence of gender dysphoria. Currently, there are only a limited number of rating scales/tools to assess gender identity. To further complicate the picture, many of these tools make the assumption that gender is a binary structure (male vs. female), and they may not properly capture the level of distress that nonbinary or agender individuals may feel.

Some scales used in assessment include the Utrecht Gender Dysphoria Scale,[59] which has the adolescent rate their agreement or disagreement to a series of 12 statements about their gender identity; the Body Image Scale,[60] which evaluates one's satisfaction with 30 different body features; the Gender Identity/Gender Dysphoria Questionnaire for Adolescents and Adults (GIDYQ-AA),[61,62] and the Gender Identity Questionnaire, a parent reported scale.[63] More research is needed to look at measures and scales that can encapsulate the diversity of gender identities and ways of expression, because many of the tools used are based on a more binary way of looking at gender. Furthermore, research looking at the use of these measures when considering the updated the DSM 5 definitions of gender dysphoria may also be important. Nevertheless, use of some of these tools can aid in stimulating conversation and discussion on the individual's experience of their gender identity. They may also be useful in helping parents reflect on their child's development and experiences, which may help in the assessment of the child.

In terms of the clinical interview, there are a variety of approaches that a provider can take in starting the assessment. Some providers choose to meet with parents initially to help determine goals and get a better understanding of where the parents are in terms of acceptance of their child's presentation or if there are additional concerns outside of issues related to gender. Other providers, particularly those who work within a multidisciplinary gender program construct, may meet with both the child and parents individually over an extended initial evaluation or over multiple sessions.[6,50] Regardless of the setup of the initial evaluation and approach, it is important to build trust with the child or adolescent to explore topics about gender that may be uncomfortable to talk about for some. In children, depending on the developmental level of the child, the interview may require methods outside of a direct interview. Exploring gender through more creative methods such as pretend play, use of toys, or artwork can be helpful to get a better sense of how the child sees themselves. It can also be helpful to explore with the child different possibilities in regards to gender identity and expression. Some children, particularly at younger ages, may present with the desire to be a different gender because they might not realize that it can be possible to still be the gender they were assigned at birth while having interests or expressions that may be considered gender nonconforming. On the other hand, some children will still continue to assert that they are a different gender than what they were assigned at birth, even when presented with this concept.

For adolescents, there can be more conversation in the assessment in exploring their gender identity and expression. It can be helpful to get an understanding of what information the adolescent already knows about gender, gender dysphoria, and various interventions. Providing psychoeducation on these topics in the assessment phase can be important because it sometimes occurs that adolescent's views and, in particular, desires for interventions may change after they are provided with accurate information. Topics that are often explored with an adolescent include the history of their experience of their gender identity (e.g., how long they realized there may have been a difference), the differences between gender identity and gender expression, which may not always line up in ways that society expects, their possible desire to transition (or history of social transition if they already have) socially, and their interest or desire to pursue medical and/or surgical interventions.

As previously mentioned, many of the current screening tools that exist ask questions about gender identity using binary definitions. Given that gender is seen as being on a spectrum and can also include no gender at all, or fluid identities that may not be static in time, it can be hard to assess these individuals with the definitions that currently exist. Future research and development into better ways to capture the diversity of gender are needed to help capture these individuals not only from a research perspective, but also to help the patients themselves and their parents understand their experience when it is difficult for them to clearly articulate it.

When assessing for gender dysphoria it is important to include multiple sources of history. Some parents may be hesitant to bring their child into see a mental health professional out of fear that it may implicate or stigmatize the child into thinking something is wrong with them. Although there is not a uniform approach, emphasizing that the role of the evaluation is more to help parents to understand and best support the child as well as helping them feel good about themselves, may help to rectify this opinion.[50] Not seeing the child in the evaluation can lead to skewed advice, because some parents may unknowingly emphasize or leave out certain parts of the history that may be in line with the desired outcome they may have for the evaluation. Having input from parents can also be helpful in better understanding not only the child, but also help to rule out other potential co-occurring psychological issues or concerns that may be contributing to the presentation.

Special Considerations for the Adolescent

See Box 3.4.

BOX 3.4 CONSIDERATIONS FOR THE ADOLESCENT

Fertility	• Providers should start discussions with both the adolescent and parents around considerations for fertility preservation as medical interventions (puberty suppression or gender affirming hormones) which can impact fertility status
Assessment for Autism Spectrum Disorder (ASD)	• Studies have shown increased rates of gender variance in ASD populations • Should be considered when assessing and working with adolescents given potential difficulties with social communication, and possible intellectual or language impairments may require additional consultation with specialists that work with ASD • Mental health providers should routinely screen for ASD when doing assessments for gender dysphoria • Diagnosis of ASD does not exclude one from treatment/interventions that would otherwise be given for gender dysphoria.
Legal	• Care should be taken when parents disagree on management and support of child, team approaches may be helpful in understanding differing perspectives • Ensure confidentiality and ask adolescent about whom they have or have not disclosed their gender identity to
School	• Providers may need to serve in the role as advocate for youth who attend schools that are uninformed on how to best support their students. • Adolescent should guide decisions about disclosure to peers or staff, as well as decisions on facilities/activities that are gender segregated (e.g., bathrooms, locker rooms, sports teams) • Providers should assess and monitor for bullying which can have negative mental health consequences
Advocacy	• Providers may be called upon to share their knowledge/expertise to help ensure settings the adolescent is involved in are supportive • Providers should become familiar with resources that they can refer community members and families to for support

---

FERTILITY

Current research shows that the use of gender-affirming hormone therapy results in reduction or loss of fertility and, although can be reversible with cessation of hormones, may also be irreversible.[64] The Endocrine Society guidelines recommend that discussions about fertility preservation should begin when considering pubertal suppression or hormone therapy given this risk.[52] Studies that have looked at the incidence of transgender youth who elect to have fertility preservation have found that this incidence is low, and most youth do not appear to preserve gametes prior to hormone therapy. Nahata et al. showed that only 2 out of 72 youth in a gender clinic pursued fertility preservation prior to hormone therapy.[65]

Discussions with adolescents and their parents are critical but can also be difficult, given that many adolescents by nature of their developmental stage are not typically considering their future reproductive plans. More recently, Strang et al. developed a questionnaire that included both transgender youth and parents in the creation process to help facilitate conversations and provide psychoeducation around the topic of fertility and fertility preservation to adolescents and their parents. Preliminary results of the questionnaire in a sample of youth found that the majority were not interested in fertility preservation, but many of the respondents also rated that their feelings about having their own biologic child may change over time.[66] The mental health provider can play a very significant role in facilitating this conversation and helping youth consider what their future thoughts on fertility and reproduction may be and the role that fertility preservation could play in their treatment plan. Studies that have looked at transgender adults have found that some individuals have desired to have biologic children in adulthood and express regret in not having done fertility preservation when younger.[67]

CONSIDERATION OF AUTISM SPECTRUM DISORDER DIAGNOSIS/COMANAGEMENT

In a 2010 study, de Vries et al. determined that the incidence of autism spectrum disorder (ASD) in children and adolescents referred to a gender identity clinic in the Netherlands was 7.8%. They noted that in a combined sample, 4.7% of children met criteria for both GID (DSM-IV) and ASD, whereas 17% met criteria for ASD and *Gender Identity Disorder*, Not Otherwise Specified (GID-NOS). The predominance of GID-NOS was postulated to be a result of the diversity of presenting symptoms in their participants with ASD, with some symptoms presenting as atypical in nature, therefore not meeting a full GID diagnosis.[68] A 2014 chart review by Strang et al. comparing the rates of gender variance in children with neurodevelopmental disorders (ASD, Attention Deficit Hyperactivity Disorder (ADHD), or medical neurodevelopmental disorder) compared with controls showed that gender variance existed in 5.4% of children with ASD and that children and adolescents with ASD were 7.5 times more likely than other study groups to report gender variance.[69]

The diagnosis of ASD itself presents a unique set of challenges for youth with co-occurring gender dysphoria because of the deficits in social communication, reciprocity, and nonverbal communication, as well as restricted and highly specific fixed interests that are associated with ASD. Accompanying intellectual and language impairments compound clinical pictures further and require careful consideration by health care providers. One concern regarding the prevalence of gender-nonconforming identification and gender variance in the ASD population is that these estimates may be lower than they truly are, given that treatment considerations for individuals with ASD are often aimed at conforming to social standards and may unknowingly limit gender expression and sexuality.[70]

Clarification and identification of gender dysphoria symptoms in the midst of symptoms more commonly seen in ASD (restricted interests, repetitive behaviors and rigidity) are essential before proceeding to treatment of gender dysphoria. Is a child not interested in playing with traditionally gender-related toys or role play, are they displaying rigidity and fixed interests, or is this interpreted as deficits in social communication? In these children, the diagnosis of gender dysphoria may take longer to develop, require several interviews with the patient, their families, and support systems (school and other treatment providers), and require additional consultation to other providers familiar with either diagnosis. In 2016, Strang et al. aimed to develop clinical guidelines that are specific to the ASD population. They recommend that gender clinic evaluations include screening for ASD and that youth being evaluated for ASD be screened for gender dysphoria. Neither diagnosis should be exclusionary to treatment and intervention, and providers should pay special attention to the presence or development of secondary psychiatric symptoms such as anxiety and mood disorders.[71]

Treatment considerations for comorbid occurrence should address concerns that are specific to each adolescent, with the ultimate goal of improving physical and mental health outcomes, encouraging healthy gender expression and identity development, and fostering independence. In cases where adaptive functioning and overall level of functioning is of concern, a question about independence and ability to make decisions can significantly hinder the transitioning process for an individual with comorbid ASD and gender dysphoria. This becomes a critical issue because all treatment options require high levels of commitment and adherence from the patient, their families, and support systems.[71]

Youth with ASD tend to be more rigid and concrete when compared with their peers, and it is possible that gender identity issues may not arise or be fully appreciated until later in development. Cognitive rigidity particularly related to autism can make coping with gender dysphoria exceptionally difficult for youth with ASD. This can result in distress and marked impairment because flexibility is a skill that is especially important to developing youth with gender dysphoria.[68] Therefore it is important to educate both patients and families about the diagnosis and course of treatment when appropriate. Individuals with ASD are diverse, and treatment should be tailored to the comfort level of the child and their families. For some, expression of gender can be as concrete as wearing the opposite gender's clothing, makeup, or hairstyle. Others may seek a much broader course of treatment; a diagnosis of ASD does not preclude an individual's ability to obtain or pursue treatment for gender dysphoria. Special consideration should be given for individuals with ASD with intellectual impairments, who may benefit from additional consultation with a child and adolescent psychiatrist, developmental pediatrics, and/or bioethicist. Developmental trajectories for children and youth with ASD are also diverse, and a consideration when comorbid gender dysphoria and ASD are present is to regularly reevaluate for symptomatology because communication and interpersonal skills may improve with skills training and treatment.

As children and adolescents with comorbid ASD and gender dysphoria and gender variance begin to explore their gender identity and expression, concrete expressions of gender that do not fully meet social/societal expectations of gender can lead to difficulties with "passing" as their idealized gender and may place them at risk for physical, sexual, or emotional victimization. It is important for parents and health care providers to always consider patient safety and foster a safe environment for youth to continue in their development.[71]

LEGAL ISSUES

When working with adolescents who are not able to consent to medical decisions on their own, difficulties can arise when parents or guardians do not agree on how to support their child with decisions on social and or medical transition. Other legal decisions where parents may not fully agree include decisions around name or gender marker changes to various documentation (e.g., birth certificates, passports, school records, social security cards). Mental health providers can play a role in helping hear from both parents and provide appropriate psychoeducation to help understand the different opinions. There may also be benefit from having a team approach, such as a family therapist who can work with parents, and an individual therapist who can maintain the work with the adolescent and continue to focus on other issues that may be concerning the adolescent.

Another special consideration is the issue of confidentiality. This can be very important given that individuals may not want to fully disclose their identity to everyone around them because of concerns about safety or fears of rejection. Similar to working with any other adolescent, it is important for mental health providers to be especially careful to follow rules of confidentiality. This can be challenging at times when parents are also looking for advice/guidance and frequently have many questions about their child. Providers should also be attuned to rules about documentation and who may have access to those records, such as parents/legal guardians. It is important to take a detailed history with the adolescent about their wishes surrounding privacy and disclosure and to respect their wishes.

Clinical Vignette #3

M is a 14-year-old assigned male at birth who is admitted to an inpatient psychiatric unit for engaging in self-injurious cutting behavior and expresses suicidal ideation in the context of frequent conflict and arguments with parents over academic performance and expectations at home. During M's hospitalization, she discloses to one of the providers that she identifies as a transgender female and desires to use a different name and feminine pronouns (she/her). The well-intentioned provider respects this but also speaks with the rest of the health care staff on the unit about this to encourage them to use her chosen name and pronouns out of respect. Later that evening, during family visiting hours, a different provider who is not as familiar with the situation calls out to M using her chosen name, not realizing that her family is not aware of her transgender identity. Angered, the parents want explanations for why the staff is using a different name and pronouns.

SCHOOL ISSUES

One of the most significant areas in most adolescents' lives is their time spent in the school environment. The school setting can create special considerations when working with an adolescent as opposed to an adult. The Gay, Lesbian, and Straight Education Network National School Climate Survey showed that out of 705 transgender students, 75% reported regular verbal harassment, 32% endorsed regular physical harassment, and 17% reported regular physical assault.[72] Another study looked at both transgender and cisgender adolescents and found much higher rates of reported bullying in the transgender youth group, as well as higher rates of substance use. The authors also found that the presence of bullying in the past 12 months mediated an increased risk of regular substance use.[73] Conversely, having the presence of positive supports has been shown to help mitigate some of these stressors. Greytak et al. showed that transgender youths who attended schools with support groups for LGBT youth and allies or with LGBT-inclusive curricula and supportive educators were less likely to be bullied.[74] As previously mentioned, bullying has been associated with increased rates of depression, anxiety, and suicidality.[75,76]

Schools vary in knowledge about how to best support a transgender child in the school setting and may look to the mental health professional for guidance. Providers should ensure that they discuss with the adolescent what will be discussed, and it can be helpful in some situations for the adolescent to be present to ensure that confidentiality and privacy are respected. Various issues can arise in the school setting, such as bathroom use, locker room use, rooming accommodations for overnight field trips, participation in sports activities that are divided by gender, and name/gender markers on records/student ID cards. The adolescent should guide school officials and providers based on their comfort level with disclosure and what types of accommodations they would like. For example, some adolescents, despite socially and/or medically transitioning, may still not feel comfortable using gendered facilities such as the bathroom or locker room, whereas others may feel comfortable doing so. The adolescent should guide these decisions and should not be put into a situation where they feel pressured into having to disclose their identity more openly or be in situations that are uncomfortable.

ADVOCACY

Medical providers can be impactful advocates and educators for individuals exploring their gender identity, not only to their families but also to the community. The WPATH provides guidelines for medical providers that strongly urge them to advocate on behalf of their patients to schools and community organizations, assisting with identity change documentation and providing support resources for individuals and families. Advocacy and support resources for individuals, parents and families, and healthcare providers have grown significantly and are accessible in-person and online. The following is a brief list of resources that can be accessed for support:

1. WPATH standards of care for medical providers: http://www.wpath.org/
2. The National Center for Transgender Equality, https://transequality.org/
3. Gender Spectrum, provides resources and education on a variety of topics https://www.genderspectrum.org/
4. PFLAG, Parents, Families and Friends of Lesbians and Gays, provides resources and education, as well as active local chapters for individuals and families to become involved, https://www.pflag.org/ourtranslovedones
5. HRC, Human Rights Campaign, provides resources and education for families and individuals, as well as opportunities to become involved in advocacy, http://www.hrc.org/explore/topic/transgender

6. ACLU, American Civil Liberties Union, provides legal support for individuals and families, https://www.aclu.org/issues/lgbt-rights/transgender-rights
7. GLAAD, Gay and Lesbian Alliance Against Defamation, provides media resources and education to individuals and families, https://www.glaad.org/transgender/resources

Role of the Multidisciplinary Team in Management of the Transgender Adolescent

Although a multidisciplinary team approach offers the optimal approach to treating youth with gender dysphoria, few individuals are able to access these needed evaluations. This has been attributed to several obstacles, such as insurance coverage and compensations, as well as the fact there are only a few centers across the country who offer these types of services. Gridley et al. reported on the perspectives of transgender youth on barriers to accessing health care and noted that primary care providers were not only poorly trained in the care of this patient population but also lacked understanding of the health care needs of transgender youth. Their survey study highlighted the lack of accessibility to qualified providers who were trained in gender-affirming treatment and services that are unique and designed specifically for youth. Provider limitations ranged from lack of knowledge about transgender issues including mental health concerns, questioning the seriousness and commitment of the individual to seek these treatments, frequently being referred to other providers, and inappropriate/inconsistent use of pronouns and chosen names.[77]

It is critical that mental health professionals collaborate with medical providers in understanding the risks, benefits, and limitations of interventions so that they can accurately assess whether the adolescent has an understanding before proceeding. There are situations where the mental health professional relies on the medical provider to help inform what interventions may be possible and what limitations may exist. For example, some adolescents present for care having completed pubertal development, and the benefits of puberty suppression may be limited. Other times, some youth and their parents may believe they are experiencing the start of puberty, but this may actually be secondary to the anxiety and distress about the prospect of starting puberty. Collaborative care between the mental health provider and medical provider can also help to ensure that the mental health provider does not miscommunicate the possible options for treatment and/or does not reinforce unrealistic expectations.

REFERENCES

1. Flores AR, Herman JL, Gates GJ, Brown TNT. *How Many Adults Identify as Transgender in the United States.* Los Angeles, CA: The The Williams Institute; 2016.
2. Gates GJ. *How Many People Are Lesbian, Gay, Bisexual, and Transgender.* Los Angeles, CA: The Williams Institute; 2011.
3. Clark TC, Lucassen MF, Bullen P, et al. The health and well-being of transgender high school students: results from the New Zealand adolescent health survey (Youth'12). *J Adolesc Health.* 2014;55(1):93–99.
4. Connolly MD, Zervos MJ, Barone 2nd CJ, et al. The mental health of transgender youth: advances in understanding. *J Adolesc Health.* 2016;59(5):489–495.
5. Almeida J, Johnson RM, Corliss HL, et al. Emotional distress among LGBT youth: the influence of perceived discrimination based on sexual orientation. *J Youth Adolesc.* 2009;38(7):1001–1014.
6. de Vries AL, Cohen-Kettenis PT. Clinical management of gender dysphoria in children and adolescents: The Dutch Approach. *J Homosex.* 2012;59(3):301–320.
7. Aitken M, VanderLaan DP, Wasserman L, et al. Self-harm and suicidality in children referred for gender dysphoria. *J Am Acad Child Adolesc Psychiatry.* 2016;55(6):513–520.
8. Chen M, Fuqua J, Eugster EA. Characteristics of referrals for gender dysphoria over a 13-year period. *J Adolesc Health.* 2016;58(3):369–371.
9. Wood H, Sasaki S, Bradley SJ, et al. Patterns of referral to a gender identity service for children and adolescents (1976–2011): age, sex ratio, and sexual orientation. *J Sex Marital Ther.* 2013;39(1):1–6.
10. Hsieh S, Leininger J. Resource list: clinical care programs for gender-nonconforming children and adolescents. *Pediatr Ann.* 2014;43(6):238–244.

11. James SE, Herman JL, Rankin S, et al. *Executive Summary of the Report of the 2015 U.S. Transgender Survey.* Washington, DC: National Center for Transgender Equality; 2016.
12. American Psychiatric Association, American Psychiatric Association DSM-5 Task Force. Diagnostic and Statistical Manual of Mental Disorders. In: *DSM-5.* 5th ed Washington, DC: American Psychiatric Association; 2013.
13. American Psychiatric Association, American Psychiatric Association. Task Force on DSM-IV. In: *Diagnostic and Statistical Manual of Mental Disorders.* 4th ed. Washington, DC: American Psychiatric Association; 2000. Text Rev. ed.
14. DSM-5 Fact Sheet. Gender Dysphoria [Internet]; 2013. Available from: https://www.psychiatry.org/File%20Library/Psychiatrists/Practice/DSM/APA_DSM-5-Gender-Dysphoria.pdf.
15. Zucker K, Bradley S, Sanikhani M. Sex differences in referral rates of children with gender identity disorder: some hypotheses. *J Abnorm Child Psychol.* 1997;25(3):217–227.
16. van Beijsterveldt CE, Hudziak JJ, Boomsma DI. Genetic and environmental influences on cross-gender behavior and relation to behavior problems: a study of Dutch twins at ages 7 and 10 years. *Arch Sex Behav.* 2006;35(6):647–658.
17. Kohlberg L. A cognitive-developmental analysis of children's sex-role concepts and attitudes. In: Maccoby EE, ed. *The Development of Sex Differences.* Stanford: Stanford University Press; 1966.
18. Ristori J. Gender dysphoria in childhood. *Int Rev Psychiatry (Abingdon, England).* 2016;28(1):13–20.
19. Wallien MS, Cohen-Kettenis PT. Psychosexual outcome of gender-dysphoric children. *J Am Acad Child Adolesc Psychiatry.* 2008;47(12):1413–1423.

20. Drummond KD, Bradley SJ, Peterson-Badali M, Zucker KJ. A follow-up study of girls with gender identity disorder. *Dev Psychol.* 2008;44(1):34–45.
21. Green R. *The "Sissy Boy Syndrome" and the Development of Homosexuality.* New Haven, CT: Yale University Press; 1987.
22. Bakwin H. Deviant gender-role behavior in children: relation to homosexuality. *Pediatrics.* 1968;41(3):620–629.
23. Lebovitz PS. Feminine behavior in boys: aspects of its outcome. *Am J Psychiatry.* 1972;128(10):1283–1289.
24. Zuger B. Early effeminate behavior in boys: outcome and significance for homosexuality. *J Nerv Ment Dis.* 1984;172(2):90–97.
25. Davenport CW. A follow-up study of 10 feminine boys. *Arch Sex Behav.* 1986;15(6):511–517.
26. Money J, Russo AJ. Homosexual outcome of discordant gender identity/role in childhood: longitudinal follow-up. *J Pediatr Psychol.* 1979;4(1):29–41.
27. Steensma TD, McGuire JK, Kreukels BPC, et al. Factors associated with desistence and persistence of childhood gender dysphoria: a quantitative follow-up study. *J Am Acad Child Adolesc Psychiatry.* 2013;52(6):582–590.
28. de Vries AL, McGuire JK, Steensma TD, et al. Young adult psychological outcome after puberty suppression and gender reassignment. *Pediatrics.* 2014;134(4):696–704.
29. Turban JL, Ehrensaft D. Research review: gender identity in youth: treatment paradigms and controversies. *J Child Psychol Psychiatry.* 2017; https://doi.org/10.1111/jcpp.12833 Epub ahead of print.
30. Marshall A. Suicide prevention interventions for sexual & gender minority youth: an unmet need. *Yale J Biol Med.* 2016;89(2):205–213.

31. Mereish EH, O'Cleirigh C, Bradford JB. Interrelationships between LGBT-based victimization, suicide, and substance use problems in a diverse sample of sexual and gender minorities. *Psychol Health Med.* 2014;19(1):1–13.

32. Spack NP, Edwards-Leeper L, Feldman HA, et al. Children and adolescents with gender identity disorder referred to a pediatric medical center. *Pediatrics.* 2012;129(3):418–425.

33. Wallien MS, Swaab H, Cohen-Kettenis PT. Psychiatric comorbidity among children with gender identity disorder. *J Am Acad Child Adolesc Psychiatry.* 2007;46(10):1307–1314.

34. Skagerberg E, Davidson S, Carmichael P. Internalizing and externalizing behaviors in a group of young people with gender dysphoria. *Int J Transgenderism.* 2013;14(3):105–112.

35. Reisner SL, Vetters R, Leclerc M, et al. Mental health of transgender youth in care at an adolescent urban community health center: a matched retrospective cohort study. *J Adolesc Health.* 2015;56(3):274–279.

36. Grossman AH, D'Augelli AR. Transgender youth and life-threatening behaviors. *Suicide Life Threat Behav.* 2007;37(5):527–537.

37. Holt V, Skagerberg E, Dunsford M. Young people with features of gender dysphoria: demographics and associated difficulties. *Clin Child Psychol Psychiatry.* 2016;21(1):108–118.

38. Olson J, Schrager SM, Belzer M, et al. Baseline physiologic and psychosocial characteristics of transgender youth seeking care for gender dysphoria. *J Adolesc Health.* 2015;57(4):374–380.

39. McConnell EA, Birkett MA, Mustanski B. Typologies of social support and associations with mental health outcomes among LGBT youth. *LGBT Health.* 2015;2(1):55–61.

40. Duncan DT, Hatzenbuehler ML. Lesbian, gay, bisexual, and transgender hate crimes and suicidality among a population-based sample of sexual-minority adolescents in Boston. *Am J Public Health.* 2014;104(2):272–278.

41. Meyer-Bahlburg HFL. Gender identity disorder in young boys: a parent- and peer-based treatment protocol. *Clin Child Psychol Psychiatry.* 2002;7(3):360–376.

42. Adelson SL, American Academy of Child and Adolescent Psychiatry (AACAP) Committee on Quality Issues (CQI). Practice parameter on gay, lesbian, or bisexual sexual orientation, gender nonconformity, and gender discordance in children and adolescents. *J Am Acad Child Adolesc Psychiatry.* 2012;51(9):957–974.

43. Menvielle EJ, Tuerk C. A support group for parents of gender-nonconforming boys. *J Am Acad Child Adolesc Psychiatry.* 2002;41(8):1010–1013.

44. Ehrensaft D. From gender identity disorder to gender identity creativity: true gender self child therapy. *J Homosex.* 2012;59(3):337–356.

45. Olson KR, Durwood L, DeMeules M, McLaughlin KA. Mental health of transgender children who are supported in their identities. *Pediatrics.* 2016;137(3):e20153223.

46. Levine DA, Committee on Adolescence. Office-based care for lesbian, gay, bisexual, transgender, and questioning youth. *Pediatrics.* 2013;132(1):e297–e313.

47. American Psychological Association. Guidelines for psychological practice with transgender and gender nonconforming people. *Am Psychol.* 2015;70(9):832–864.

48. Coolhart DD, Shipman DL. Working toward family attunement: family therapy with transgender and gender-nonconforming children and adolescents. *Psychiatr Clin North Am.* 2017;40(1):113–125.

49. Coleman E, Bockting W, Botzer M, et al. Standards of care for the health of transsexual, transgender, and gender-nonconforming people, Version 7. *Int J Transgenderism.* 2012;13(4):165–232.

50. Menvielle E. A comprehensive program for children with gender variant behaviors and gender identity disorders. *J Homosex.* 2012;59(3):357–368.

51. Hill DB, Menvielle E. "You have to give them a place where they feel protected and safe and loved": the views of parents who have gender-variant children and adolescents. *J LGBT Youth.* 2009;6(2–3):243–271.

52. Hembree WC, Cohen-Kettenis PT, Gooren L, et al. Endocrine treatment of gender-dysphoric/gender-incongruent persons: an endocrine society clinical practice guideline. *J Clin Endocrinol Metab.* 2017;102(11):3869–3903.

53. Cohen-Kettenis PT, van Goozen SH. Pubertal delay as an aid in diagnosis and treatment of a transsexual adolescent. *Eur Child Adolesc Psychiatry.* 1998;7(4):246–248.

54. Delemarre-van de Waal HA, Cohen-Kettenis PT. Clinical management of gender identity disorder in adolescents: a protocol on psychological and paediatric endocrinology aspects. *Eur J Endocrinol.* 2006;155(suppl 1):S131–S137.

55. de Vries AL, Steensma TD, Doreleijers TA, Cohen-Kettenis PT. Puberty suppression in adolescents with gender identity disorder: a prospective follow-up study. *J Sex Med.* 2011;8(8):2276–2283.

56. de Vries AL, McGuire JK, Steensma TD, et al. Young adult psychological outcome after puberty suppression and gender reassignment. *Pediatrics.* 2014;134(4):696–704.

57. Kreukels BP, Cohen-Kettenis PT. Puberty suppression in gender identity disorder: the Amsterdam experience. *Nat Rev Endocrinol.* 2011;7(8):466–472.

58. Edwards-Leeper L, Spack NP. Psychological evaluation and medical treatment of transgender youth in an interdisciplinary "Gender Management Service" (GeMS) in a major pediatric center. *J Homosex.* 2012;59(3):321–336.

59. Schneider CC, Cerwenka S, Nieder TO. Measuring gender dysphoria: a multicenter examination and comparison of the utrecht gender dysphoria scale and the gender identity/gender dysphoria questionnaire for adolescents and adults. *Arch Sex Behav.* 2016;45(3):551–558.

60. Lindgren TW, Pauly IB. A body image scale for evaluating transsexuals. *Arch Sex Behav.* 1975;4(6):639–656.

61. Singh D, Deogracias JJ, Johnson LL, et al. The gender identity/gender dysphoria questionnaire for adolescents and adults: further validity evidence. *J Sex Res.* 2010;47(1):49–58.

62. Deogracias JJ, Johnson LL, Meyer-Bahlburg HF, et al. The gender identity/gender dysphoria questionnaire for adolescents and adults. *J Sex Res.* 2007;44(4):370–379.

63. Johnson LL, Bradley SJ, Birkenfeld-Adams AS, et al. A parent-report gender identity questionnaire for children. *Arch Sex Behav.* 2004;33(2):105–116.

64. Seal LJ. A review of the physical and metabolic effects of cross-sex hormonal therapy in the treatment of gender dysphoria. *Ann Clin Biochem.* 2016;53(1):10–20.

65. Nahata L, Tishelman AC, Caltabellotta NM, Quinn GP. Low fertility preservation utilization among transgender youth. *J Adolesc Health.* 2017;61(1):40–44.

66. Strang JF, Jarin J, Call D, et al. Transgender youth fertility attitudes questionnaire: measure development in nonautistic and autistic transgender youth and their parents. *J Adolescent Health.* 2018;62(2):128–135.

67. Wierckx K, Van Caenegem E, Pennings G, et al. Reproductive wish in transsexual men. *Hum Reprod.* 2012;27(2):483–487.

68. de Vries AL, Noens IL, Cohen-Kettenis PT, et al. Autism spectrum disorders in gender dysphoric children and adolescents. *J Autism Dev Disord.* 2010;40(8):930–936.

69. Strang JF, Kenworthy L, Dominska A, et al. Increased gender variance in autism spectrum disorders and attention deficit hyperactivity disorder. *Arch Sex Behav.* 2014;43(8):1525–1533.

70. Moreno A, Laoch A, Zasler ND. Changing the culture of neurodisability through language and sensitivity of providers: creating a safe place for LGBTQIA+ people. *NeuroRehabilitation.* 2017;41(2):375–393.

71. Strang JF, Meagher H, Kenworthy L, et al. Initial clinical guidelines for co-occurring autism spectrum disorder and gender dysphoria or incongruence in adolescents. *J Clin Child Adolesc Psychol.* 2018;47(1):105–115.

72. Kosciw J, Greytak E, Bartkiewicz MJ, et al. *The 2011 National School Climate Survey: The Experiences of Lesbian, Gay, Bisexual, and Transgender Youth in Our Nation's Schools.* New York, NY: Gay, Lesbian, and Straight Education Network; 2012.

73. Reisner SL, Greytak EA, Parsons JT, Ybarra ML. Gender minority social stress in adolescence: disparities in adolescent bullying and substance use by gender identity. *J Sex Res.* 2015;52(3):243–256.

74. Greytak EA, Kosciw JG, Boesen MJ. Putting the "T" in "Resource": the benefits of LGBT-related school resources for transgender youth. *J LGBT Youth.* 2013;10(1–2):45–63.

75. Sourander A, Jensen P, Rönning JA, et al. What is the early adulthood outcome of boys who bully or are bullied in childhood? The Finnish "From a Boy to a Man" study. *Pediatrics.* 2007;120(2):397–404.

76. Kim YS, Leventhal BL, Koh Y, et al. School bullying and youth violence: causes or consequences of psychopathologic behavior? *Arch Gen Psychiatry.* 2006;63(9):1035–1041.

77. Gridley SJ, Crouch JM, Evans Y, et al. Youth and caregiver perspectives on barriers to gender-affirming health care for transgender youth. *J Adolesc Health.* 2016;59(3):254–261.

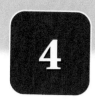

4

Disorders of Sexual Development

PAURUSH BABBAR | ANUP SHAH | BENJAMIN ABELSON | AUDREY C. RHEE

Introduction

Disorders of sexual development (DSD)—a less derogatory term than intersex—are a heterogenous group of conditions characterized by aberrant chromosomal, gonadal, and/or anatomic sex with widely varying genotypic and phenotypic manifestations. Sexual differentiation comprises three successive steps: (1) genotypic events determined at conception in regard to chromosomal composition; (2) phenotypic events driven from the chromosomal makeup, which induce gonadal differentiation; and (3) gender identity formation, which can be a lifelong, evolving paradigm predicated on issues such as hormonal induction, external genitalia, and psychologic factors, to name a few.[1,2] Patients with DSD are generally identified at birth, usually based on physical exam; then a multidisciplinary approach is used to manage these complex issues surgically, psychologically, and socially. These patients are treated by pediatric specialists who are rigorously trained to handle the complex pathophysiology of DSD conditions.

In contrast, transgender patients are genotypically and phenotypically "normal" but have a gender identity that is not congruent with their biologic sex. These patients are usually first evaluated by the physician as adolescents or adults, whereas most DSD patients are plugged into the medical system from a much earlier age. Transgender patients historically have had a much tougher time finding physicians trained in the nuances of their care and only recently have found more holistic and inclusive medical services to meet their needs.

This chapter provides an overview of DSD and the special considerations for these patients. The medical intricacies of DSD and their nuanced treatment is beyond the scope of this chapter. Instead, it delves into a historical overview of sex assignment with special focus on the current guidelines; it concludes by looking at the role of karyotyping in the transgender population.

Embryologic Basis of Sexual Differentiation

An understanding of the embryologic development of the internal and external genitalia is crucial in discussing DSD. We will first discuss the basic steps of normal sexual differentiation so that we can then explain the mechanisms that may alter normal development. Chromosomal gender is determined at the time of conception, as XY chromosomes will lead to male development and XX chromosomes will progress to female development. Early in development, primordial undifferentiated germ cells are arranged in the yolk sac; they will later migrate, become primitive testicles or ovaries, and assist in sexual development.

Two components of the embryo are the precursors to the internal reproductive organs—the paramesonephric (or Müllerian) ducts and the mesonephric (or Wolffian) ducts. Female development is essentially the "default" pathway of development, as the absence of components of the Y chromosome allow for the development of ovaries, fallopian tubes, the uterus, and vagina from the paramesonephric ducts. The so-called testis-determining factor, encoded on the short arm of the Y chromosome (the SRY, or sex-determining region of the Y chromosome) induces growth of the sex cords into primitive testes, where Sertoli cells begin producing Müllerian inhibiting substance (MIS).[3] Without SRY, the sex cords differentiate into ovarian follicles. MIS causes regression of the Müllerian system and stimulates testosterone production from the testicle around the eighth week of gestation, which causes regression of the Müllerian system and stimulates development of the mesonephric duct into the epididymis, vas deferens, and seminal vesicles.[4]

External genitalia remain undifferentiated until the third month of gestation. As shown in Fig. 4.1, urogenital folds fuse anteriorly to form the genital tubercle and lateral swellings form the labioscrotal folds. Testosterone is converted to dihydrotestosterone (DHT), which acts on the external genitalia to enlarge the tubercle into the penis and fuse the urogenital and labioscrotal folds in the midline.[4]

Without androgens, the genital tubercle forms the clitoris and the perineal structures do not fuse in the midline, allowing formation of the vaginal opening.[5] In summary, the production of testosterone and dihydrotestosterone (DHT) is central to the formation of the internal male structures, the involution of the internal female structures, and the development of the male external genitalia. This provides a framework within which most cases of DSD can be understood. There are XX individuals who are virilized as well as XY individuals who are undervirilized due to exposure to androgens or lack of exposure, respectively.

Historical Overview of Sex Assignment at Birth and in Childhood: Current Guidelines

Sex assignment for DSD is a critical medical, social, and legal event that is expected to occur at birth and is often revisited in childhood. Many practitioners argue that this event is of central importance to the care of individuals with DSD.[6–8] In particular, immediately postpartum, parents of DSD children find it particularly distressing to be uncertain regarding the gender assignment of their child, as gender role determines naming, rearing behaviors, and social interactions with other family members. The onus on the medical and surgical teams is to provide guidance in the sex assignment process, and early

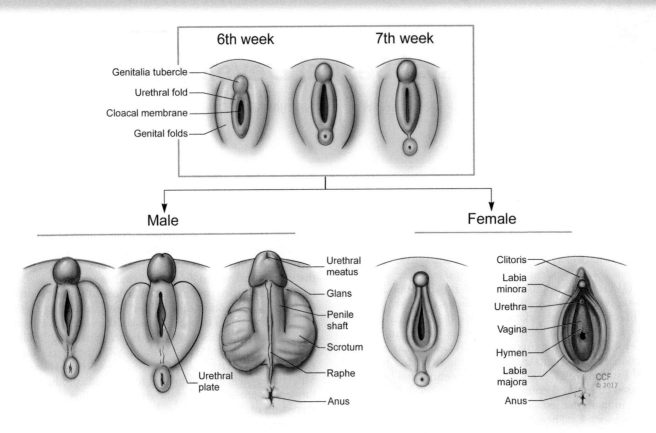

Fig. 4.1   Male–female genital development. DHT is vital factor in the development of the external genitalia. *(Reprinted with permission, Cleveland Clinic Center for Medical Art & Photography © 2017. All Rights Reserved.)*

incorporation of DSD-specialized physicians is encouraged. Specialists typically include pediatric endocrinologists, pediatric surgeons and urologists, gynecologists, pediatric psychologists, geneticists, and neonatologists.

Historically, sex assignment was primarily driven by phenotypic examination of the newborn, followed by the most current techniques in surgical reconstruction for gender assignment.[9–11] The construction of female genitalia is more feasible than the creation of male genitalia[12]; as a result, more DSD patients have been reared as females. Early work to standardize this decision-making process can be traced back to John William Money and colleagues at the Johns Hopkins Hospital in the 1950s.[10,11,13] Money, a psychologist by training, conducted a decades-long clinical practice alongside pediatric endocrinologists and surgeons and developed a clear guideline for determining sex, based on the feasibility of surgical reconstruction of the external genitalia. Money states the following in his 1957 manuscript:[13]

Our findings point to the extreme desirability of deciding, with as little diagnostic delay as possible, on the sex of assignment and rearing when a hermaphroditic baby is born. Thereafter, uncompromising adherence is desirable. The chromosomal sex should not be the ultimate criterion, nor should the gonadal sex. By contrast, a great deal of emphasis should be placed on the morphology of the external genitals and the ease with which these organs can be surgically reconstructed to be consistent with the assigned sex.

Money subscribes to the theory of a blank psychologic slate of gender at birth. Implicitly, Money's research holds two postulates as central to his unifying theory of gender assignment,

and these were articulated in a 1997 review of sex assignment at birth.[12] Money's work was predicated on two fundamental beliefs: (1) that "individuals are psychosexually neutral at birth" and (2) that "healthy psychosexual development is intimately related to the appearance of the genitals." In effect, Money's work not only adhered to a standard that guided the sex assignment of DSD individuals but also implied that gender identity was a predominantly psychologic and social construct that was not rooted in biology. These two postulates have been strongly challenged in recent decades, and a more critical determination of sex assignment is now in practice that takes into account a DSD individual's specific chromosomal, genetic and gondal status in assigning gender at birth.

These changed views have led to the development of consensus guidelines to address the evaluation and management of DSD individuals at birth.[6,14,15] A central theme of these guidelines is that only a minority (20%) of DSD newborns will have a definitive genetic or molecular diagnosis. Evaluation begins with careful physical examination of the newborn by an experienced clinician to evaluate the external genitalia, including a detailed investigation of the labioscrotal folds and their fusion; the presence or absence of gonads in the abdominal, inguinal, or scrotal position; the size of the phallus and the site of the urinary meatus.[14] These landmarks may not be readily apparent on external examination and thus may require surgical exploration. Prior to any exploration, however, the clinician should follow a well-established algorithm that attempts to specify the chromosomal, molecular, and/or anatomic diagnosis of the DSD. A reformatted algorithm to establish the chromosomal or molecular etiology of each specific DSD is shown in Fig. 4.2; it begins with karyotyping to

Genetic Evaluation of DSD

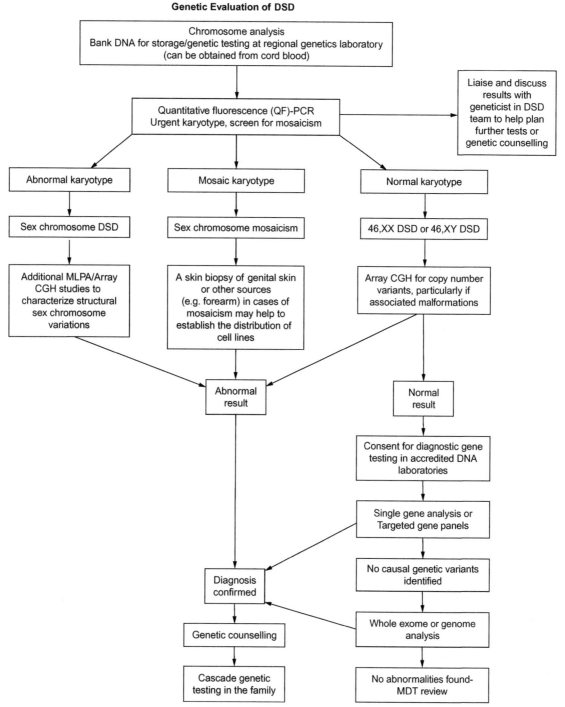

Fig. 4.2 **Genetic evaluation of disorders of sexual development (DSD).** *(From Ahmed SF, Achermann JC, Arlt W, et al. Society for endocrinology UK guidance on the initial evaluation of an infant or an adolescent with a suspected disorder of sex development (revised 2015). Clin Endocrinol (Oxf).* 2016;84(5):771–788.) PCR polymerase chain reaction. MLPA multiplex ligation-dependent probe. CGH comparative genomic hybridization. MDT multi-disciplinary team.

establish the distinction between an overvirilized 46XX-chromosomal female versus an undervirilized 46XY male, or chromosomal mosaicism. Further investigation includes hormonal testing, including 17-OH progesterone, testosterone, gonadotropin-releasing hormone (GnRH), anti-Müllerian hormone, an electrolyte panel, and urinalysis. Abdominal and pelvic ultrasound should be performed to determine the presence or absence of Wolffian or Müllerian structures. Hormonal stimulation tests can be performed as well, including

human chorionic gonadotropin (hCG) and adrenocorticotrophic hormone (ACTH) stimulation. Last, specific genetic determination, although rare, as mentioned earlier, can be performed by microarray or full-sequencing technologies of known sex-determining genes in an attempt to identify a specific genetic defect. Notably, other than the physical exam and imaging, all these laboratory tests take more than a week to be completed. This delay can cause additional stress to the family, and, as providers, we should be sensitive to this.

Given the relative frequency of specific etiologies of DSD, the consensus guidelines can help in assigning gender for these conditions. In a 2006, the "Consensus Statement on Management of Intersex Disorders" by Hughes et al. was published, providing guidelines for sex assignment in cases of DSD.[15] These guidelines recommend that 46XX females with congenital adrenal hyperplasia (CAH) and clitoromegaly be reared as females, with surgical correction for the most virilized of cases. Similarly, patients with 46XY with complete gonadal dysgenesis and 46XY patients with complete androgen insensitivity syndrome (CAIS) should also be reared as females. Contrary to previous recommendations, 46XY males with a micropenis are to be reared as males.[16] Similarly, patients with isolated 46XY hypospadias should be reared as males. A particularly interesting DSD example is the 46XY patient with 5-alpha reductase (5-AR) type 2 deficiency. The majority of these individuals identify as males later in life; however, prior to puberty, many are reared as females because of their phenotype. A nuanced view should be taken with these patients, as studies suggest that individuals with 5-AR-type 2 deficiency who have a phallic length greater than 6 cm report satisfactory sexual function as males.[17]

Per the consensus statement, the majority of patients with DSD (including conditions such as 17-beta-hydroxysteroid dehydrogenase [HSD]-3 deficiency, partial androgen insensitivity syndrome [PAIS], incomplete gonadal dysgenesis, cloacal exstrophy, and ovotesticular DSD) do not have specific recommended gender assignments. Instead, anatomic variances, gonadal function after puberty, as well as social and parental influences should be considered when assigning gender to these patients. A comprehensive multidisciplinary evaluation with endocrinologic, pediatric, and urologic providers may assist in the early determination of gender in these patients.

Overview of Disorders of Sexual Development

DSD can be broadly divided into two categories: undervirilization of 46XY males and virilization of 46XX females.[5] The following text considers some of the more common DSDs that providers should be aware of and specifically focuses on issues of gender identity with regard to each condition. More specific medical and technical surgical issues as they pertain to the listed DSDs are beyond the scope of this chapter; the reader is therefore directed to specialized pediatric urologic reconstruction studies.

UNDERVIRILIZATION OF 46XY MALES

Undervirilization of a male with karyotype 46XY can be due to the defective production of testosterone from the testes during the critical period of sexual differentiation, a receptor defect in detecting testosterone, a defect in the conversion of testosterone to other necessary hormones needed for masculinization, or the impaired action or production of MIS.

Disorders of Androgen Synthesis or Action

Androgen Insensitivity Syndrome (Complete or Partial). Androgen insensitivity syndrome, previously termed "testicular feminization syndrome," can be divided into complete and partial forms. In CAIS, patients are characterized as having a 46XY karyotype with female external genitalia, bilateral testes, and absence of the Müllerian structures. From a genetic perspective, CAIS is

an X-linked condition with an incidence of 1 in 20,000 to 1 in 64,000.[18] Many genetic mutations (e.g., deletions, substitutions, transitions) have been identified in CAIS, but in all cases there is a defect in the gene encoding the androgen receptor, which impairs the target organs' ability to detect and/or process testosterone.[19] CAIS patients will exhibit normal-appearing external female characteristics with the exception of appropriate secondary pubic and axillary hair. Interestingly, at puberty these patients will have breast development secondary to increased plasma estradiol; as a result, they develop a feminine body habitus.[2] CAIS is one of the DSDs that may not be identified at birth, as these patients phenotypically appear like normal female neonates. However, with the increasing adoption of prenatal genetic screening, more of these patients can be identified at birth. Often, they are diagnosed when they are incidentally found to have testes during inguinal hernia repair surgery or during evaluation for primary amenorrhea in early adolescence.[2] At this age, patients present with diminished pubic and axillary hair and a genital exam that is notable for a blind-ended vagina and absence of a cervix. Imaging will confirm complete absence of the Müllerian structures. Diagnosis of CAIS is further confirmed with karyotype testing, as these patients are always 46XY.

Surgical management of these patients is predicated on the optimal timing of gonadectomy. Historically, patients underwent gonadectomy shortly after birth, when pediatric anesthesia was deemed safe, so as to mitigate the increased risk of testicular malignancy. The downside to early gonadectomy is the postoperative need for exogenous estrogen therapy to induce puberty and the need for yearly dual energy x-ray absorptiometry (DEXA) scans to screen for compromised bone mineral density.[20] Consensus guidelines have recently changed and experts now recommend that the gonadectomy be delayed until after puberty to allow peripheral aromatization of testosterone to estradiol, which would then facilitate appropriate pubertal physiologic changes. Studies have found that the risk of testicular malignancy in CAIS is much lower than previously thought; the incidence is now estimated to be at approximately 2%. Most cases are seminomas and occur in adolescence or later in life.[20] CAIS patients have been thought to have a female gender identity, but recent studies have found that their gender identities are variable, with a higher than expected proportion of patients reporting a nonandrophile sexual orientation.[21]

PAIS is a collection of X-linked disorders characterized by a wide array of phenotypic manifestations of incomplete masculinization including the presence of ambiguous genitalia. These patients have a 46XY karyotype but unlike their CAIS counterparts, they are often identified at birth. Classically, patients are found to have some combination of hypospadias, rudimentary Wolffian duct remnants, gynecomastia, and infertility. Hundreds of mutations have been identified in PAIS but most commonly, patients have a reduced number of androgen receptors or decreased binding affinity in these receptors for testosterone.[2] Treatment for patients with PAIS is predicated on the inevitable virilization of the ambiguous genitalia and their subsequent appearance. If raised as male, patients with cryptorchid testes undergo orchidopexy; gynecomastia is addressed and genital reconstruction is performed. Surveillance of the testicles by a urologist is important, as there is an increased risk of testicular malignancy in these patients. Contrary to CAIS patients, patients with PAIS are considered at high risk for testicular malignancy. Therefore in those patients who are raised as female, early gonadectomy is recommended. In these patients, genital reconstruction with procedures such as bowel

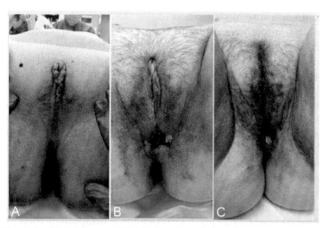

Fig. 4.3 (A) Labioscrotal folds fused at the midline with a shallow dimple along the perineum. Preputial skin around the phallic structure and hypospadiac meatus. (B) Three weeks postoperatively from bowel vaginoplasty and labioplasty. (C) Eight weeks postoperatively from bowel vaginoplasty and labioplasty.

vaginoplasty with labioplasty is an option, and we report excellent outcomes at our institution (Fig. 4.3). Last, patients raised as females will need adjunctive hormone therapy starting at puberty. Gender identity in patients with PAIS is an intriguing topic, and there is evidence showing that brain androgen receptors have the same mutation for partial androgen insensitivity as the other end-organ targets.[2] Studies have found that the gender in which a PAIS child is reared often correlates with that individual's gender identity when he or she is an adult.[22]

5-alpha-Reductase Deficiency. 5-AR deficiency involves a mutation in the 5-AR enzyme, which catalyzes the conversion of testosterone to DHT. DHT is broadly responsible for male phenotypic development and pubertal androgen-mediated tissue growth. As a result, patients with 5-AR deficiency are 46XY karyotype and have varying presentations of their external genitalia ranging from a microphallus with degrees of hypospadias to a phenotypic female with clitoromegaly. Often these patients have a bifid scrotum and a diminutive phallus, which, in the infant presenting with this condition, can be mistaken for female genitalia with clitoromegaly. On exam, these patients have a blind-ended vagina with the presence of testes and epididymides in the labia majora, inguinal canals, or abdomen. At puberty these patients can experience a marked increase in phallic size with male-pattern muscular development, and there are reports of spermatogenesis in some patients and the achievement of fertility through assisted reproductive techniques.[23] Virilization after puberty occurs as a result of the higher levels of in vivo testosterone that eventually overwhelms the androgen receptors and because there is an isoform of 5-AR that is usually inactive. At puberty, however, this acts as the catalyst that converts some of the high levels of testosterone to DHT, which accounts for many of the aforementioned postpubertal changes. Patients with 5-AR deficiency are diagnosed prepubertally with an hCG stimulation test, which results in an elevated plasma testosterone:DHT ratio.

In patients diagnosed in the neonatal period who are to be reared as males, androgen supplementation can be initiated immediately to augment penile growth and aid in surgical genital repair.[24] During puberty these patients undergo typical virilization, as seen in patients with 5-AR deficiency; phenotypically these patients are indistinguishable from natal males in their muscular development and body hair distribution. Surgically,

these patients may require phalloplasty, scrotoplasty, urethroplasty, extirpation of the vaginal pouch, and orchidopexy.[25]

Patients who are not diagnosed early in life are often raised as female until they reach puberty, at which point the disorder is usually recognized; then a bilateral orchiectomy is performed and estrogen supplementation is initiated. If they self-identify as female, these patients will require feminizing genitoplasty and clitoroplasty to achieve satisfactory cosmesis of their ambiguous genitalia. However, not all of these individuals will identify as female. There are case reports of some who were initially reared as female but, at puberty, self-identified as male. Clearly gender assignment and identification remain challenging issues in this patient population, and consideration to identity should be given when these patients are being treated medically and surgically.

Disorders of Gonadal (Testicular) Development

Complete Gonadal Dysgenesis. First described in 1955 by Swyer,[26] complete gonadal dysgenesis (Swyer syndrome) describes a normal phenotypic female, with female internal and unambiguous external genitalia, tall stature, and primary amenorrhea with a 46XY karyotype.[27] With an incidence of 1 in 80,000 births and an autosomal recessive inheritance pattern, patients with complete gonadal dysgenesis have streak gonads that do not produce testosterone. As a result, there is no differentiation of the Wolffian structures or secretion of anti-Müllerian hormone (which is the key agent in the regression of Müllerian structures). Although these disorders can easily be mistaken for one another, CAIS differs from gonadal dysgenesis since CAIS patients usually have bilateral testes and produce anti-Müllerian hormone; as a result, they lack internal female pelvic organs. Approximately 90% of patients with complete gonadal dysgenesis are diagnosed at puberty, when they present for the evaluation of primary amenorrhea.[28] Once the diagnosis of complete gonadal dysgenesis has been made, they are started on exogenous estrogen therapy in order to induce pubertal changes, and the streak gonads are surgically removed to reduce the risk of gonadal tissue malignancy. Patients with complete gonadal dysgenesis are reared as females and tend to maintain this gender identity throughout life.

Ovotesticular Disorders of Sexual Development. Ovotesticular disorder of sexual development, or true hermaphroditism, broadly describes patients who have both ovarian and testicular tissue on histologic examination.[29] When a gonad contains both ovarian follicles and testicular seminiferous tubules, it is called an "ovotestis." Patients with ovotesticular DSD can present with bilateral ovotestis, one ovotestis and a contralateral ovary or testis, or an ovary with a contralateral testis.[29] The karyotype of these patients can vary: the majority are 46XX and the remainder are various mosaic forms. Most commonly, patients with some degree of ambiguous genitalia and undescended gonads as well as inguinal hernias are diagnosed at birth. Very rarely, patients have well-differentiated external genitalia and are diagnosed at puberty, when they present with inguinal hernias, undescended gonads, gynecomastia, cyclic hematuria, or amenorrhea.[29] Most patients with ovotesticular DSD have a uterus, but in many cases it is rudimentary.[24]

Gender assignment in these cases is dependent on factors such as the presence of a uterus and the stage of its development, the size of the phallus, the amount of testicular tissue present, and whether the hypospadias is surgically correctable.[24] Female gender assignment is considered in patients with a uterus and if sufficient ovarian tissue is present. These patients will need a partial gonadectomy to remove all testicular tissue and reduce risk of malignant transformation. There may be a need for exogenous estrogen therapy depending on the amount and functionality of the ovarian tissue. There are case reports of successful pregnancies in patients reared as female who had a well-developed uterus and ovaries. Many leading authorities advocate that in patients who present with the possibility of future fertility, consideration should be given to assigning these individuals as female and rearing them as such. For patients with sufficient phallic length, a correctable degree of hypospadias, and viable testicular tissue, male gender assignment may be a good choice, although there are no published reports of fertility in these patients.

VIRILIZATION OF 46XX FEMALES

Androgen Excess

Congenital Adrenal Hyperplasia. CAH is group of autosomal recessive enzyme deficiencies that are responsible for the most common cause of virilization in the 46XX female. It is also the most common cause of ambiguous genitalia in the newborn. Many enzymatic deficiencies can cause CAH, but the three most common are 21-hydroxylase (21-OH) deficiency (~90%), 11-beta-hydroxylase deficiency (5% to 8%), and 3-beta-HSD (1% to 2%). These enzymes are critical in the cortisol biosynthetic pathway; with a deficiency in them, one will see impaired production of hydrocortisone and a resultant increase in ACTH. This will ramp up the production of adrenal steroids proximal to the enzymatic defect, which can in turn upregulate the secondary production of testosterone, causing the virilization and ambiguous genitalia seen in patients with a 46XX karyotype (Fig. 4.5).

CAH secondary to 21-OH deficiency comprises over 90% of cases and is related to mutations on the short arm of chromosome 6 in the *CYP21* gene. From a clinical perspective, there is a classic salt-wasting form (75% of patients) that presents with electrolyte imbalances and virilization; a simple virilizing form (25% of patients); and a very rarely observed nonclassic form, which of late onset with neither salt wasting nor virilization.

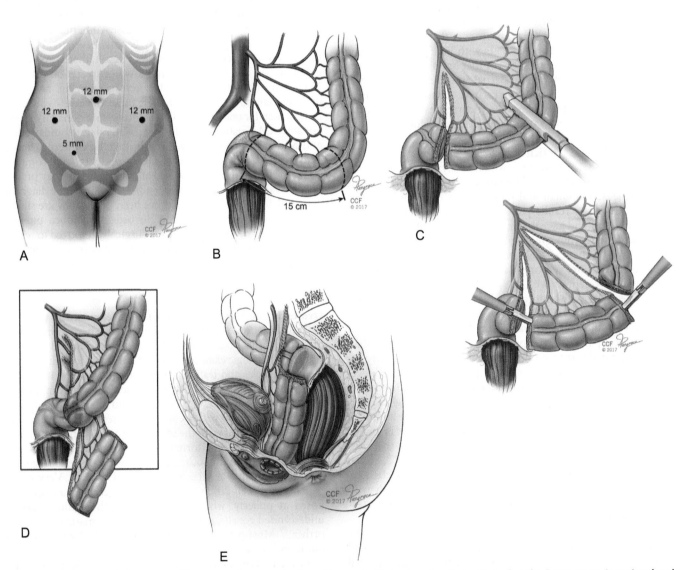

Fig. 4.4   (A) Suggested placement of laparoscopic trocars for bowel harvest of bowel vaginoplasty. Note that the 5 mm trocar is optional and can be used for aiding in removal of a prostatic utricle. (B) Position of bowel segment. (C) Stapling devices are used. Care is taken to ensure sufficient length of mesentery is obtained. (D) Care is taken to ensure adequate blood supply to the segment of bowel used. (E) A neovaginal introitus is created along the perineum where the segment of bowel is anastomosed. *(Reprinted with permission, Cleveland Clinic Center for Medical Art & Photography © 2017. All Rights Reserved.)*

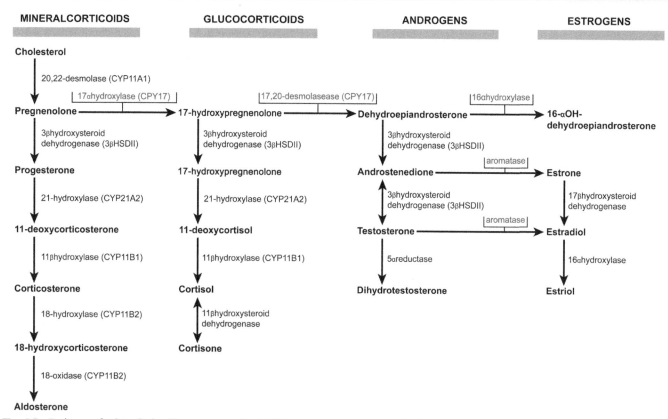

Fig. 4.5 Pathway of adrenal gland hormone synthesis. Most common enzymes with clinical relevance in the disorder of congenital adrenal hyperplasia are noted.

In females with the classic salt-wasting and simple virilizing forms of CAH, some degree of virilization is present and there are findings of ambiguous genitalia such as clitoromegaly, labial fusion, and a common urogenital sinus between the urethra and vagina. In the most severe forms (often associated with the salt-wasting form), there are findings of a hypospadiac penis from the grossly enlarged clitoris and bilateral undescended gonads. The nonclassic form may present in adolescence or adulthood with precocious puberty, clitoromegaly, oligomenorrhea, hirsutism, and infertility. Patients with CAH from 21-OH deficiency have an elevation in basal plasma 17-hydroxyprogesterone, the substrate upstream from the deficient enzyme. In general, patients with 21-OH deficiency will have decreased aldosterone (although this can be normal), decreased cortisol, and excess androgen (Table 4.1). In neonates with the salt-wasting form of CAH, there can be symptoms of failure to thrive, weight loss, lethargy, vomiting, and dehydration from adrenal crises. There have been reports of death from hyperkalemia and severe dehydration in the most severe cases. In female

patients, the finding of masculinization and ambiguous genitalia will suggest to the astute clinician further investigation for CAH; however, this can be delayed in males who appear phenotypically normal.

The second most common enzymatic defect causing CAH is 11-beta-hydroxylase (11-beta-OH) deficiency, which has an incidence of 1 in 100,000 live births and is associated with a mutation in the *CYP11B1* gene. There is a classical form that presents with severe virilization in females; such individuals appear at birth to be phenotypically normal males and are often not recognized at that time. The nonclassical form is generally diagnosed in childhood and adolescence with premature adrenarche, penile growth/clitoromegaly, hypertension, advanced skeletal age, hirsutism, oligomenorrhea, and infertility. Interestingly, these patients will not present with life-threatening symptoms of adrenal crisis because salt wasting generally does not occur. 11-beta-OH deficiency is diagnosed with selective elevation of 11-deoxycorticosterone (DOC) and 11-deoxycortisol, which are the two steroids upstream from the 11-beta-OH. As in patients with 21-OH deficiency, glucocorticoid levels in these patients are decreased and androgen levels are increased. The mineralocorticoid levels are increased as a result of an elevation in 11-DOC, a potent mineralocorticoid. Such an elevation in mineralocorticoids can cause hypertension, hypernatremia, and hypokalemia in patients with 11-beta-OH deficiency.

Rarely, patients will have an enzymatic deficiency of 3-beta-HSD, which causes CAH. These patients generally have low mineralocorticoid and glucocorticoid levels, which can cause a salt-wasting diathesis with hyperkalemia. These patients will generally have low levels of sex steroids, but their dehydroepiandrosterone (DHEA) levels are elevated, which can in turn

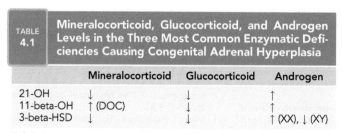

TABLE 4.1	Mineralocorticoid, Glucocorticoid, and Androgen Levels in the Three Most Common Enzymatic Deficiencies Causing Congenital Adrenal Hyperplasia		
	Mineralocorticoid	Glucocorticoid	Androgen
21-OH	↓	↓	↑
11-beta-OH	↑ (DOC)	↓	↑
3-beta-HSD	↓	↓	↑ (XX), ↓ (XY)

DOC, Deoxycorticosterone; *HSD,* hydroxysteroid dehydrogenase; *OH,* hydroxylase.

cause mild hypervirilization in the female fetus but undervirilization in the male fetus due to the relatively weak effect of DHEA. The diagnosis of 3-beta-HSD is made by elevated serum levels of 17-hydroxypregnenolone and DHEA.

Although the medical management of CAH is predicated on the replacement and optimization of mineralocorticoids, glucocorticoids, and androgens, the surgical management presents a unique challenge. Many advocate that 46XX individuals with CAH and hypervirilization should be reared as females and that feminizing genitoplasty with procedures such as clitoroplasty, vaginoplasty, and labioplasty should be performed to assist with gender assignment. However, the timing of these procedures remains controversial. Recently surgeons have been optimizing the surgical technique used for genitoplasty so as to offer procedures resulting in good cosmesis and also functionality. Zucker and colleagues found that of 26 female CAH patients who underwent genital reconstruction, 60% were very satisfied and 32% were moderately satisfied with the cosmetic outcomes.[30,31] Lesma et al. found that 34.8% of female patients who underwent surgical intervention for CAH required revision vaginoplasty for vaginal stenosis.[32] There is still much work to be done with regards to whether reconstructive procedures are necessary and to optimizing the time of and outcomes these procedures to ensure patient satisfaction.

Disorders of Gonadal (Ovarian) Development

Ovotesticular Disorders of Sexual Development. The earlier text includes a discussion of ovotesticular DSD.

Gonadal Dysgenesis. The earlier text includes a discussion of gonadal dysgenesis.

Role of Karyotyping in the Transgender Population

Of particular interest is the study of gender identity and gender dysphoria and its relationship with DSD. The ICD-10 (International Classification of Diseases) criteria for gender dysphoria or transgenderism in childhood specifically state that inclusion into these diagnoses must preclude any separate diagnosis of DSD. Specifically, the ICD-10 64.0 criteria state that "the disorder is not a symptom of another mental disorder or a genetic, intersex, or chromosomal abnormality." Providers seeing young patients presenting with persistent gender-nonconforming behaviors should consider including a DSD workup if the clinical scenario indicates that this is warranted.

To our knowledge, the largest published study that examined the relationship between DSD and gender identity was published by Inoubli et al., who studied a cohort of 368 transgender individuals (251 male-to-female, 117 female-to-male) and found that 3.19% of male-to-female patients and 0.85% of the female-to-male patients had an abnormal karyotype.[33] Of the male-to-female cohort, three patients were diagnosed with Klinefelter disease (XXY) and four were found to have translocations not associated with the sex-chromosomes. In the female-to-male group, one patient had a translocation not associated with sex chromosomes. The authors noted that that the incidence of Klinefelter syndrome in this cohort (1.2%) was higher than that in the general population. Additionally, the incidence of any karyotyping abnormality in the entire cohort (2.45%) was also higher than that in the general population (0.63%).[33,34] Nevertheless, the authors argue that the utility of universal karyotyping in the treatment and management of patients with gender dysphoria is limited and that patients with DSD will typically have other clinical or hormonal signs that would point to a DSD diagnosis. We believe that karyotyping should be performed in select patients, such as phenotypic females with primary amenorrhea or phenotypic males with hypogonadism. In the absence of these signs, karyotyping can be omitted from the initial evaluation of patients presenting with gender dysphoria.

Conclusion

The care of patients with DSD is extremely nuanced and must be handled with the utmost care. At this time a multidisciplinary team approach is employed by most large academic centers. This ensures that patients and their families receive an integrated approach to care at a centralized location. Having specialists trained in the intricacies of DSD is crucial to the short- and long-term well-being of patients on the medical, surgical, psychologic, social, and spiritual levels. The general recommendation is for early coordination of care with a designated clinical lead so that new diagnostic and clinical information can be shared with the patient and his or her family.[14]

The medical community has made progress in the evaluation and treatment of patients with DSD. It is important to be cognizant of the differences between transgender patients and those with DSD. We must recognize that gender identity is separate from phenotypic presentation, but it remains an important part of the conversation, especially with regard to gender assignment.

REFERENCES

1. Jost A, Vigier B, Prépin J, Perchellet JP. Studies on sex differentiation in mammals. *Recent Prog Horm Res.* 1973;29:1–41.
2. Diamond DA, Yu RN. Disorders of sexual development: etiology, evaluation, and medical management. In: Wein AJ, Kavoussi LR, Partin AW, Peters CA, eds. *Campbell-Walsh Urology.* 11th ed. Philadelphia, PA: Elsevier; 2016:3469–3497.
3. Park JM. Embryology of the genitourinary tract. In: Wein AJ, Kavoussi LR, Partin AW, Peters CA, eds. *Campbell-Walsh Urology.* 11th ed. Philadelphia, PA: Elsevier; 2016:2823.
4. Cuckow P. Embryology of the urogenital tract. In: Gearhard J, Rink R, Mouriquand P, eds. *Pediatric Urology.* 2nd ed. Philadelphia, PA: Elsevier; 2009:1.
5. Bouvattier C. Disorders of sex development: endocrine aspects. In: Gearhart J, Rink R, Mouriquand P, eds. *Pediatric Urology.* 2nd ed. Philadelphia, PA: Elsevier; 2009.
6. Fisher AD, Ristori J, Fanni E, et al. Gender identity, gender assignment and reassignment in individuals with disorders of sex development: a major of dilemma. *J Endocrinol Invest.* 2016;39(11):1207–1224.
7. Meyer-Bahlburg HF. Sex steroids and variants of gender identity. *Endocrinol Metab Clin North Am.* 2013;42(3):435–452.
8. Houk CP, Lee PA. Approach to assigning gender in 46,XX congenital adrenal hyperplasia with male external genitalia: replacing dogmatism with pragmatism. *J Clin Endocrinol Metab.* 2010;95(10):4501–4508.
9. DiSandro M, Merke DP, Rink RC. Review of current surgical techniques and medical management considerations in the treatment of pediatric patients with disorders of sex development. *Horm Metab Res.* 2015;47(5):321–328.
10. Hampson JG, Money J, Hampson JL. Hermaphrodism: recommendations concerning case management. *J Clin Endocrinol Metab.* 1956; 16(4):547–556.
11. Money J, Hampson JG, Hampson JL. Hermaphroditism: recommendations concerning assignment of sex, change of sex and psychologic management. *Bull Johns Hopkins Hosp.* 1955;97(4):284–300.

12. Diamond M, Sigmundson HK. Sex reassignment at birth. Long-term review and clinical implications. *Arch Pediatr Adolesc Med.* 1997;151 (3):298–304.

13. Money J, Hampson JG, Hampson JL. Imprinting and the establishment of gender role. *AMA Arch Neurol Psychiatry.* 1957;77(3):333–336.

14. Ahmed SF, Achermann JC, Arlt W, et al. Society for endocrinology UK guidance on the initial evaluation of an infant or an adolescent with a suspected disorder of sex development (revised 2015). *Clin Endocrinol (Oxf).* 2016;84(5):771–788.

15. Hughes IA, Houk C, Ahmed SF, Lee PA. Lawson Wilkins Pediatric Endocrine Society/European Society for Paediatric Endocrinology Consensus Group. Consensus statement on management of intersex disorders. *J Pediatr Urol.* 2006;2 (3):148–162.

16. Bin-Abbas B, Conte FA, Grumbach MM, Kaplan SL. Congenital hypogonadotropic hypogonadism and micropenis: effect of testosterone treatment on adult penile size why sex reversal is not indicated. *J Pediatr.* 1999;134 (5):579–583.

17. Cheon CK. Practical approach to steroid 5alpha-reductase type 2 deficiency. *Eur J Pediatr.* 2011;170(1):1–8.

18. Ahmed SF, Cheng A, Dovey L, et al. Phenotypic features, androgen receptor binding, and mutational analysis in 278 clinical cases reported as androgen insensitivity syndrome. *J Clin Endocrinol Metab.* 2000;85(2):658–665.

19. Saranya B, Bhavani G, Arumugam B, et al. Three novel and two known androgen receptor gene mutations associated with androgen insensitivity syndrome in sex-reversed XY female patients. *J Genet.* 2016;95(4):911–921.

20. Patel V, Casey RK, Gomez-Lobo V. Timing of gonadectomy in patients with complete androgen insensitivity syndrome-current recommendations and future directions. *J Pediatr Adolesc Gynecol.* 2016;29(4):320–325.

21. Brunner F, Fliegner M, Krupp K, et al. Gender role, gender identity and sexual orientation in CAIS ("XY-women") compared with subfertile and infertile 46,XX women. *J Sex Res.* 2016;53 (1):109–124.

22. Gangaher A, Chauhan V, Jyotsna VP, Mehta M. Gender identity and gender of rearing in 46 XY disorders of sexual development. *Indian J Endocrinol Metab.* 2016;20(4):536–541.

23. Kang HJ, Imperato-McGinley J, Zhu YS, et al. The first successful paternity through in vitro fertilization-intracytoplasmic sperm injection with a man homozygous for the 5 alpha-reductase-2 gene mutation. *Fertil Steril.* 2011;95 (6):2125.e5–2125.e8.

24. Gearhart JG, Rink RC, Mouriquand PDE. *Pediatric Urology.* 2nd ed. Philadelphia: Elsevier; 2009.

25. Costa EM, Domenice S, Sircili MH, et al. DSD due to 5alpha-reductase 2 deficiency—from diagnosis to long term outcome. *Semin Reprod Med.* 2012;30(5):427–431.

26. Swyer GI. Male pseudohermaphroditism: a hitherto undescribed form. *Br Med J.* 1955;2 (4941):709–712.

27. King TF, Conway GS. Swyer syndrome. *Curr Opin Endocrinol Diabetes Obes.* 2014;21(6): 504–510.

28. Michala L, Goswami D, Creighton SM, Conway GS. Swyer syndrome: presentation and outcomes. *BJOG.* 2008;115(6):737–741.

29. Irkilata HC, Basal S, Taslipinar A, et al. Ovotesticular disorder of sex development with a prostatic gland and review of literature. *Andrologia.* 2009;41(6):387–391.

30. Zucker KJ, Bradley SJ, Oliver G, et al. Self-reported sexual arousability in women with congenital adrenal hyperplasia. *J Sex Marital Ther.* 2004;30(5):343–355.

31. Wang LC, Poppas DP. Surgical outcomes and complications of reconstructive surgery in the female congenital adrenal hyperplasia patient: what every endocrinologist should know. *J Steroid Biochem Mol Biol.* 2017;165:137–144. Pt A.

32. Lesma A, Bocciardi A, Montorsi F, Rigatti P. Passerini-glazel feminizing genitoplasty: modifications in 17 years of experience with 82 cases. *Eur Urol.* 2007;52(6):1638–1644.

33. Inoubli A, De Cuypere G, Rubens R, et al. Karyotyping, is it worthwhile in transsexualism? *J Sex Med.* 2011;8(2):475–478.

34. Maeda T, Ohno M, Matsunobu A, et al. A cytogenetic survey of 14,835 consecutive liveborns. *Jinrui Idengaku Zasshi.* 1991;36(1):117–129.

Hormone Treatment for the Adult Transgender Patient

RAY QIAN, JR. | JOSHUA D. SAFER

Introduction

Transgender medicine is a developing field of medicine that spans multiple subspecialties. Transgender individuals are defined as those whose gender identity differs from the assigned sex recorded for them at birth based on external sexual characteristics. Gender identity includes an innate biologic component in humans,[1] rather than a reversible trait developed from societal constructs.

This chapter will provide an overview of the different modalities of medical therapy available for transgender individuals. Medicines, mostly in the form of sex hormones, are able to effectively modulate the various endocrine pathways of the human body responsible for sex characteristics considered traditionally male and female. With appropriate supervision, it is now feasible for both transgender men and women who are interested in modifying their physical characteristics to have their body appearance better align with their gender identity.

The Biologic Nature of Gender Identity

The hypothesis that gender identity is of a biologic origin is supported by multiple studies.[1] Research that validates this includes observational studies of genetically male individuals born with congenital abnormalities who were assigned and raised either as males or females,[2] with a proportion undergoing surgical feminization.[1,3] Individuals who were raised as males were found to have more comfort with their gender identities than those raised as females,[1] findings that went against the long-held belief that gender identity was established through societal or parental influences.

Neuroanatomically, certain regions of the brain in transgender individuals appear more in-line with their gender identity.[4,5] In a post-mortem analysis of six transgender women[4] (male to female, MTF) and one transgender man[5] (female to male, FTM), the size of the bed nucleus of the stria terminalis of the hypothalamus was similar to the expected size of typical females and males, respectively. This was the case, independent of exposure to sex hormone treatment or sexual orientation. A neuroimaging study with magnetic resonance imaging (MRI) scans of living transgender individuals showed transgender women prior to beginning hormone therapy with larger, "feminized" regional gray matter within the right putamen,[6] whereas therapy-naïve transgender males had "masculinized" gray matter of the right putamen.[7] In another study, positron emission tomography (PET) scans of individuals' hypothalamus during exposure to 4,16-androstadiene3-one, a compound that reportedly provokes hypothalamus responses in a sexual dimorphic manner, showed that treatment-naïve transgender females had hypothalamus activity responses similar to nontransgender female controls.[8]

Typical Hormone Regimens for Transgender Men

Testosterone replacement is the mainstay therapy for transgender men desiring a more masculine appearance.[9,10] The treatment regimen very much resembles therapies for males with hypogonadism, with the goal of therapy to achieve testosterone levels within the normal male physiological range (300 to 1000 ng/dL). Patients typically will notice signs of male sexual maturation (increased facial and body hair, muscle mass, acne, and libido), as well as amenorrhea within the first several months after initiating testosterone therapy. Other changes, such as male pattern hair loss, voice deepening, redistribution of fat away from the waist and hips, and clitoromegaly, are also usually seen within the first year of therapy.

Hormone regimens for transgender men are listed in Table 5.1. Testosterone can be administered via several routes: through daily transdermal patches (2.5 to 7.5 mg/day) and gels (2.5 to 10 g/day); weekly via subcutaneous or intramuscular injections of testosterone enanthate or testosterone cypionate (50 to 200 mg/week or 100 to 200 mg/2 weeks); quarterly via testosterone undecanoate (1000 mg/12 weeks); and orally with oral testosterone undecanoate (160 to 240 mg/day).[a] Regimens may be initiated at half the estimated effective dose and then titrated quickly to achieve physiological testosterone levels. Although transgender men often use lower doses than required for other men in general, due to being smaller, it is also safe to start regimens at the full effective dose.

Typical Hormone Regimen for Transgender Women

Hormone regimens for transgender women are listed in Table 5.2. Due to their ease of administration and wide availability, oral formulations of conjugated estrogens (2.5 to 7.5 mg) and 17-beta estradiol (2 to 8 mg) are the typical first line estrogens used. Estrogens may also be administered topically or intramuscularly. However, the regimen for transgender women desiring to achieve female sex characteristics is more complicated, as supplementing exogenous estrogen alone is not usually sufficient in decreasing endogenous testosterone levels to female levels (30 to 100 ng/dL) to achieve feminization.

In conjunction with estrogen therapy, spironolactone, an aldosterone receptor antagonist with diuretic properties known for decreasing mortality in patients with advanced heart failure,[11] is commonly prescribed for its antiandrogen effects for transgender women (similar to its use for treatment of hirsutism and polycystic ovarian syndrome). Spironolactone can be prescribed at

---

[a]Oral formulations currently not available in the United States.

TABLE 5.1	Hormone Regimens for Transgender Men

TRANSDERMAL

Patch 2.5–7.5 mg/day
Gel 1% 2.5–10 g/day

SUBCUTANEOUS/INTRAMUSCULAR

Testosterone enanthate, cypionate
50–200 mg/week
100–200 mg/2 weeks

Testosterone undecanoate
1000 mg/12 weeks

ORAL

Testosterone undecanoate
160–240 mg/day

TABLE 5.2	Hormone Regimens for Transgender Women

ESTROGEN THERAPY

Transdermal
17-beta estradiol 0.1–0.4 mg 1 or 2 times/week

Oral
Conjugated estrogens 2.5–7.5 mg/day
17-beta estradiol 2–8 mg/day

Intramuscular
Estradiol valerate 5–30 mg/2 weeks

ANTIANDROGEN THERAPY

Spironolactone (PO) 100–400 mg/day
Leuprolide (IM) 3.75–7.5 mg/month
Histrelin acetate (SC implant) 50 mg/12 months
Goserelin acetate (SC implant) 3.6 mg/month
Cyproterone acetate (PO) 50–100 mg/day

IM, Intramuscular; *PO*, oral; *SC*, subcutaneous; *TD*, transdermal.

100 to 200 mg daily, with a maximum of 400 mg as tolerated. Potential side effects in addition to urinary frequency that should be monitored with each dose change include hyperkalemia and orthostatic hypotension. Alternate antiandrogen adjuncts to estrogens include GnRH agonists like leuprolide and goserelin acetate and progestins such as cyproterone acetate which may also be added as part of medical therapy. The goal of combination therapy is to achieve female testosterone levels without supraphysiologic levels of estrogen in the body and the potentially dangerous side effects thought to be associated with high-dose estrogens.

Physical changes are typically observed during the first several months of therapy and include decreased libido and spontaneous erections, decreased facial and body hair, atrophy of muscle mass, decreased skin oiliness, redistribution of body fat to the hips, waist, and thighs, and increase in breast tissue growth. After several years of hormone therapy, the prostate and testes may atrophy, and breast tissue will achieve its maximal growth.

Treatment Safety, Risks of Hormone Therapy, and Monitoring of Adverse Effects

Overall, hormone therapy for transgender men and women is safe, effective, and well tolerated.[12] Despite reported concerns, data do not suggest increased incidence of cancer in transgender

patients treated with hormone therapy.[13–16] While there is an association with estrogen therapy and venous thromboembolism (VTE), there does not appear to be an increased incidence of myocardial infarction or transient ischemic attack among transgender individuals compared to nontransgender controls.[17,18,19]

TRANSGENDER MEN

Guidelines propose the following contraindications to testosterone therapy: individuals who are pregnant, have symptoms of unstable coronary artery disease, or have untreated polycythemia.[20] It is not possible for testosterone therapy to unmask polycythemia and hyperlipidemia, both of which should be monitored and treated accordingly. Current data do not suggest that patients undergoing testosterone therapy are at increased risk for malignancies of the uterus and ovaries.[14,21–25]

Transgender men on testosterone therapy should have routine monitoring approximately every 3 months during the first year of therapy (meaning with each dose change), and then every 6 to 12 months thereafter for both efficacy of therapy and for potential side effects. Testosterone levels should be checked at these intervals, as well as hemoglobin/hematocrit and other labs, such as a lipid profile as needed. A baseline bone mineral density evaluation can be performed before initiating testosterone therapy when there is concern and appropriate cancer screening should be continued for all organs and tissues present (e.g. cervix, breast).

TRANSGENDER WOMEN

As with all individuals on estrogen therapy, there is a possible risk of developing a VTE[13,17] due to the procoagulant effects of estrogen. This can lead to significant morbidity and mortality and there is fear that the risk could be compounded by other hypercoagulable factors. All patients, if initiated on exogenous estrogen therapy, should be counseled on this risk, as well as screened for personal and family history of VTE, tobacco smoking, and active malignancy. It is reasonable to avoid prescribing ethinyl estradiol due to its particular high risk of thrombogenicity.[9]

Monitoring is typically performed approximately every 3 months (meaning with each dose change) during the first year of treatment and 6 to 12 months thereafter. The goal is to achieve testosterone levels that fall within the female range (<100 ng/dL) while avoiding supraphysiologic estradiol levels (>200 ng/mL). For those individuals who are prescribed spironolactone, potassium should be monitored to avoid hyperkalemia. Individual bone mineral densities and lipid profiles, both of which can be affected by estrogen, can be monitored when there is concern. Routine screening for all organs and tissues present (e.g. prostate, breast) should also be undertaken. Some practitioners also monitor prolactin levels, although this may not be needed when the adjunctive testosterone lowering agent is spironolactone.[26]

Adjustment of Hormone Therapy Postsurgery

Gender affirmation surgery for transgender women usually involves orchiectomy. Once the gonads are removed, patients can discontinue antiandrogen therapy and can reduce estrogen treatment doses to conventional replacement levels (e.g., perhaps half the dose required to keep testosterone in the female range).

Other Considerations

MENTAL HEALTH

To provide comprehensive care for the transgender patient, it is imperative that there be strong mental health support available to those that need it. Prior to starting hormone therapy, patients should be screened for comorbid psychiatric conditions that may impair an individual's ability to undergo hormone therapy and for rare confounding psychiatric disorders that may be mistaken for gender dysphoria.[27] Due to profound social stigma,[28] there is a high incidence of mental health morbidity among the transgender population, which should be adequately addressed prior to and then in parallel with hormone therapy.

CHILDREN AND ADOLESCENTS

In children, unlike with adults, transgender identity is not always clear. Regardless, no medical intervention is required until adolescence.[29,30] GnRH analogs can be given in early adolescence (usually at Tanner stage 2) to delay complete sexual maturation. These medications serve a two-fold purpose: to allow time for an individual's sexual identity to become more apparent, and to allow the transgender individual to avoid an unwanted puberty experience.[30] Later in adolescence, hormonal treatment can be considered. Additionally, irreversible procedures and surgeries are not typically performed until patients are of age of majority to legally consent independently.[10]

REFERENCES

1. Saraswat A, Weinand JD, Safer JD. Evidence supporting the biologic nature of gender identity. *Endocr Pract.* 2015;21(2):199–204.
2. Reiner WG, Gearhart JP. Discordant sexual identity in some genetic males with cloacal exstrophy assigned to female sex at birth. *N Engl J Med.* 2004;350:333–341.
3. Meyer-Bahlburg HFL. Gender identity outcome in female-raised 46,XY persons with penile agenesis, cloacal exstrophy of the bladder, or penile ablation. *Arch Sex Behav.* 2005;34:423–438.
4. Zhou J-N, Hofman MA, Gooren LJG, Swaab DF. A sex difference in the human brain and its relation to transsexuality. *Nature.* 1995;378:68–70.
5. Kruijver FP, Zhou JN, Pool CW, et al. Male-to-female transsexuals have female neuron numbers in a limbic nucleus. *J Clin Endocrinol Metab.* 2000;85:2034–2041.
6. Luders E, Sánchez FJ, Gaser C, et al. Regional gray matter variation in male-to-female transsexualism. *Neuroimage.* 2009;46:904–907.
7. Zubiaurre-Elorza L, Junque C, Gómez-Gil E, et al. Cortical thickness in untreated transsexuals. *Cereb Cortex.* 2013;23:2855–2856.
8. Berglund H, Lindström P, Dhejne-Helmy C, Savic I. Male-to-female transsexuals show sex-atypical hypothalamus activation when smelling odorous steroids. *Cerebr Cortex.* 2008;18:1900–1908.
9. World Professional Association for Transgender Health. *Standards of Care for the Health of Transsexual, Transgender, and Gender Nonconforming People.* 7th version. <https://www.wpath.org/publications/soc>; 2011. Accessed 14.11.18.
10. Joint meeting of the International Society of Endocrinology and the Endocrine Society: ICE/ENDO 2014. <https://endo.confex.com/endo/2014endo/webprogram/Paper14354.html>; 2014. Accessed 01.08.16.
11. Nagarajan V, Chamsi-Pasha M, Tang WHW. The role of aldosterone receptor antagonists in the management of heart failure: an update. *Cleve Clin J Med.* 2012;79:631–639.
12. Weinand JD, Safer JD. Hormone therapy in transgender adults is safe with provider supervision; a review of hormone therapy sequelae for transgender individuals. *J Clin Transl Endocrinol.* 2015;2(2):55–60.
13. Wierckx K, Elaut E, Declercq E, et al. Prevalence of cardiovascular disease and cancer during cross-sex HRT in a large cohort of trans persons: a case-control study. *Eur J Endocrinol.* 2013;169(4):471–478.
14. Miller N, Bédard Y, Cooter N, Shaul D. Histological changes in the genital tract in transsexual women following androgen therapy. *Histopathology.* 1986;10(7):661–669.
15. Jacobeit J, Gooren L, Schulte H. Safety aspects of 36 months of administration of long-acting intramuscular testosterone undecanoate for treatment of female-to-male transgender individuals. *Eur J Endocrinol.* 2009;161(5):795–798.
16. Kuroda H, Ohnisi K, Sakamoto G, Itoyama S. Clinicopathological study of breast tissue in female-to-male transsexuals. *Surg Today.* 2008;38(12):1067–1071.
17. Wierckx K, Mueller S, Weyers S, et al. Long-term evaluation of cross-sex hormone treatment in transsexual persons. *J Sex Med.* 2012;9:2641–2651.
18. Ott J, Kaufmann U, Bentz E, et al. Incidence of thrombophilia and venous thrombosis in transsexuals under cross-sex HRT. *Fertil Steril.* 2010;93(4):1267–1272.
19. Getahun D, Nash R, Flanders WD, et al. Cross-sex hormones and acute cardiovascular events in transgender persons: a cohort study. *Ann Intern Med.* 2018;169(4):205–213.
20. Coleman E, Bockting W, Botzer M, et al. Standards of care for the health of transsexual, transgender, and gender-nonconforming people, version 7. *Int J Transgenderism.* 2012;13(4):165–232.
21. Baldassarre M, Giannone F, Foschini M, et al. Effects of long-term high dose testosterone administration on vaginal epithelium structure and estrogen receptor-α and -β expression of young women. *Int J Impot Res.* 2013;25(5):172–177.
22. Mikhaĭlichenko V, Fesenko V, Khmelnitskiĭ N, et al. Morphological and functional changes of organs of female and male reproductive systems at change of sex. *Urologiia.* 2013;3:18–23.
23. Ikeda K, Baba T, Noguchi H, et al. Excessive androgen exposure in female-to-male transsexual persons of reproductive age induces hyperplasia of the ovarian cortex and stroma but not polycystic ovary morphology. *Hum Reprod.* 2013;28(2):453–461.
24. Turo R, Jallad S, Prescott S, Cross W. Metastatic prostate cancer in transsexual diagnosed after three decades of estrogen therapy. *Can Urol Assoc J.* 2013;7(7–8):E544–E546.
25. Dorff T, Shazer R, Nepomuceno E, Tucker S. Successful treatment of metastatic androgen-independent prostate carcinoma in a transsexual patient. *Clin Genitourin Cancer.* 2007;5(5):344–346.
26. Bisson JR, Chan KJ, Safer JD. Prolactin levels do not rise among transgender women treated with estradiol and spironolactone. *Endocr Pract.* 2018;24(7):646–651.
27. Safer DL, Bullock KD, Safer JD. Obsessive-compulsive disorder presenting as gender dysphoria/gender incongruence: a case report and literature review. *AACE Clinical Case Reports.* 2016;2(3):e268–e271.
28. Bockting WO, Miner MH, Swinburne Romine RE, et al. Stigma, mental health, and resilience in an online sample of the US transgender population. *Am J Public Health.* 2013;103:943–951.
29. Wallien MSC, Cohen-Kettenis PT. Psychosexual outcome of gender-dysphoric children. *J Am Acad Child Adolesc Psychiatry.* 2008;47:1413–1423.
30. Cohen-Kettenis PT, Delemarre-van de Waal HA, Gooren LJG. The treatment of adolescent transsexuals: changing insights. *J Sex Med.* 2008;5:1892–1897.

Hormone Treatment for the Adolescent Transgender Patient

STEPHANIE ROBERTS | JEREMI CARSWELL

Foreword

While it is still a different era than anyone born before 1965 can remember, much is left to be done to optimize care of transgender youth. Whether to include *Gender Dysphoria* as a psychiatric diagnosis in the next version of the *Diagnostic and Statistical Manual of Psychiatric Diseases* (DSM) remains controversial.[1] This is reminiscent of 1973, when homosexuality was removed from the DSM as a psychiatric disease.[2] Only within the past 5 years has *Gender Identity Disorder* been expunged from the DSM and replaced with *Gender Dysphoria*, which had helped to soften the view of this diagnosis being seen as a psychological illness.[3] Previously, transgender youth were only able to obtain insurance coverage for mental health services for their diagnosis of *Gender Dysphoria*. Neither medical therapy to suppress unwanted natal puberty nor gender-affirming hormones were covered under this diagnosis. The most expensive treatments of gender-affirmative care, including "top surgery" in transgender men and feminizing genitoplasties in transgender women were limited to those who could afford high out-of-pocket expenses. This created a privileged environment for those who could afford medical and surgical transition. Thankfully, more insurance companies are recognizing the medical and surgical necessity of these treatments to alleviate gender dysphoria and its associated comorbid depression and anxiety.

It has not been an easy road to the current state of caring for transgender youth. Current guidelines have recommended delaying medical transition until the age of 16 and, until then, mental health counseling was the mainstay of treatment.[4,5] If transgender youth have to wait until age 16 for medical intervention, little can be done for trans men who complete full female puberty, with their final height unable to be influenced by medical treatment and a need for a complicated mastectomy to remove breast tissue. If intervention could be done earlier, weekly testosterone could stop menses and induce masculinization including virilizing the body, face and scalp hair, muscle development, and changes in fat distribution. Trans women who reach 16 years without intervention may develop a full male voice, facial hair, or Adam's apple. These young patients would have benefited from the typical antiandrogen treatment of spironolactone to suppress the pilosebaceous unit associated with hair growth, as well as high-dose oral estrogen in order to suppress serum testosterone levels to the low physiologic female range. Pushing the estrogen dose to these high doses increases the risk of thromboembolism; however, without this type of dosing, virilization may continue, necessitating some to pursue expensive electrolysis while others may be dissatisfied with their breast growth prompting them to seek augmentation surgery.

There are many medical and surgical consequences associated with delay in treatment, but the greatest morbidity in adolescents is the consequence associated with the persistent disconnect between their gender identity and their ability to live in their affirmed gender social role. One statistic says it best: there is a 41% risk of suicide attempt in young adults who are 18 to 24 years old if their affirmed identity is not supported or treated psychologically or medically.[6] When one of the pioneers of transgender medicine, Dr. Louis Gooren, from Amsterdam's Gender Clinic retrospectively studied the causes of death of approximately 1200 individuals from his cohort, he found that the risk of mortality was 51% higher than the general population. The psychological causes, mainly suicide and drug abuse, were unrelated to the use of hormonal therapy.[7] All patients in this cohort had started hormonal treatment as adults. The authors concluded that delayed treatment resulted in patients feeling unable to fit in physically and socially and this played a significant role in the cause of death of many of the patients studied. These data provided the impetus for the Dutch to try an earlier more effective treatment, now affectionately termed "the Dutch protocol" on which our current approach to transgender youth is based.

Norman Spack, MD

Introduction

Since ancient times there has been recognition of gender variance. Classical mythology abounds with examples of the gender variant; the most well-known is the Greek Olympian god Dionysus, who was male in figure but frequently described as androgynous. Hermaphroditus, the son of Hermes and Aphrodite, fell in love with the water nymph Salmacis, who had their physical forms joined to form an androgynous being. Agdistis, a multigendered and powerful god, was created by the mating of Zeus with Mother Earth.[8,9] In more modern times, the acceptance and recognition of gender nonconformity has been increasing at an unprecedented rate, with subsequent expansion of dedicated medical and mental health specialists all over the world.[10–13] Accurate estimates of the number of people defining themselves as gender variant is unknown but historically varies from 1 in 4000 to 1 in 50,000, but the actual prevalence is likely to be much higher.[14] It is currently estimated that there are about 700,000 adults in the United States who are transgender, although the true number is not currently known.[15]

Cross-sex hormonal therapy for adults has been available for many years but its use is not always able to completely alter the natal physiologic changes that occurred at the time of puberty, leading many patients to seek surgical procedures to help them with their transition. Suppressive therapy to prevent unwanted and often distressing secondary sex characteristics with gonadotropin-releasing hormone (GnRH) agonists to block the natal puberty was first described by the Dutch in 1998 but is now widely used and part of the standards of care for adolescents.[4,5,16] The incorporation of these agents, casually called "blockers," has revolutionized the care of transgender adolescents, allowing them to much more easily pass in society as their self-identified gender. Available evidence suggests that hormonal transition is an effective treatment for gender dysphoria,[17] and blockers have become a mainstay treatment for younger patients.

The model for transgender adolescent care in the United States was first established by our group at Boston Children's Hospital based on practices pioneered by Amsterdam's Gender Clinic. In standard practice, children are given a GnRH agonist for pubertal blockade in early puberty followed by consideration for cross-sex hormones at age 16 years and gender affirmation surgery after age 18.[18] While practices for cross-sex hormone therapy have mostly been extrapolated from adult transgender care pathways, the timing of puberty in adolescents requires special consideration. Puberty onset varies in each individual and may be less apparent in natal boys as testicular enlargement without outward androgenic signs is the first sign of puberty and is often unrecognized by parents. Additionally, arresting puberty causes a return to a prepubertal growth rate and proceeding with or altering the dosing regimen of cross-sex hormones may need to be hastened in order to avoid the development of poor bone density and to take into account desired adult height. If the above-mentioned standard practice is followed, (implementing cross-sex hormones closer to 16 years of age), adolescents on GnRH agonists may suffer from remaining in a prepubertal body while their peers undergo their normally timed natal puberty.

This chapter will review the current hormonal therapy options available for the adolescent with particular emphasis on pubertal blockade and subsequent gender-affirming hormone therapy.

Guidelines and Requirements for Hormone Therapy

The approach to treating children and adolescents is complex, as available evidence suggests that the majority of children who behave in a "cross gender role" prepubertally may later identify with their natal gender during or after adolescence, a phenomenon known as "desistance."[19–21] Looking retrospectively it appears that there is a link between the intensity of the gender dysphoria and continued identification into adolescence and adulthood.[22,23] That is, children who are highly persistent, insistent, and consistent in their identity are likely to be stable in their trans-identity into adulthood. Additionally, when the physical signs of puberty appear, the dysphoria worsens. Despite this knowledge, being able to accurately identify these "persistent" children during the prepubertal phase is a challenge. The decision to initiate hormone therapy, therefore, has been recommended to be not only measured and multidisciplined, but also timed to start after the first signs of puberty.

Similar to the adult patient, guidelines for the diagnosis and treatment of adolescents are available from both the Endocrine Society and the World Professional Association for Transgender Health (WPATH) standards of care, both of which rely on the DSM for guidance in establishment of the diagnosis.[4,5] A skilled mental health professional must first make the diagnosis of Gender Dysphoria.[24] Rationale for this recommendation is that it is important to be able to identify and parse out other conditions that may obscure the correct diagnosis as well as ensuring that there is continued mental health support during social and medical transition.

The DSM 5 has revised its nomenclature, replacing the diagnosis Gender Identity Disorder with the term Gender Dysphoria. This emphasizes that the clinically important element is distress surrounding the condition, while making the distinction that gender nonconformity is not itself a disorder.[25,26] As an example, hormone therapy may provide significant relief to an individual who has gender dysphoria but not necessarily to someone who has gender nonconformity without distress. While it is controversial and potentially stigmatizing to have gender-related issues fall under the realm of mental health, advocates point out that its inclusion allows for medical and mental health treatment to be covered by insurance using this diagnosis. The International Classification of Diseases, 11th edition (ICD 11) will likely use the term Gender Incongruence and move this diagnosis out of the chapter of mental and behavioral disorders.[27,28]

The administration of gender-affirming exogenous hormones is considered essential to the treatment of gender dysphoria by current standards of care.[4,5] Hormone therapy must be balanced based on its risk/benefit ratio, the patient's coexisting medical conditions, social concerns, and cost. The efficacy of hormonal therapy has been well studied and documented, although many of these studies include patients who have also undergone gender affirmation surgery. A meta-analysis conducted by Murad and colleagues of 28 studies of both hormone therapy as well as gender affirmation surgery found significant improvement in gender dysphoria, quality of life, and psychological symptoms after therapy, albeit from relatively low quality studies.[17] One prospective study assessing 57 patients at varying time points following treatment for diagnosed Gender Dysphoria found that the most substantial decrease in psychoneurotic distress occurred after the initiation of cross-sex hormones.[29] The corollary is that the risk of suicidality is decreased with better access to medical treatment.[30]

The rationale for hormonal therapy is based on the observation that young prepubertal children are typically gender-identified by their clothing, mannerisms, and activities. The ability to prevent the physical characteristics that typically associate with what is feminine or masculine would allow for the trans-identifying individual to avoid the permanent secondary sexual characteristics that are often distressing. For the adolescent in early puberty there is the potential for two phases for hormone therapy: the suppression of natal hormones to prevent the secondary sexual characteristics of the assigned gender, and the initiation of gender-affirming or "cross-sex" hormones.

Guidelines for GnRH agonist treatment as outlined by the Endocrine Society (Table 6.1) state that adolescents should fulfill criteria for a diagnosis of Gender Dysphoria (DSM 5) and that they should be in early puberty, as the emotional reaction to physical changes of puberty has diagnostic value. Additionally, they must not have a psychiatric comorbidity that interferes with diagnosis or treatment. They must also have adequate psychological and social support and they must demonstrate understanding of the purpose of the GnRH agonist and its role in the larger picture of gender transition. Current guidelines advocate for use of GnRH agonists in all adolescents prior to cross-sex hormone administration; however, this may not be required in late-presenting adolescents, especially trans men who can effectively virilize with exogenous testosterone treatment. As previously mentioned, GnRH agonist therapy can be expensive and it is currently covered in a limited number of states.[31]

TABLE 6.1	Criteria for Gender Affirming Hormone Therapy for Adolescents

Adolescents are eligible for GnRH agonist treatment if:
1. A qualified mental health professional has confirmed that the adolescent has a diagnosis of Gender Dysphoria consistent with DSM 5 criteria with symptoms worsening with the onset of puberty, and that any co-existing psychological, medical or social problems that could interfere with treatment have been addressed.
2. The adolescent is informed of the treatment risks and side effects and both the adolescent and guardian(s) have provided consent for treatment.
3. A pediatric endocrinologist or other clinician experienced in pubertal assessment agrees with the indication for treatment, has confirmed that Tanner Stage 2 or greater of puberty has occurred, and has confirmed that there are no medical contraindications to treatment.

Adolescents are eligible for cross-sex hormone treatment if:
1. They fulfill the criteria for GnRH agonist treatment and there is persistence of gender dysphoria.
2. The adolescent has sufficient mental capacity to estimate the risks and benefits of treatment and both the adolescent and guardian(s) have provided consent for treatment.

Adapted from Hembree WC, Cohen-Kettenis PT, Gooren L, et al. Endocrine treatment of gender-dysphoric/gender-incongruent persons: an Endocrine Society clinical practice guideline. J Clin Endocrinol Metab. 2017;102(11):3869–3903.

Per the guidelines, an adolescent should fulfill all of the above criteria and have the capacity to make an informed decision to receive gender-affirming hormones. It is important to note that since publication of the 2011 guidelines, the age of initiation of gender-affirming hormones has steadily decreased, with some centers starting as young as 12 or 13 years of age in selected cases. In our practice, the youngest we typically start cross hormone therapy is 14 years. The newest guidelines were published in 2017 and do not restrict providers to a minimum age. It is also worth noting that although there is a stipulation for adults to have "real life experience" as living in their affirmed gender (they live full-time in this gender), there is no such recommendation specific to the adolescent for either puberty blocker treatment or cross-sex hormone administration.

As the field of transgender medicine has evolved, it has become evident that not every adolescent has a "classic" presentation of *Gender Dysphoria*; they may be quite comfortable with their current state of physical development but still maintain a strong desire to move forward with GnRH agonist or gender-affirming hormones. This is something that should not necessarily preclude hormonal therapy, particularly as GnRH agonists are reversible. When assessing a gender nonconforming child or adolescent with dysphoria who desires a neutral gender, their identity as such should not be overlooked. The withholding or delay of therapy is by itself an unfavorable option with potentially severe psychosocial and permanent physical health consequences. These scenarios can be quite challenging if the adolescent and parents are not in agreement, which emphasizes the need for a multidisciplinary team approach to caring for these patients.

Considerations in the Adolescent Patient Population

Providing medical treatment to the transgender adolescent carries an increased complexity compared to the treatment of adults. Family dynamics and need for guardian consent in the absence of clear factors to identify those youth who will persist in their affirmed gender identity must be balanced within the co-occurrence of an unwanted natal puberty, which if left untreated, can worsen gender dysphoria. Transgender youth often feel that they are suffering from precocious puberty of an unwanted natal puberty and delayed puberty of their self-affirmed gender. Medical providers also struggle with the lack of long-term safety data on current standards in medical care of transgender youth in an era of evidence-based medicine.[32] Evolving practices in caring for transgender youth include meeting patients' needs as the prevalence of nonbinary gender identity increases, where adolescents may exhibit gender fluidity.[33] Additionally, increasing medical complexity, such as the increasing prevalence of autism spectrum disorder in transgender youth, can complicate the assessment of gender identity and obtainment of assent for treatment.[34–36]

Newer publications have highlighted the protective role that parental support and acceptance may have on the development of mental health disorders and high-risk behaviors such as substance abuse in transgender youth.[37–39] Parental support has been associated with significantly higher satisfaction in life and fewer depressive symptoms including a lower rate of suicidal ideation.[40] It is widely known that suicide attempts in transgender youth are alarmingly high. In one study of trans youth 12 to 24 years of age, nearly one-fourth had mild-to-moderate depression and one-tenth had severe to extreme depression. Half of the youth had reported contemplating suicide and one-third had attempted suicide at least once. These rates have been supported by other studies at other centers caring for transgender children and adolescents. In addition, high-risk behaviors are prevalent among trans youth with many reporting alcohol, tobacco, marijuana, and other illicit drug use.[41] Transgender youth require ongoing monitoring for depressive symptoms as they may be at risk for developing suicidal ideation as they get older, which can be independent of behavioral and emotional problems.[42]

Ethical issues in treating adolescents include respecting an adolescent's autonomy and right to assent to treatment while requiring the consent of his or her parents or guardians for moving forward with medical treatment.[43] Providers struggle with how best to proceed with treatment in cases where one or both parents are not in support of the diagnosis of gender dysphoria and/or certain treatments for medical transition. Very challenging cases may require the consult of an ethics committee or involvement of a legally appointed guardian to advise on the child's best interest.

Adequate consent for gender affirming hormones must include the unknown long-term risks to fertility. Increased awareness for the need for adequate fertility education, access to care, and treatment options for this population is growing.[44] This was previously thought to be an issue concerning only adults, but children are significantly affected as well.[45] Data from the literature on central precocious puberty have shown that GnRH agonist treatment confers no risk to fertility.[46] Fertility preservation options will vary based on the pubertal stage at the time of gender-affirming hormone initiation.[47] Families should be offered a consultation with a fertility specialist if available in the medical community and future studies are needed to clarify how opinions on parenthood and fertility vary as the adolescent ages. We have data that show that transgender adults who have pursued parenthood have been able to reimagine having a child under different terms and have resisted accepting current cultural norms of parenthood.[48]

Finally, while there is relative consensus on how to support and treat adolescents, social transition in prepubertal children is more controversial.[49] Increasing attention has been given to the role of the provider in advising parents of transgender youth and support has been mounting for a gender affirmative model.[49] Some argue that prepubertal children should be treated to reduce gender dysphoria and increase acceptance of their assigned sex.[50] Newer studies show the positive effects that are associated with supporting the affirmed gender of gender nonconforming prepubertal children. These studies show that those children who are allowed to socially transition have similar rates of depression and only minimally increased rates of anxiety when compared to cischildren of the same age.[51,52] Further prospective studies are needed.

Pubertal Suppression

The prevention of the secondary sexual characteristics of an individual's natal gender has become standard of care in the treatment of gender nonconforming individuals and is recommended by both WPATH and the Endocrine Society in the treatment of these patients, and has been published as part of the Dutch protocol.[53–55] This relatively simple intervention has revolutionized the experience for many individuals, allowing them to avoid many of the secondary sexual characteristics of their biologic sex, thus giving them in essence a "tabula rasa" for the hormone therapy of their affirmed gender and allowing them to "pass" in society more easily in their affirmed gender, which has been associated with better psychological adjustment and outcomes in adulthood.[56]

While the benefit of GnRH agonists is the reversibility of the treatment, medical providers and psychologists caring for transgender youth share concerns about the psychological impact of removing sex hormones via GnRH agonist therapy during a critical time of sex steroid exposure in adolescence. However, proponents of GnRH agonist therapy assert that this treatment offers much needed relief from the development of natal puberty and allows the adolescent, their family, and mental health and medical providers additional time to explore the adolescent's gender identity, extent of dysphoria, and appropriate treatment plan.

From a physiologic standpoint, the hypothalamic-pituitary-gonadal (HPG) axis undergoes a period of quiescence in childhood and is subsequently reactivated at the onset of puberty. This reactivation is due to a complex interplay of genetic, environmental, and nutritional factors. Puberty is initiated by the release of tonic inhibition of pulsatile secretion of GnRH from the hypothalamus in the setting of increased stimulatory factors on GnRH secretion. These pulses cause release of luteinizing hormone (LH) and follicular-stimulating hormone (FSH) from the pituitary gland. These pituitary gonadotropins then circulate to the gonads and stimulate production of sex steroids, predominantly estrogen from the ovary and testosterone from the testes (Fig. 6.1).[57]

With the use of GnRH agonists, there is loss of endogenous GnRH pulsatility. GnRH agonists bind to the GnRH receptor, initially stimulating the pituitary gonadotrophs to produce and secrete LH and FSH and downstream gonadal sex steroids. Following this initial response, there is desensitization and downregulation of the GnRH receptor and subsequent inhibition of the HPG axis including loss of natal sex steroids. One of the most important issues to counsel patients about is the

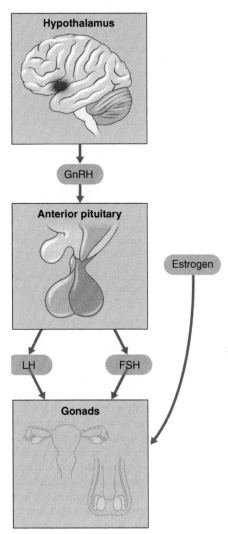

Fig 6.1 The hypothalamus secretes gonadotropin-releasing hormone, which during puberty signals the pituitary gland to release luteinizing hormone *(LH)* and follicular-stimulating hormone *(FSH)*. These gonadotropins then signal the gonads (either testes or ovaries) to make sex steroids. The gonadotropin-releasing hormone *(GnRH)* agonist works at the level of the hypothalamus and pituitary gland, causing a downregulation of GnRH receptors in the pituitary gland and desensitization of the pituitary gonadotropes, thus decreasing levels of LH and FSH. (Adapted from Du Plessis SS, Cabler S, McAlister DA, Sabanegh E, Agarwal A. The effect of obesity on sperm disorders and male infertility. *Nat Rev Urol.* 2010;7:153–161.)

potential for a surge in pubertal signs and symptoms that occurs because of the initial agonist action of the medication. Measurement of LH and FSH immediately following the first dose of GnRH agonist will yield an elevation of LH/FSH and gonadal steroids. These should, however, return to low normal or prepubertal levels.[58]

In prepubertal transgender youth who are determined to be good candidates for therapy, GnRH agonists are administered in the early stages of puberty, classified as Tanner stage 2 breast development in natal girls and 4 mL testicular size in natal boys (Fig. 6.2A and B). In Caucasian US youths, this typically occurs at around age 10 years for both boys and girls (data from National Health and Nutrition Examination Survey (NHANES) collected 1988–94), although this has been the subject of some debate.[59] It is important to distinguish central puberty from

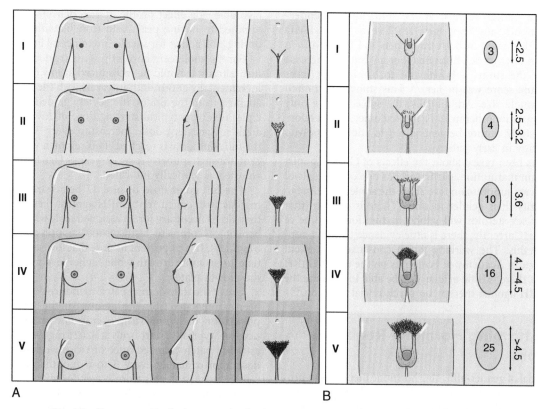

Fig. 6.2 Tanner staging for breast and pubic hair. (A) Female. (B) Male. (By Michal Komorniczak.)

adrenarche, which is the awakening of the adrenal glands that promotes growth and development at the pilosebaceous units of the skin.[60,61] Adrenarche is responsible for apocrine odor, axillary hair, acne, and pubic hair. This distinction is particularly important as adrenarche and puberty are often temporally related but are different axes entirely, and adrenarche may precede central puberty by several years.[62-64] This distinction can be determined by clinical and biochemical assessment by an experienced clinician.

GnRH agonists can also be used in transgender adolescents in late or completed puberty. While generally tolerated, this may lead to perimenopausal symptoms, such as low energy, hot flashes, and decreased libido due to the sudden loss of sex hormones. Linear growth will also be affected for the duration of the blockade; children will be expected to grow at a prepubertal velocity, which is much lower than the sex-steroid–fueled growth spurt of adolescence. In the late pubertal child, GnRH agonist therapy may be appropriate for a natal female who has developed some breast tissue but remains premenarchal or in the natal male who is has enlarged testicles but has not yet developed facial hair or a more angular face shape.

GnRH agonists are available as an intramuscular injection or as a subcutaneous implant. A daily intranasal spray is available but not widely used in this population. Leuprolide is available as a once-monthly or every-3-month injection, while histrelin acetate is available as a subcutaneous implant that releases medication daily. In our clinical practice, we often use the latter given its high level of effectiveness, rapid onset of action, lack of need for repeated injections, and long-term effect.[65] While approved for one year by the Food and Drug Administration (FDA), many patients benefit from a longer duration of use, up to 2 to 3 years in our experience.

Once implemented, GnRH agonist therapy is typically continued until gender-affirming hormones are at desired levels, or until continuing therapy with a GnRH agonist is no longer indicated (e.g. natal male undergoes gonadectomy). Treatment with gender-affirming hormones may require higher doses if not used concomitantly with a GnRH agonist, especially in natal males. With the increased prevalence of gender fluidity, some individuals desire pubertal blockade but do not desire to move forward with gender-affirming hormones and this can be challenging to manage without a clear endpoint of treatment in the setting of adverse effects (e.g. decreasing bone density) associated with not having circulating sex steroids.

Despite having years of experience with GnRH agonists in the central precocious puberty population, in which it has been shown to be safe and effective as well as reversible, little is known about potential long-term effects in the transgender population.[66-70] It has, however, been shown to be an effective therapy for cessation of puberty in these patients.[71] Regardless, there are specific concerns about the longer-term use of these agonists on bone health, psychological maturation, and long-term adjustment.

Approximately 40% of bone mass accrual occurs during puberty with the increase of sex steroids as one of the major drivers of this process.[72] Children who have early puberty have a higher bone mineral density (BMD) and the corollary is also true: children with delayed puberty have decreased BMD.[73-75] Long-term treatment with GnRH agonists does not appear to be detrimental.[76,77] This information, however, should be applied with caution in the transgender population. There has been only one study published looking at the BMD effect of GnRH agonist on a population of treated individuals. This study compared pre- and post-treatment BMD Z-scores at the start of therapy with a GnRH agonist, at the initiation of gender-affirming hormones, and then again at 22 years of age. BMD Z-scores were decreased in both trans men and trans women at the initiation of cross-sex hormone therapy but did increase by the end of the study, although not to baseline for trans women (absolute score was higher).[78] This study was limited by its small sample size. Additionally, the subjects were only on GnRH agonist monotherapy for a limited time, and therefore results of the study cannot be generalized to adolescents who may start therapy in early puberty.

Concern has been raised about the effects of GnRH agonist therapy on brain maturation, particularly as one of the goals of providing puberty suppression is to allow the adolescent time to solidify or clarify their gender identity. There is concern that suppression of sex steroids will inhibit maturation of some of these processes. Currently, there is little evidence to either support or refute this. The working group consensus statement from the American Academy of Pediatrics on the use of GnRH agonists is that there is little evidence to be able to evaluate the impact of GnRH agonist therapy on psychosocial function.[66]

Gender-Affirming Hormone Regimens and Options

The primary goal of gender-affirming hormone therapy is to provide the attainment of desirable secondary sexual characteristics. Ideally, the patient's desired affirmed puberty will closely mimic physiologic puberty; however, youth must be counseled about having realistic expectations of anticipated changes from gender-affirming hormones, especially with regard to timing of those changes. This is achieved by starting hormones at low doses with a gradual increase until adult doses are reached. Dosing is tailored based on pubertal stage at initiation of therapy and response to treatment. Patients will require lifetime hormone therapy to maintain their secondary sexual characteristics. An understanding of the transient and permanent secondary sexual characteristics that ensue once treatment is initiated is an important part of informed consent for gender affirming hormones.

FEMINIZING HORMONES

Estrogen is available in oral, transdermal topical, and parenteral forms (Table 6.2). Note that ethinyl estradiol is no longer recommended for feminizing therapy due to the increased risk of thromboembolic disease associated with this formulation of estrogen.[79] In our clinical practice, we recommend considering use of transdermal-beta-estradiol. Transdermal estrogen bypasses first-pass metabolism and therefore has a more favorable side effect profile. It also delivers a constant dose as opposed to having peaks and troughs with oral or parenteral dosing, and allows for smaller incremental increases in dosing.[80]

For the adolescent currently being treated with a GnRH agonist, estradiol should be introduced at low doses and increased incrementally at 6-month intervals with the following guideline adapted from the Endocrine Society guidelines.[4] General principles involve a typical starting dose of 25% to 50% of the full adult replacement dose, increasing every 3 to 6 months until the full adult dose is reached. This regimen will bring an adolescent through puberty over 2 years. The time frame may be adjusted as clinically indicated.

The full adult dose of oral 17-beta estradiol (Estrace) is 2 mg/day with concurrent GnRH agonist therapy which is lower than doses necessary for an assigned male who does not have the benefit of complete testosterone suppression (typically 2 to 8 mg/day). It is important to note that low serum estrogen levels tend to promote growth while higher levels will cause fusion of the growth plates.[72,81]

Use of the transdermal patch to induce puberty has primarily been extrapolated from the literature in the hypogonadal patient population, including Turner syndrome patients.[80] In our practice, we typically start with a 0.025 mg/24-hour transdermal estradiol patch changed once or twice weekly and increase the dose approximately every 3 to 6 months based on hormone replacement protocols from cisgender girls.[82]

In adolescents there is less clinical experience with other forms of estradiol such as those that are injectable (estradiol valerate) or alternative topical preparations. Special consideration is given to complicated clinical scenarios such as trans girls desiring estrogen treatment with a coexisting prolactinoma, increased risk of breast cancer (e.g. BRCA mutation), family history of a clotting disorder, or active liver disease, and will require consensus through an interdisciplinary approach. Titration of estrogen more quickly to cause fusion of the growth plates should be considered for patients who desire a shorter height than predicted by bone age or midparental height.

When implementing feminizing hormones without concurrent use of a GnRH agonist, antiandrogen therapy can be used as an adjunct. In the United States, spironolactone is commonly used. Spironolactone is a weak diuretic that is FDA approved for hypertension and hyperkalemia. Its mechanism of action is to inhibit aldosterone action in the distal renal tubules. It was first described as an effective antiandrogen in women with polycystic ovary syndrome in 1980.[83] Sebum and hair production is under the influence of androgens, primarily dihydrotestosterone, catalyzed by 5α-reductase of testosterone.[84] Giltay and Gooren studied the effect of androgen deprivation on facial hair growth by measurement of hair growth rate (mm/day),

TABLE 6.2	Hormone Regimens: Transfeminine Patients			
Medications	How Supplied	Initial Dose	Comments
Estrogens Transdermal (once or twice weekly)	0.025, 0.0375, 0.05, 0.075, 0.1 mg/24 hr patches	0.025 mg/24 hr for induction and increase dose as tolerated	Mimics physiology closest; bypasses first-pass metabolism of the liver Several brands with various sizes/adhesives Concentration Max (Cmax) highest when applied to buttocks
Oral	0.5, 1, 2 mg tablets	0.5 mg/day and increase dose as tolerated	Undergoes first-pass metabolism through the liver, circulated as estrone sulfate
Antiandrogens Spironolactone	25, 50, 100 mg tablets	50 mg/day and increase dose as tolerated	Mild diuretic and may cause hyperkalemia, hyponatremia, hypomagnesemia

density, and diameter for a period of 12 months in subjects on antiandrogen and estrogen therapy. Hair diameter fell sharply at 4 months then remained constant, while the growth rate and density fell more slowly but progressively. This may explain why beard growth continues (albeit lighter and finer) after full suppression of endogenous androgens and may take time once spironolactone is initiated.[85]

Spironolactone exerts its antiandrogenic effect by being a weak inhibitor of testosterone synthesis and receptor binding. It may also weakly block 5-alpha-reductase and 17-hydroxysteroid dehydrogenase and increase sex hormone binding globulin and aromatase levels, thus increasing estrogen levels. This agent has been used for over three decades in patients who have Polycystic Ovarian Syndrome (PCOS), acne, and hirsutism with varying degrees of success. Because spironolactone inhibits aldosterone action, it has the potential to increase potassium levels and decrease sodium levels. It is important to recognize that it is also a weak diuretic and therefore patients will have increased urinary output and may have decreased blood pressure. Orthostatic symptoms, breast tenderness, and gynecomastia can result with increased dosing. Spironolactone dosing is typically 100 to 200 mg divided twice daily and it may take up to 6 to 9 months to see complete antiandrogen effects.[4] It should not be taken when patients have gastrointestinal illness (vomiting, diarrhea, or inability to take fluids).

MASCULINIZING HORMONES

Oral testosterone is not FDA-approved in the United States due to the associated risk of liver toxicity. Transdermal systems for delivering testosterone include a nongenital patch and gel formulations and solution. The scrotal patch is no longer available in the United States. Gel formulations must be used with care. When applied daily, these transdermal systems result in similar testosterone concentrations to those seen in normal young men in magnitude and diurnal variation; however use of the patch is often limited by skin irritation. Care must be taken in children trying gel preparations with good handwashing and covering treated areas of the body so as not to transfer testosterone to other individuals, including cis women (Table 6.3).[86]

The Endocrine Society guidelines recommend that testosterone doses escalate every 3 to 6 months, starting with testosterone cypionate or enanthate 25 mg intramuscularly every 1 to 2 weeks, with a goal full adult dose of 100 mg intramuscularly every 1 to 2 weeks.[4] There is growing clinical experience with these preparations of testosterone given subcutaneously

weekly.[87] The typical dose for this is 50 mg weekly, although some patients do require higher doses, up to 80 mg weekly.

Given that testosterone cypionate and enanthate are both viscous solutions, made in cottonseed oil and sesame oil, respectively, we typically advise using a 25-gauge needle for subcutaneous administration.

Postmenarchal females may be started on 50 mg subcutaneous or intramuscular weekly from the onset with a final adult dose ranging from 50 to 100 mg weekly.[87] Initiation, or arrival at the typical dose quickly, is important for its estrogen "blocking" action. The use of an adjunctive progestin, such as norethindrone or medroxyprogesterone, may be used for unwanted uterine bleeding from endometrial sloughing as a result of aromatization of testosterone to estrogen. Other available testosterone formulations (for which there is little clinical evidence in the pediatric population) include nasal testosterone spray which must be administered several times per day, buccal tablets, and subcutaneous testosterone pellets.

Anatomic, Physiologic, and Phenotypic Effects of Hormone Therapy

FEMINIZING HORMONES

Goals of estrogen-based therapy are to decrease spontaneous erections, further reduce testicular size, increase the ratio of body fat to muscle mass, and induce breast development. The time table for these effects are to some degree determined by individual factors as well as dosing, but typically changes are noted within the first 6 months and may take up to 5 years for full feminization.[4] Within the first 3 months, most adolescents will notice softening of the skin, decrease in muscle mass and increase in body fat, redistribution of fat to the hips and thighs, decrease in libido and erections. More gradual changes include nipple and breast growth, slowing of facial and body hair, and decrease in testicular size. Estrogen therapy cannot reverse some changes associated with masculinization. For example, facial hair growth will not completely cease without electrolysis or laser hair removal.[85] Bony facial features, low-pitched voice, and testicular size will also not change once there is testosterone exposure.

Clinicians should set expectations about adult breast size following pubertal induction with estrogen which will likely lead to a small breast size. No clear studies have explored the superiority of oral versus transdermal 17-beta estradiol in the breast

TABLE 6.3	Hormone Regimens: Transmasculine Patients			
Testosterone Formulation	**How Supplied**	**Starting Dose**		**Comments**
Testosterone cypionate	100 and 200 mg/mL in 1 and 10 mL multiuse vials	20–25 mg/week subcutaneous or intramuscular and increase dose as tolerated		Excipient is sesame oil; allergic reaction possible
Testosterone enanthate	200 mg/mL in 1 and 10 mL multiuse vials	20–25 mg/week subcutaneous or intramuscular and increase dose as tolerated		
Testosterone gel	1.62% (20.2 mg/pump press) or 20.25 or 40.5 mg/packet	2.5 g gel (1 packet or 1 pump)		Must be applied to upper shoulders/back. Beware of contact transfer
Testosterone gel	1% (25 or 50 mg/packet)	5 g gel (1 packet)		Must be applied to upper shoulders/back. Beware of contact transfer. Requires a large surface area

development of cis- or transgender girls; however most clinicians agree that a gradual dose escalation is preferable to optimize breast growth. Perceived breast size may also vary due to underlying adiposity which can enhance breast size but this tissue does not contain true glandular breast tissue. During pubertal development, estrogen stimulates proliferation of the ductal epithelium and surrounding connective tissue. Progesterone, which rises in late stages of puberty, promotes mammary gland development and contributes to breast fullness in the later stages of puberty.[88] There is inconclusive evidence about the adjunctive use of progestins to promote breast development.[89] Breast augmentation is an option; however long-term data on rates of satisfaction with breast size after pubertal induction do not exist.

MASCULINIZING HORMONES

Testosterone, when given to fully estrogenized females, will have the desired effects of masculinization. Initial changes in the first 3 months typically include oilier skin and acne, increased growth and thickness of body hair, increased muscle mass and strength, redistribution of fat from the hips to the central abdomen, increase in libido, clitoral growth, and vaginal dryness. Three to six months after starting testosterone, the voice may begin lowering. Growth of facial hair typically takes 1 to 4 years to reach full growth. Irreversible effects associated with testosterone therapy include clitoral growth (typically to a maximum of 4 cm stretched length), facial hair growth, voice change, and protrusion of the Adam's apple.[4] Female breast size is relatively unchanged with testosterone administration. Testosterone may be damaging to endogenous oocytes and long-term data on the impact of fertility are needed; however, cases of trans men contributing and/or carrying viable pregnancies are reported.[90]

Hormone Surveillance

Gender-affirming, or cross-sex, hormones are thought to confer the same risks associated with sex-hormone replacement in cisgendered individuals; however this has not been rigorously studied in adolescents. Risks are higher in individuals abusing or using unsupervised gender-affirming hormone therapy leading to supraphysiologic doses or, conversely, inadequate doses leading to inadequate replacement. Current recommendations for monitoring while on cross-sex hormones are based largely on expert opinion. Additionally, guidelines for treating hypogonadal adult cis men with testosterone have been integrated into current surveillance recommendations.[91] Currently, the approach to monitoring has not been differentiated between approach in adolescents and adults; however, risks for adolescents may be lower and the clinician should tailor the approach to the individual.

A thorough medical history, including current medications, should be obtained prior to prescribing hormones with particular attention to risk factors of the anticipated hormone use. For example, atypical antipsychotics can significantly increase the baseline prolactin level. A family history of any clotting disorders or thromboembolic events should be obtained. Baseline monitoring should include weight, height, and body mass index in addition to blood pressure and a full physical exam including Tanner staging for puberty. Monitoring of baseline complete blood count, renal and liver function, lipid and glucose, insulin, and glycosylated A1C are recommended.[4] However in clinical practice, only a baseline hematocrit and liver function are

typically needed for female-to-male adolescents beginning testosterone and little baseline testing for male-to-female adolescents starting estrogen is obtained in our clinical practice.

FEMINIZING HORMONES

The consensus guidelines recommend a clinical assessment every 2 to 3 months in the first year followed by clinical evaluation every 6 to 12 months for monitoring of feminization and development of any adverse reactions. For adolescents, the initiation and pubertal induction with gender-affirming hormones is a highly anticipated time, however, with many mixed emotions as the adolescent adjusts to their new body and new manifestations, including mood changes, of their affirmed gender identity. The importance of frequent clinical visits with the treating transgender health providers as well as ongoing psychotherapy cannot be overstated during this time.

Laboratory monitoring includes LH, FSH, a serum total testosterone level, and estradiol every 3 months. In adolescents receiving GnRH agonist therapy, these labs are of little utility. In settings where high-dose estrogen is given in the absence of a GnRH agonist, monitoring serum testosterone and estradiol levels may be of more value. Overall goals should aim for serum testosterone levels less than 55 ng/dL and peak serum estradiol levels less than 200 pg/mL.[4] Supraphysiologic doses of serum estradiol should be avoided to minimize the risk of hypertension, liver disease, and thromboembolic disease. The exact risk of developing these conditions in adolescence are unclear. It should be noted that serum estradiol levels can be used to monitor oral, transdermal, and parenteral estradiol as they are bioequivalent. Other forms of estradiol, such as conjugated estrogens, are not detected by the assay and are not recommended.

While not included in the current practice guidelines from the Endocrine Society, baseline and subsequent screening of serum prolactin levels may be considered. Some practitioners advocate incorporating this into one's practice.[92] Estrogen therapy can increase the growth of lactotroph cells in the pituitary gland which make prolactin. While routine monitoring of serum prolactin levels are not included in the guidelines, there has historically been some concern about prolonged, high-dose estrogen exposure leading to hyperprolactinemia. In transgender women, up to 20% may have elevations in prolactin levels associated with enlargement of the pituitary gland. To date, five cases of macroprolactinomas have been reported in trans women; however, these were mostly in the setting of supraphysiological doses of estrogen administration, some of which were unsupervised self-administration.[92–98] While monitoring of serum prolactin levels in adolescents on estrogen is not routinely recommended, it may be considered in relevant clinical circumstances.

MASCULINIZING HORMONES

Serum total testosterone levels should be measured every 2 to 3 months until levels are in the normal male range, generally between 350 and 700 ng/dL.[4] For testosterone enanthate or cypionate injections given every 2 weeks the testosterone level is ideally measured midway between injections; however peak or trough levels can be drawn and interpreted in the context of the last administered testosterone dose. Transdermal, weekly intramuscular or subcutaneous testosterone administration allows for more stable levels, so measurements may be done any time after a steady state has been reached. Serum estradiol levels are also recommended to be measured during the first 6 months or until there has been cessation of uterine bleeding for 6 months, with goal estradiol levels less than 50 pg/mL. Serum monitoring of estradiol may not be necessary if uterine bleeding resolves quickly after the onset of cross-sex hormones with testosterone.

Additional laboratory monitoring recommended by the guidelines includes complete blood count and liver function testing at baseline and every 3 months for the first year, then every 6 to 12 months. Once on a therapeutic dose of testosterone, yearly total testosterone level and hematocrit is recommended. Erythrocytosis and polycythemia are the most adverse effects of testosterone administration. The exact mechanism responsible for the stimulatory effect of erythropoiesis by testosterone is not fully understood. Polycythemia can lead to an increased risk of clotting, heart failure, and splenomegaly. In our clinical practice, we tolerate hemoglobin elevations up to 16.5 g/dL before

considering a reduction or cessation in the testosterone dose. In severe cases, polycythemia may require therapeutic phlebotomy as performed in those patients with primary polycythemia.

Routine liver function monitoring is typically required in those youth on oral testosterone, which is no longer available in the United States. However, the guidelines still maintain their recommendation for liver function testing based on a study showing that 15% of trans men on testosterone therapy developed transient elevations in liver function enzymes.[99] Testosterone administration leads to a more atherogenic lipid profile including higher triglyceride values and lower high-density lipoprotein cholesterol as well as insulin resistance. However, testosterone therapy has not been shown to be associated with a higher risk of cardiovascular disease or type 2 diabetes.[100–102] In trans men, testosterone has not been shown to have an effect on total and cause-specific mortality compared to the general population not on exogenous testosterone therapy.[103]

REFERENCES

1. Lev A. Gender dysphoria: two steps forward, one step back. *Clin Soc Work J.* 2013;41(3):288.
2. Drescher J. Out of DSM: depathologizing homosexuality. *Behav Sci (Basel).* 2015;5(4):565–575.
3. Drescher J. Queer diagnoses revisited: the past and future of homosexuality and gender diagnoses in DSM and ICD. *Int Rev Psychiatry.* 2015;27(5):386–395.
4. Hembree WC, Cohen-Kettenis P, Delemarre-van de Waal HA, et al. Endocrine treatment of transsexual persons: an Endocrine Society clinical practice guideline. *J Clin Endocrinol Metab.* 2009;94(9):3132–3154.
5. World Professional Association for Transgender Health. *Standards of Care for the Health of Transsexual, Transgender, and Gender Nonconforming People.* 7th version Minneapolis: WPATH; 2001.
6. Haas A, Rodgers P, Herman J. *Suicide Attempts Among Transgender and Gender Non-Conforming Adults: Findings of the National Transgender Discrimination Survey.* New York, NY: American Foundation for Suicide Prevention; 20141–18. Los Angeles, CA: The Williams Institute, UCLA School of Law.
7. Asscheman H, Giltay EJ, Megens JA, de Ronde WP, van Trotsenburg MA, Gooren LJ. A long-term follow-up study of mortality in transsexuals receiving treatment with cross sex hormones. *Eur J Endocrinol.* 2011;164(4):635–642.
8. Guirand F. Greek mythology. In: *New Larousse Encyclopedia of Mythology.* London: Paul Hamlyn; 1968:85–198.
9. Servi K. The Gods. In: *Greek Mythology.* Athens: Ekdotike Athenon S.A; 1997.
10. Bonifacio HJ, Rosenthal SM. Gender variance and dysphoria in children and adolescents. *Pediatr Clin North Am.* 2015;62(4):1001–1016.
11. Drescher J, Byne W. Gender dysphoric/gender variant (GD/GV) children and adolescents; summarizing what we know and what we have yet to learn. *J Homosexuality.* 2012;59(3):501–510.
12. Sherer I, Rosenthal S, Ehrensaft D, Baum J. Child and adolescent gender center: a multidisciplinary collaboration to improve the lives of gender nonconforming children and teens. *Pediatr Rev.* 2012;33(6):273–275.

13. Leibowitz SF, Spack NP. The development of a gender identity psychosocial clinic: treatment issues, logistical considerations, interdisciplinary cooperation, and future initiatives. *Child Adolesc Psychiatr Clin N Am.* 2011;20(4):701–724.
14. Deutsch MB. Making it count: improving estimates of the size of transgender and gender nonconforming populations. *LGBT Health.* 2016;3(4):181–185.
15. Gates G. How many people are lesbian, gay, bisexual, and transgender? williamsinstitute.law.ucla.edu. Accessed 9/15/16.
16. Cohen-Kettenis PT, van Goozen S. Pubertal delay as an aid in diagnosis and treatment of a transsexual adolescent. *Eur Child Adolesc Psychiatry.* 1998;7(4):246–248.
17. Murad MH, Elamin MB, Garcia MZ, et al. Hormonal therapy and sex reassignment: a systematic review and meta-analysis of quality of life and psychosocial outcomes. *Clin Endocrinol.* 2010;72:214–231.
18. Spack NP, Edwards-Leeper L, Feldman HA, et al. Children and adolescents with gender identity disorder referred to a pediatric medical center. *Pediatrics.* 2012;129(3):418–425.
19. Drummond KD, Bradley SJ, Peterson-Badali M, Zucker KJ. A follow-up study of girls with gender identity disorder. *Dev Psychol.* 2008;44:34–45.
20. Wallien MS, Cohen-Kettenis PT. Psychosexual outcome of gender-dysphoric children. *J Am Acad Child Adolesc Psychiatry.* 2008;47:1413–1423.
21. Zucker KJ. On the "natural history" of gender identity disorder in children. *J Am Acad Child Adolesc Psychiatry.* 2008;47:1361–1363.
22. Steensma TD, McGuire JK, Kreukels BPC, Beekman AJ. Cohen-Kettenis PT. Factors associated with desistance and persistence of childhood gender dysphoria: a quantitative follow-up study. *J Am Acad Child Adolesc Psychiatry.* 2013;52(6):582–590.
23. Steensma TD, Biemond R, de Boer F, Cohen-Kettenis PT. Desisting and persisting gender dysphoria after childhood: a qualitative follow-up study. *Clin Child Psychol Psychiatry.* 2011;16(4):499–516.
24. American Psychiatric Association. *Diagnostic and Statistical Manual of Mental Disorders.* 5th ed. Arlington, VA: American Psychiatric Publishing; 2013.

25. Zucker KJ, Cohen-Kettenis PT, Drescher J, Meyer-Bahlburg HFL, Pfäfflin F, Womack WM. Memo outlining evidence for change for gender identity disorder in the DSM-5. *Arch Sex Behav.* 2013;42:901–914.
26. Byne W, Bradley S, Coleman E, et al. Report of the American Psychiatric Association task force on treatment of gender identity disorder. *Am J Psychiatry.* 2012;41(4):759–796.
27. Drescher J, Cohen-Kettenis PT, Reed GM. Gender incongruence of childhood in the ICD-11: controversies, proposal, and rationale. *Lancet Psychiatry.* 2016;3:297–304.
28. Drescher J, Cohen-Kettenis P, Winter S. Minding the body: situating gender identity diagnoses in the ICD-11. *Int Rev Psychiatry.* 2012;24:568–577.
29. Heylens G, Verroken C, De Cock S, T'Sjoen G, De Cuypere G. Effects of different steps in gender reassignment therapy on psychopathology: a prospective study of persons with a gender identity disorder. *J Sex Med.* 2014;11(1):119–126.
30. Bauer GR, Scheim AI, Pyne J, Travers R, Hammond R. Intervenable factors associated with suicide risk in transgender persons: a respondent driven sampling study in Ontario, Canada. *BMC Public Health.* 2015;15:525.
31. Stevens J, Gomez-Lobo V, Pine-Twaddell E. Insurance coverage of puberty blocker therapies for transgender youth. *Pediatrics.* 2015;136(6):1029–1031.
32. Feldman J, Brown GR, Deutsch MB, et al. Priorities for transgender medical and healthcare research. *Int Rev Psychiatry.* 2016;28(1):95–102.
33. Richards C, Bouman WP, Seal L, Barker MJ, Nieder TO, T'Sjoen G. Non-binary or genderqueer genders. *Int Rev Psychiatry.* 2016;28(1):95–102.
34. Shumer DE, Reisner SL, Edwards-Leeper L, Tishelman A. Evaluation of Asperger syndrome in youth presenting to a gender dysphoria clinic. *LGBT Health.* 2015;3(5):387–390.
35. VanderLaan DP, Leef JH, Wood H, Hughes SK, Zucker KJ. Autism spectrum disorder risk factors and autistic traits in gender dysphoric children. *J Autism Dev Disorder.* 2015;45(6):1742–1750.
36. Jacobs LA, Rachlin K, Erickson-Schroth L, Janssen A. Gender dysphoria and co-occurring

Autism Spectrum Disorders: review, case examples and treatment considerations. *LGBT Health.* 2014;1(4):277–282.

37. Wilson EC, Chen YH, Arayasirikul S, Raymond HF, McFarland W. The impact of discrimination on the mental health of trans*-female youth and the protective effect of parental support. *AIDS Behav.* 2016;20(10): 2203–2211.

38. Le V, Arayasirikul S, Chen YH, Jin H, Wilson EC. Type of social support parental acceptance among transfemale youth and their impact on mental health, sexual debut, history of sex work and condomless anal intercourse. *J Int AIDS Soc.* 2016;19(3 suppl 2):20781.

39. Ryan C, Russell ST, Huebner D, Diaz R, Sanchez J. Family acceptance in adolescence and the health of LGBT young adults. *J Child Adolesc Psychiatr Nurs.* 2010;23(4):205–213.

40. Simons L, Schrager SM, Clark LF, Belzer M, Olson J. Parental support and mental health among transgender adolescents. *J Adolesc Health.* 2013;53(6):791–793.

41. Olson J, Schrager SM, Belzer M, Simons LK, Clark LF. Baseline physiologic and psychosocial characteristics of transgender youth seeking care for gender dysphoria. *J Adolesc Health.* 2015;57(4):374–380.

42. Aitken M, VanderLaan DP, Wasserman L, Stojanovski S, Zucker KJ. Self-harm and suicidality in children referred for gender dysphoria. *J Am Acad Child Adolesc Psychiatry.* 2016;55 (6):513–520.

43. Shumer DE, Tishelman AC. The role of assent in the treatment of transgender adolescents. *Int J Transgend.* 2015;16(2):97–102.

44. Ethics Committee of the American Society for Reproductive Medicine. Access to fertility services by transgender persons: an Ethics Committee opinion. *Fertil Steril.* 2015;104(5): 1111–1115.

45. Nahata L, Quinn GP, Tishelman A. A call for fertility and sexual function counseling in pediatrics. *Pediatrics.* 2016;137(6).

46. Lee PA, Houk CP. Gonadotropin-releasing hormone analog therapy for central precocious puberty and other childhood disorders affecting growth and puberty. *Treat Endocrinol.* 2006;5(5):287–296.

47. De Roo C, Tilleman K, T'Sjoen G, De Sutter P. Fertility options in transgender people. *Int Rev Psychiatry.* 2016;28(1):112–119.

48. von Doussa H, Power J, Riggs D. Imagining parenthood: the possibilities and experiences of parenthood among transgender people. *Cult Health Sex.* 2015;17(9):1119–1131.

49. Olson KR. Prepubescent transgender children: what we do and do not know. *J Am Acad Child Adolesc Psychiatry.* 2016;55(3):155–156.

50. Drescher J, Pula J. Ethical issues raised by the treatment of gender-variant prepubescent children. *Hastings Cent Rep.* 2014;44(suppl 4):S17–S22.

51. Zucker KJ, Wood H, Singh D, Bradley SJ. A developmental, biopsychosocial model for the treatment of children with gender identity disorder. *J Homosex.* 2012;59(3):369–397.

52. Olson KR, Durwood L, DeMeules M, McLaughlin KA. Mental health of transgender children who are supported in their identities. *Pediatrics.* 2016;137(3). e20153223.

53. Delemarre-van de Waal H, Cohen-Kettenis P. Clinical management of gender identity disorder in adolescents: a protocol on psychological and paediatric endocrinology aspects. *Eur J Endocrinol.* 2006;155(suppl 1):S131–S137.

54. Cohen-Kettenis PT, van Goozen SH. Pubertal delay as an aid in diagnosis and treatment of a transsexual adolescent. *Eur Child Adolesc Psychiatry.* 1998;7:246–248.

55. De Vries AL, Steensma TD, Doreleijers TA, Cohen-Kettenis PT. Puberty suppression in adolescents with gender identity disorder: a prospective follow-up study. *J Sex Med.* 2011;8(8):2276–2283.

56. Lawrence AA. Sexual orientation versus age of onset as bases for typologies (subtypes) for gender identity disorder in adolescents and adults. *Arch Sex Behav.* 2010;39(2):514–545.

57. Abreu AP, Kaiaser UB. Pubertal development and regulation. *Lancet Diabetes Endocrinol.* 2016;4(3):254–264.

58. Boepple PA, Mansfield MJ, Wierman ME, et al. Use of a potent, long acting agonist of gonadotropin-releasing hormone in the treatment of precocious puberty. *Endocr Rev.* 1986;7(1):24–33.

59. Roche AF, Wellens R, Attie KM, Siervogel RM. The timing of sexual maturation in a group of US white youths. *J Pediatr Endocrinol Metab.* 1995;8(1):11–18.

60. Rich BH, Rosenfield RL, Lucky AW, Helke JC, Otto P. Adrenarche: changing adrenal response to adrenocorticotropin. *J Clin Endocrinol Metab.* 1981;52(6):1129–1136.

61. Rosenfield RL. Clinical practice. *Hirsutism* N Engl J Med. 2005;353(24):2578–2588.

62. Illig R, DeCampo C, Lang-Muritano MR, et al. A physiological mode of puberty induction in hypogonadal girls by low dose transdermal 17β-oestradiol. *Eur J Pediatr.* 1990;150(2):86–91.

63. Herman-Giddens ME, Slora EJ, Wasserman RC, et al. Secondary sexual characteristics and menses in young girls seen in office practice: a study from the Pediatric Research in Office Settings network. *Pediatrics.* 1997;99 (4):505–512.

64. Ducharme JR, Forest MG, DePeretti E, Sempe M, Collu R, Bertrand J. Plasma adrenal and gonadal sex steroids in human pubertal development. *J Clin Endocrinol Metab.* 1976;42(3):468–476.

65. Kumar P, Sharma A. Gonadotropin-releasing hormone analogs: understanding advantages and limitations. *J Human Sci Reproduction.* 2014;7(3):170–174.

66. Carel JC, Eugster EA, Rogol A, et al. Consensus statement on the use of gonadotropin-releasing hormone analogs in children. *Pediatrics.* 2009;123(4):e752–e762.

67. Pasquino AM, Pucarelli I, Accardo F, Demiraj V, Segni M, Di Nardo R. Long-term observation of 87 girls with idiopathic central precocious puberty treated with gonadotropin-releasing hormone analogs: impact on adult height, body mass index, bone mineral content, and reproductive function. *J Clin Endocrinol Metab.* 2008;93(1):190–195.

68. Mul D, Bertelloni S, Carel JC, Saggese G, Chaussain JL, Oostdijk W. Effect of gonadotropin-releasing hormone agonist treatment in boys with central precocious puberty: final height results. *Horm Res.* 2002;58(1):1–7.

69. Tanaka T, Niimi H, Matsuo N, et al. Results of long-term follow-up after treatment of central precocious puberty with leuprorelin acetate: evaluation of effectiveness of treatment and recovery of gonadal function. The TAP-144-SR Japanese Study Group on Central Precocious Puberty. *J Clin Endocrinol Metab.* 2005;90(3):1371–1376.

70. Heger S, Partsch CJ, Sippell WG. Long-term outcome after depot gonadotropin-releasing hormone agonist treatment of central precocious puberty: final height, body proportions, body composition, bone mineral density, and reproductive function. *J Clin Endocrinol Metab.* 1999;84(12):4583–4590.

71. Schagen SE, Cohen-Kettenis PT, Delemarre-van de Waal HA, Hannema SE. Efficacy and safety of gonadotropin-releasing hormone agonist treatment to suppress puberty in gender dysphoric adolescents. *J Sex Med.* 2016;13 (7):1125–1132.

72. Albin AK, Kiklasson A, Westgren U, Norjavaara E. Estradiol and pubertal growth in girls. *Horm Res Paediatr.* 2012;78 (4):218–225.

73. Saggese G, Bertelloni S, Baroncelli GI. Sex steroids and the acquisition of bone mass. *Horm Res.* 1997;48(suppl 5):65–71.

74. Yilmaz D, Ersoy B, Bilgin E, Gumuser G, Onur E, Pinar ED. Bone mineral density in girls and boys at different pubertal stages: relation with gonadal steroids, bone formation markers, and growth parameters. *J Bone Miner Metab.* 2005;23(6):476–482.

75. Finkelstein JS, Neer RM, Biller BM, Crawford JD, Klibanski A. Osteopenia in men with a history of delayed puberty. *N Engl J Med.* 1992;326(9):600–604.

76. Bertelloni S, Baroncelli GI, Sorrentino MC, Perri G, Saggese G. Effect of central precocious puberty and gonadotropin-releasing hormone analogue treatment on peak bone mass and final height in females. *Eur J Pediatr.* 1998; 157(5):363–367.

77. Alessandri SB, Pereira Fde A, Villela RA, et al. Bone mineral density and body composition in girls with idiopathic central precocious puberty before and after treatment with a gonadotropin-releasing hormone agonist. *Clinics (Sao Paolo).* 2012;67(6):591–596.

78. Klink D, Caris M, Heijboer A, van Trotsenburg M, Rotteveel J. Bone mass in young adulthood following gonadotropin releasing hormone analog treatment and cross sex hormone treatment in adolescents with gender dysphoria. *J Clin Endocrinol Metab.* 2015;100(2):E270–E275.

79. Gooren LJ, Giltay EJ, Bunck MC. Long-term treatment of transsexuals with cross-sex hormones: extensive personal experience. *J Clin Endocrinol Metab.* 2008;93(1):19–25.

80. Torres-Santiago L, Mericq V, Taboada M, et al. Metabolic effects of oral versus transdermal 17β-estradiol (E₂): a randomized clinical trial in girls with Turner syndrome. *J Clin Endocrinol Metab.* 2013;98(7):2716–2724.

81. MacGillivray MH, Morishima A, Conte F, Grumbach M, Smith EP. Pediatric endocrinology update: an overview. The essential roles of estrogens in pubertal growth, epiphyseal fusion and bone turnover: lessons from mutations in the genes for aromatase and the estrogen receptor. *Horm Res.* 1998;49(suppl 1):2–8.

82. DiVasta AD, Gordon CM. Hormone replacement therapy for the adolescent patient. *Ann N Y Acad Sci.* 2008;1135:204–211.

83. Shapiro G, Evron S. A novel use of spironolactone: treatment of hirsutism. *J Clin Endocrinol Metab.* 1980;51(3):429–432.

84. Imperato-McGinley J, Gautier T, Cai LQ, Yee B, Epstein J, Pochi P. The androgen control of sebum production. Studies of subjects with dihydrotestosterone deficiency and complete

androgen insensitivity. *J Clin Endocrinol Metab*. 1993;76(2):524–528.

85. Giltay EJ, Gooren LJ. Effects of sex steroid deprivation/administration on hair growth and skin sebum production in transsexual males and females. *J Clin Endocrinol Metab*. 2000;85(8):2913–2921.

86. Shoskes JJ, Wilson MK, Spinner ML. Pharmacology of testosterone replacement therapy preparations. *Transl Androl Urol*. 2016;5 (6):834–843.

87. Spratt DI, Stewart I, Savage C, et al. Subcutaneous injection of testosterone is an effective and preferred alternative to intramuscular injection: demonstration in female-to-male transgender patients. *J Clin Endocrinol Metab*. 2017;102(7):2349–2355.

88. Javed A, Lteif A. Development of the human breast. *Semin Plast Surg*. 2013;27(1):5–12.

89. Wierckx K, Gooren L, T'Sjoen G. Clinical review: breast development in trans women receiving cross-sex hormones. *J Sex Med*. 2014;11(5):1240–1247.

90. Light AD, Obedin-Maliver J, Sevelius JM, Kerns JL. Transgender men who experienced pregnancy after female-to-male gender transitioning. *Obstet Gynecol*. 2014;124(6):1120–1127.

91. Bhasin S, Cunningham GR, Hayes FJ, et al. Testosterone therapy in men with androgen deficiency syndromes: an Endocrine Society clinical practice guideline. *J Clin Endocrinol Metab*. 2010;95(6):2536–2559.

92. Bunck MC, Debono M, Giltay EJ, Verheijen AT, Diamant M, Gooren LJ. Autonomous prolactin secretion in two male-to-female transgender patients using conventional oestrogen dosages. *BMJ Case Rep*. 2009; https://doi.org/10.1136/bcr.02.2009.

93. Cunha FS, Domenice S, Câmara VL, et al. Diagnosis of prolactinoma in two male-to-female transsexual subjects following high-dose cross-sex hormone therapy. *Andrologia*. 2015; 47(6):680–684.

94. Asscheman H, Gooren LJ, Assies J, Smits JP, de Slegte R. Prolactin levels and pituitary enlargement in hormone-treated male-to-female transsexuals. *Clin Endocrinol (Oxf)*. 1988;28(6): 583–588.

95. Gooren LJ, Assies J, Asscheman H, de Slegte R, van Kessel H. Estrogen-induced prolactinoma in a man. *J Clin Endocrinol Metab*. 1988;66 (2):444–446.

96. García-Malpartida K, Martín-Gorgojo A, Rocha M, Gómez-Balaguer M, Hernández-Mijares A. Prolactinoma induced by estrogen and cyproterone acetate in a male-to-female transsexual. *Fertil Steril*. 2010;94(3):1097.

97. Serri O, Noiseux D, Robert F, Hardy J. Lactotroph hyperplasia in an estrogen treated male-to-female transsexual patient. *J Clin Endocrinol Metab*. 1996;81(9):3177–3179.

98. Goh HH, Ratnam SS. Effect of estrogens on prolactin secretion in transsexual subjects. *Arch Sex Behav*. 1990;19(5):507–516.

99. van Kesteren PJ, Asscheman H, Megens JA, Gooren LJ. Mortality and morbidity in transsexual subjects treated with cross-sex hormones. *Clin Endocrinol (Oxf)*. 1997;47(3):337–342.

100. Wierckx K, Elaut E, Declercq E, et al. Prevalence of cardiovascular disease and cancer during cross-sex hormone therapy in a large cohort of trans persons: a case-control study. *Eur J Endocrinol*. 2013;169(4):471–478.

101. Wierckx K, Mueller S, Weyers S, et al. Long-term evaluation of cross-sex hormone treatment in transsexual persons. *J Sex Med*. 2012;9(10):2641–2651.

102. Elbers JM, Giltay EJ, Teerlink T, et al. Effects of sex steroids on components of the insulin resistance syndrome in transsexual subjects. *Clin Endocrinol (Oxf)*. 2003;58(5):562–571.

103. Asscheman H, Giltay EJ, Megens JA, de Ronde WP, van Trotsenburg MA, Gooren LJ. A long-term follow-up study of mortality in transsexuals receiving treatment with cross-sex hormones. *Eur J Endocrinol*. 2011;164(4): 635–642.

7

Overview of Surgery for Transgender Patients

TONYA N. THOMAS

Introduction

Gender affirmation surgery (formerly called sex reassignment surgery) may be sought by transgender individuals to physically change their sexual characteristics to affirm their gender identity. While not all transgender individuals choose to undergo gender affirmation surgery, surgical treatment is a medically necessary, standard-of-care intervention for gender dysphoria for many transgender patients.[1] Gender affirmation surgery helps transgender patients transition both physically and socially, and helps alleviate the physical and emotional distress caused by gender dysphoria.[1,2] Many surgical procedures including breast/chest (top) surgery, genital (bottom) surgery, and other masculinizing or feminizing facial and body procedures may be offered according to the individual's transition goals (Table 7.1). In this chapter, a brief history and the epidemiology of gender affirmation surgery are reviewed, as well as the World Professional Association for Transgender Health (WPATH) criteria for surgical treatment, recommended surgeon qualifications and training, a brief overview of the most common surgical procedures, and other perioperative considerations specific to transgender patients.

History of Gender Affirmation Surgery

Historically, Lili Elbe is regarded as one of the earliest transgender women to undergo gender affirmation surgery, and sadly died from complications related to her final surgery, a uterine transplant, in the early 1930s in Germany.[3] The earliest accounts of a transgender man undergoing gender affirmation surgery are from the 1940s, when Michael Dillon underwent gender affirmation surgery by Sir Harold Gillies, who performed a phalloplasty using tubed abdominal flaps.[3,4] In 1953, Christine Jorgenson, an American World War II veteran, drew wide media attention after she underwent male-to-female vaginoplasty in Copenhagen, Denmark, using a full-thickness penile skin graft.[5,6] Shortly afterward in 1956, Dr. Georges Burou first performed the anteriorly pedicled penile inversion male-to-female vaginoplasty technique, which has since been modified and remains the primary surgical technique for male-to-female vaginoplasty.[5,6]

It was not until the 1960s to 1970s when Johns Hopkins University, followed by other academic medical centers, began to offer treatment and surgery to transgender patients through its Gender Identity Clinic.[7] Johns Hopkins University later closed the clinic in 1979 following reports of controversial outcomes, and other academic centers followed suit.[7,8] Following the closure of these academic programs, gender affirmation surgery became largely privatized during the 1980s.[7]

The radial forearm free flap for phalloplasty was first described by Song et al. around this time in 1982, and shortly afterward the technique was modified by Chang and Hwang to the current tube-within-a-tube phalloplasty and urethroplasty technique.[5,9,10] In recent years, gender affirmation surgery has experienced a resurgence in academic medical centers, with hospitals now forming centers for transgender care and providing gender affirmation surgery in high-volume, academic settings.

Epidemiology

Studies that have attempted to assess the prevalence of transgenderism in the population have been methodologically complicated by changing diagnostic criteria and terminology, the level of cultural acceptance of transgender individuals in the time and place in which the studies occurred, and access to clinical care settings for transgender patients.[11] The vast majority of studies have been performed in the Western world (mainly Europe), with fewer studies performed in the East, and have shown widely variable prevalence of transgenderism, ranging from 0.45 to 23.6 per 100,000 people.[11–13] A systematic review and meta-analysis of the available literature by Arcelus et al. showed an overall prevalence of transgenderism of 4.6 in 100,000 people; 6.8 transgender women (transwomen, assigned male sex at birth, feminine gender identity) in 100,000 people, and 2.6 transgender men (transmen, assigned female sex at birth, masculine gender identity) in 100,000 people (2.6:1 ratio of transwomen to transmen), with the overall prevalence increasing over the past 50 years.[11] As data collection methods improve, more rigorous studies need to be undertaken to assess the prevalence of transgender people in the general population outside of clinical care settings.

In clinical experience, not all transgender patients who seek medical or hormonal care also seek surgical treatment, and individuals may choose to undergo any combination of counseling, hormonal, and surgical treatments they desire to meet their individual transition goals and needs. In a cross-sectional survey of 350 eligible transgender participants in Virginia, 57% reported receiving hormonal treatment, and only 22% reported having had chest/breast surgery (19%) or genital surgery (9%).[14] Relatedly, the National Transgender Discrimination Survey reported 61% of 6456 eligible participants had undergone medical transition (any type of hormonal treatment), while 33% reported having undergone surgical transition (some type of transition-related surgical procedure). The majority of participants reported the desire to have some form of gender affirmation surgery in the future.[15] In an analysis of data from the National Inpatient Sample, Canner et al. found that the incidence of genital gender-affirming surgery has increased over

TABLE 7.1	Surgical Procedures for Treatment of Gender Dysphoria			
FEMALE-TO-MALE SURGICAL PROCEDURES		**MALE-TO-FEMALE SURGICAL PROCEDURES**		
Breast/Chest (Top) Surgery	Genital (Bottom) Surgery	Breast/Chest (Top) Surgery	Genital (Bottom) Surgery	Other Masculinizing or Feminizing Surgical Procedures
Subcutaneous mastectomy Creation of a male chest	Hysterectomy Oophorectomy Metoidioplasty Vaginectomy Phalloplasty Scrotoplasty Erection and/or testicular prostheses	Augmentation mammoplasty (implants, lipofilling)	Penectomy Orchiectomy Vaginoplasty Vulvoplasty Clitoroplasty Labiaplasty	Facial surgery Thyroid chondroplasty Voice modification surgery Liposuction/body contouring Body implants (e.g., pectoral, gluteal)

Adapted from the World Professional Association for Transgender Health Standards of Care for the Health of Transsexual, Transgender, and Gender Nonconforming People 7th Version (2011).

time, and that while most patients continue to self-pay, coverage for gender affirmation surgery by Medicare and Medicaid has increased over time.[16] These reports, while limited by the inherent weaknesses of survey studies and large de-identified data-sets, demonstrate the need for continued study into the surgical needs and preferences of transgender patients, and highlight the need for improvement in access to care, coverage for necessary gender affirmation surgical procedures, and the need for formalized training of qualified surgeons and health professionals to meet the increasing demand.

Criteria for Surgery

The WPATH (formerly the Harry Benjamin International Gender Dysphoria Association) criteria for surgical treatment are published by the association in the *Standards of Care for the Health of Transsexual, Transgender, and Gender Nonconforming People*.[1] The *Standards of Care* (SOC) are evidence-based, multidisciplinary best practice guidelines, formulated to assist health professionals in the care of transgender people. The WPATH SOC guide health-care professionals when determining an individual's candidacy for gender affirmation surgery, and are intended to serve as a flexible framework that may be individualized to fit a specific patient's needs. Criteria specific to breast/chest (top) and genital (bottom) surgery are outlined in Table 7.2, adapted from the SOC. A referral letter from one or two (depending on the surgical procedure) qualified mental health professionals documenting the patient's history, assessment, treatment course, and eligibility for surgery is required for breast/chest (top) and genital (bottom) surgery.[1] While no explicit criteria exist, and no referral letter is required for other masculinizing or feminizing surgeries (e.g., facial surgery, thyroid chondroplasty, voice modification, liposuction, body contouring, body implants), a mental health professional may assist in counseling a person considering these surgeries. A thorough surgical counseling and informed consent process should always take place prior to proceeding with any surgical procedure.

Importantly, surgical candidates must have persistent, well-documented gender dysphoria, well-controlled comorbidities, and be of age and capacity to be fully informed and to consent to surgery. Additional criteria related to the use of hormone therapy and experience living in the patient's desired gender role may also exist, depending on the procedure. Hormone therapy may be individualized or deferred in some instances if a person has a medical contraindication to hormone therapy or is unable or unwilling to take hormones. Emphasis is placed on 12 continuous months of living in the gender role congruent with the individual's gender identity prior to undergoing genital surgery (female-to-male metoidioplasty or phalloplasty, or male-to-female vaginoplasty) to allow patients considering these procedures the opportunity to experience the social, emotional, and interpersonal changes that may occur while living in their desired gender role, prior to undergoing irreversible genital surgery.

The surgical consult visit and informed consent process for surgery should include a conversation about the individual's goals and expectations for surgery, the risks of surgery, and the anticipated outcomes of surgery. Patients are advised that the goal of surgery is to achieve good cosmetic appearance and function; however, every patient's body is different, and surgical results will vary from person to person. The risks of any gender-affirming surgical procedure may include bleeding or hemorrhage, the potential need for transfusion of blood products, hematoma, seroma, wound infection or abscess, wound healing issues, injury to surrounding organs, venous thromboembolism, medical complications including cardiopulmonary complications, and risks related to anesthesia. Other risks specific to the planned procedure should be emphasized, and are briefly examined in this chapter in the overview of surgical procedures section.

Surgeon Competency

While formal fellowship training programs in gender affirmation surgery are beginning to emerge, the WPATH SOC recommend that surgeons performing gender affirmation surgery be board-certified urologists, gynecologists, plastic surgeons, or general surgeons who have undergone additional specialized training and have competence in genital reconstruction.[1] Documented, supervised training in breast/chest and genital techniques with a more experienced surgeon is required, and surgeons are recommended to regularly attend professional meetings, and formally audit and publish their outcomes. Surgeons should ideally be trained in multiple techniques to offer the most appropriate surgery for the individual patient; however, if the technique in which a surgeon is trained and competent is not appropriate, then referral to another surgeon

TABLE 7.2	World Professional Association for Transgender Health Criteria for Surgery		
Criteria for Breast/ Chest (Top) Surgery	**Criteria for Genital (Bottom) Surgery**		
One Referral[a]	Two Referrals[a]		
Female-to-male mastectomy and creation of a male chest *Male-to-female augmentation mammoplasty*	*Female-to-male hysterectomy and oophorectomy* *Male-to-female orchiectomy*	*Female-to-male metoidioplasty and phalloplasty* *Male-to-female vaginoplasty[b]*	
1. Persistent, well-documented gender dysphoria 2. Capacity to make a fully informed decision and to consent for treatment 3. Age of majority in a given country[c] 4. If significant medical or mental health concerns are present, they must be reasonably well controlled	1. Persistent, well-documented gender dysphoria 2. Capacity to make a fully informed decision and to consent for treatment 3. Age of majority in a given country[c] 4. If significant medical or mental health concerns are present, they must be well controlled 5. 12 continuous months of hormone therapy as appropriate to the patient's gender goals (unless the patient has a medical contraindication or is otherwise unable or unwilling to take hormones)	1. Persistent, well-documented gender dysphoria 2. Capacity to make a fully informed decision and to consent for treatment 3. Age of majority in a given country[c] 4. If significant medical or mental health concerns are present, they must be well controlled 5. 12 continuous months of hormone therapy as appropriate to the patient's gender goals (unless the patient has a medical contraindication or is otherwise unable or unwilling to take hormones) 6. 12 continuous months of living in a gender role that is congruent with their gender identity	
Hormone therapy is not a prerequisite for female-to-male mastectomy and creation of a male chest Feminizing hormone therapy recommended for male-to-female breast augmentation (minimum 12 months) to maximize breast growth to optimize surgical results	*Aim of hormone therapy is to induce a period of reversible estrogen or testosterone suppression prior to irreversible surgery Criteria do not apply to patients having surgery for medical indications other than gender dysphoria*	*Regular visits with a mental health or other medical provider are recommended*	

[a]From qualified mental health professional(s).
[b]Includes penectomy, orchiectomy (if not previously performed), vaginoplasty, vulvoplasty, clitoroplasty, labiaplasty.
[c]If younger follow Standards of Care for children and adolescents.
Adapted from the World Professional Association for Transgender Health. *Standards of Care for the Health of Transsexual, Transgender, and Gender Nonconforming People*. 7th Version. WPATH; 2011.

well versed in an alternative technique is advised. As academic centers continue to build programs that focus on the care of transgender patients, more formalized surgical training programs are expected to develop, and will offer more structured training in the care of transgender patients and surgical techniques of gender affirmation surgery.

Overview of Surgical Procedures for Treatment of Gender Dysphoria

Various surgical procedures (see Table 7.1) may be offered for the treatment of gender dysphoria including breast/chest surgery (top surgery), genital surgery (bottom surgery), and other non-breast/chest and nongenital masculinizing or feminizing surgeries (e.g., facial surgery, thyroid chondroplasty, voice modification surgery, liposuction, body contouring, body implants). Transgender men may choose to undergo subcutaneous mastectomy and creation of a male chest, hysterectomy, oophorectomy, metoidioplasty, vaginectomy, phalloplasty, scrotoplasty, and placement of erection and/or testicular prostheses. Surgeries including breast augmentation, penectomy, orchiectomy, vaginoplasty, vulvoplasty, clitoroplasty, and labiaplasty may be sought by transgender women. The combination and extent of surgical procedures a transgender person may choose to undergo varies according to the individual person's gender identity and transition goals. WPATH does not designate an order in which surgeries must occur, and individuals are not required to undergo both top and bottom surgery.[1]

NONBREAST/CHEST AND NONGENITAL SURGERY

Masculinizing or feminizing surgeries (e.g., facial surgery, thyroid chondroplasty, voice modification surgery, liposuction, body contouring, body implants) may be performed to help achieve a more feminine or masculine outward appearance. These surgeries may improve the individual's ability to interact and be accepted socially in their desired gender role, and should not be considered purely aesthetic.[2] Many factors contribute to perception of the face as male or female, including features such as the brow, jawline, chin, and eyes, the configuration of facial features, and facial dimension.[17–19] Procedures including contouring of the forehead, chin, and jaw, blepharoplasty, rhinoplasty, cheek augmentation, and other facial procedures are often undertaken to feminize the facial characteristics, and are commonly known as *facial feminization surgery*. Surgical complications appear to be rare, with high patient satisfaction, improvement in quality of life, and excellent aesthetic outcomes.[20,21]

Chondrolaryngoplasty (commonly known as thyroid cartilage reduction or Adam's apple reduction) is performed to reduce the laryngeal prominence or Adam's apple, an obvious male feature of the neck. In order to achieve a more feminine contour, the superior thyroid notch and rim are excised. Common postoperative issues may include voice hoarseness, weakness, or odynophagia, but more serious complications, including hematoma, infection, loss of voice, swelling or edema, superior laryngeal nerve injury, and laryngeal cutaneous fistula, can occur.[21–23] Voice feminization surgery is a distinctly different procedure from chondrolaryngoplasty, which does not change a person's vocal pitch. Lower tone or deepening of the voice is often achieved through masculinizing hormone therapy for female-to-male transgender patients, whereas feminizing hormone therapy does not result in a more feminine tone of voice for adult male-to-female transgender patients.[1,24] Voice and communication therapy by a licensed and credentialed speech therapist or speech language pathologist is recommended for any patient undergoing voice feminization surgery, and may also be offered to any transfemale or transmale patient desiring treatment.[1] In addition to changes in voice, transmen receiving masculinizing hormonal therapy also achieve a more male outward appearance through redistribution of adipose tissue, increase in muscle mass, increase in the growth of body and facial hair, and male pattern baldness in some cases, therefore making other non-chest/breast and nongenital masculinizing procedures less common.[25]

BREAST/CHEST (TOP) SURGERY

Creation of a masculine chest is often considered one of the most important procedures in surgical transition for a female-to-male transgender individual, given that breasts are a visible and distinctly feminine characteristic.[26] Prior to surgery, many transmen may practice breast binding to give a more masculine appearance to the chest. Male-to-female mastectomy should create an aesthetic contour of the chest, reduce and properly position the nipple-areola complex, obliterate the inframammary crease, and avoid significant chest wall scarring.[27] To achieve an ideal masculine chest, the surgeon must be knowledgeable of the anatomic differences between the male and female chest, as well as the variations in natal female anatomic breast configurations.[27,28] Different mastectomy and contouring techniques have been proposed, and are well summarized in an algorithm by Monstrey et al., where semicircular, transareolar, concentric circular, extended concentric, and free nipple graft techniques are selected depending on breast size, ptosis, and skin elasticity.[28] In a systematic review of masculinizing top surgery techniques and outcomes, Wilson et al. aimed to identify the most common techniques and to quantify associated outcomes including quality of life.[26] Out of a total of 2138 breasts (1069 patients), the most common techniques utilized were those without skin resection (semicircular or transareolar 8.0%), periareolar skin resection (concentric circular, extended concentric 34.1%), inferior pedicle mammoplasty (15.7%), and inframammary resection with free nipple grafting (42.2%). Acute reoperation was lowest in the free nipple grafting group (4.8%). Secondary operations were highest in the periareolar skin resection group (37.5%). Patient satisfaction was overall high, with little difference between surgical groups.

Augmentation mammoplasty for male-to-female transgender patients is performed following at least 12 months of feminizing hormone therapy to allow time for breast growth and development prior to surgery. Breast growth usually occurs within 2 to 3 months, and continues for up to 2 years after starting therapy. Often, hormone therapy alone does not result in sufficient breast development, and 60% to 70% of transwomen seek augmentation.[29,30] Surgical technique for breast augmentation in male-to-female transgender patients must take into consideration the anatomic differences between the male and female chest, including the wider chest, greater muscle mass, and smaller nipple-areolar complex, but is similar to augmentation in natal women. Larger implants are often used, and placed subpectorally through an inframammary incision.[31] Complications of breast augmentation may include implant visibility or palpability, rippling, malposition, rupture, rotation, or contracture.[32] Reoperation does not appear common, but indications for implant exchange or removal among 24 transgender women who were included in a 10-year retrospective review of 230 patients included contracture ($n=7$, 29.1%), size ($n=11$, 45.8%), capsular contracture and size ($n=1$, 4.1%), asymmetry/malposition ($n=4$, 16.6%), and shape ($n=1$, 4.1%).[33]

GENITAL (BOTTOM) SURGERY

According to Hage and De Graaf, the ideal female-to-male neophallus should be aesthetic, provide tactile and erogenous sensation, and allow standing urination and penetrative intercourse, while avoiding major morbidity in the donor area.[34] Using the hypertrophied clitoris resulting from androgenic hormonal stimulation, metoidioplasty creates a microphallus by releasing the clitoral ligaments to lengthen the neophallus, and uses local labial or vaginal flaps or grafts to lengthen the urethra.[35,36] While the procedure may be completed in one stage with minimal surgical morbidity, drawbacks of the procedure include creation of a small neophallus, often not capable of standing urination or penetrative intercourse.[36,37] Total phalloplasty and urethroplasty may be performed using a variety of flap techniques, most commonly the radial forearm free flap. The radial flap is harvested from the forearm and formed into the tube-within-a-tube structure while still connected on its vascular supply, and a penile glans and corona are also formed from the flap. The urethra is lengthened and the groin vessels are dissected; then the free flap is transferred and anastomosed. The clitoris is kept intact to allow for stimulation. The donor site is grafted with split-thickness skin grafts. Scrotoplasty is performed, and testicular and erectile prosthetics can be implanted at a later time.[38] In a series of 287 consecutive radial forearm free flap phalloplasties performed from 1992 to 2007, Monstrey et al. described their outcomes following surgery. Early anastomic revision was required in 34 patients, and there was complete flap loss in two patients. Urologic complications occurred in 41%, including fistula ($n=72$), stricture ($n=21$), and both fistula and stricture in 26 patients. Revision urethroplasty procedures were required in 49 patients.[39]

The ideal male-to female vaginoplasty according to Karim et al. should create a moist, elastic, and hairless neovagina with a depth of at least 10 cm and diameter of 3 cm. The neourethra should be shortened to provide a downward urinary stream, and the clitoris should be sensitive and functional. These goals should be achieved without major surgical intervention, extensive postoperative treatment, or significant scaring or morbidity to the donor area.[40] While no vaginoplasty technique is yet ideal, the procedure is most commonly performed using the penile inversion technique, using local penile flaps and scrotal split-thickness skin grafts to line the neovagina. Briefly, the procedure is performed by harvesting a scrotal graft and performing an orchiectomy, disassembling the penis into a ventral urethral flap that is spatulated and formed into the neourethra and neourethral meatus, and a dorsal neurovascular flap that is shaped and positioned to form the sensate neoclitoris. The neovaginal cavity is created by dissecting the rectovesical space, then lining the space with the scrotal graft and inverted penile skin. The labia majora and labia minora are created using local flaps to form an aesthetic vulva. Advantages of the penile inversion vaginoplasty are the use of available local penile flaps and scrotal grafts, while disadvantages include the need for postoperative dilation, no natural lubrication, and the risks of vaginal stricture in 12% (4.2% to 15%), rectal injury in 2% to 4.2%, rectovaginal fistula in 1% (0.8% to 17%), and urethral meatal stenosis in 5% (1% to 6%).[41] Alternative vaginoplasty procedures involve the use of nongenital cutaneous flaps, or intestinal vaginoplasty using ileum or sigmoid. Due to the increased risks and morbidity associated with these surgeries, they are often used only as secondary procedures for failed penile inversion vaginoplasty, or in cases of penoscrotal hypoplasia where adequate penoscrotal skin is not present (usually in young patients on puberty suppression).[42,43] Grafts may contract, and bowel vaginoplasty involves risks related to abdominal surgery and bowel resection, as well as stenosis and excessive mucus production.[41,44]

Perioperative Considerations Specific to Transgender Patients

Prior to any surgery that will permanently eliminate a transgender patient's natural ability to reproduce genetically related children, patients must be thoroughly counseled on options for fertility preservation. Ideally, counseling should occur prior to any hormonal therapy, which may impair fertility.[1] Patients may be referred to a reproductive endocrinology and infertility specialist or urologic fertility specialist for a fully informed discussion of the options of oocyte or embryo freezing, or sperm preservation/banking.

To promote a safe, patient-centered environment, hospital staff who will be interacting with patients during their surgical experience, including admitting staff, preoperative and postoperative recovery unit staff, operating room staff, and appropriate nursing floor staff, should receive training in gender and sexuality related terminology and the use of patient-preferred names and pronouns to encourage sensitivity and to avoid misgendering patients. Patients should be called by their preferred name and pronouns, and gender identity should not be assumed by a patient's appearance. Patients should be assigned to hospital floors or rooms congruent with their gender identity. For example, male-to-female transgender patients may be assigned to a women's floor or room, and female-to-male patients may be assigned to a men's floor or room. Private rooms, when available, may also help promote confidentiality and privacy for transgender patients.

Special consideration should be given by the surgical team to perioperative venous thromboembolism prophylaxis (especially in patients on estrogen who are at increased risk), appropriate antibiotic selection for surgical procedures, surgical positioning (as many gender affirming surgeries may require extended time under anesthesia), and postoperative activity restrictions specific to the surgical procedures.[45,46] The use of preoperative bowel preparation, urinary catheters, drains, and packing is individualized according to the specific surgery being performed and according to surgeon preference. Postoperatively, close in-person follow-up with the surgeon who performed the procedure is essential to assess healing, cosmetic outcome, function, and the presence of any complications. Often, transgender patients may travel from another state or country for surgery, and in this situation, a local care provider able to assist in the event of any unexpected or emergent postoperative issues should be prearranged. In the event of complications, the patient should be referred back to the original surgeon, or to another surgeon with expertise in the procedure. Virtual visits may also be a clinically useful adjunct for follow up of nonurgent issues.

Conclusions

Gender affirmation surgery is a medically necessary intervention for gender dysphoria, and should be offered to patients who desire surgery and meet the WPATH SOC criteria for surgery. A wide range of surgical procedures are available, including chest/breast (top) surgery, genital (bottom) surgery, and non-chest/breast, nongenital masculinizing or feminizing facial and body procedures. The type and number of surgical procedures performed can be tailored to the individual patient's preferences and transition goals. Each procedure and surgical technique carries different risks and benefits, which should be openly and fully discussed with the patient beforehand in consultation. In addition, patients should receive fertility counseling, and the surgical team should be aware of the special perioperative considerations specific to transgender patients and the planned procedure. Gender affirmation surgery has evolved since its inception, and as the need for access to care increases in the transgender population, the need for specialized centers, certified training programs, and qualified surgeons and health professionals specializing in transgender care will continue to rise.

REFERENCES

1. The World Professional Association for Transgender Health. *Standards of Care for the Health of Transsexual, Transgender, and Gender Nonconforming People*. https://www.wpath.org/publications/soc. Accessed 30.01.17.
2. Hage JJ, Karim RB. Ought GIDNOS get nought? Treatment options for nontranssexual gender dysphoria. *Plast Reconstr Surg*. 2000;105 (3):1222–1227.
3. Nair R, Sriprasad S. 1129 Sir Harold Gillies: pioneer of phalloplasty and the birth of uroplastic surgery. *J Urol*. 2010;183(4). e437.
4. Rashid M, Tamimy MS. Phalloplasty: the dream and the reality. *Indian J Plast Surg*. 2013;46 (2):283–293.
5. Frey JD, Poudrier G, Thomson JE, Hazen A. A historical review of gender-affirming medicine: focus on genital reconstruction surgery. *J Sex Med*. 2017;14(8):991–1002.

6. Hage JJ, Karim RB, Laub Sr DR. On the origin of pedicled skin inversion vaginoplasty: life and work of Dr Georges Burou of Casablanca. *Ann Plast Surg*. 2007;59(6):723–729.
7. Meyer JK, Reter DJ. Sex reassignment. Follow-up. *Arch Gen Psychiatry*. 1979;36(9):1010–1015.
8. Abramowitz SI. Psychosocial outcomes of sex reassignment surgery. *J Consult Clin Psychol*. 1986;54(2):183–189.
9. Song R, Gao Y, Song Y, Yu Y, Song Y. The forearm flap. *Clin Plast Surg*. 1982;9(1):21–26.
10. Chang TS, Hwang WY. Forearm flap in one-stage reconstruction of the penis. *Plast Reconstr Surg*. 1984;74(2):251–258.
11. Arcelus J, Bouman WP, Van Den Noortgate W, Claes L, Witcomb G, Fernandez-Aranda F. Systematic review and meta-analysis of prevalence studies in transsexualism. *Eur Psychiatry*. 2015;30(6):807–815.

12. Tsoi WF. The prevalence of transsexualism in Singapore. *Acta Psychiatr Scand*. 1988;78(4): 501–504.
13. Walinder J. Incidence and sex ratio of transsexualism in Sweden. *Br J Psychiatry*. 1971;119 (549):195–196.
14. Bradford J, Reisner SL, Honnold JA, Xavier J. Experiences of transgender-related discrimination and implications for health: results from the Virginia Transgender Health Initiative Study. *Am J Public Health*. 2013;103(10): 1820–1829.
15. Grant JM, Mottet LA, Tanis J, Harrison J, Herman JL, Keisling M. Injustice at every turn: a report of the national transgender discrimination survey. Washington: National Center for Transgender Equality and National Gay and Lesbian Task Force, 2011.
16. Canner JK, Harfouch O, Kodadek LM, et al. Temporal trends in gender-affirming surgery

among transgender patients in the United States. *JAMA Surg.* 2018;153(7):609–616.

17. Ousterhout Dr DK. Paul Tessier and facial skeletal masculinization. *Ann Plast Surg.* 2011;67(6): S10–S15.

18. Bruce V, Burton AM, Hanna E, et al. Sex discrimination: how do we tell the difference between male and female faces? *Perception.* 1993;22(2):131–152.

19. Brown E, Perrett DI. What gives a face its gender? *Perception.* 1993;22(7):829–840.

20. Raffaini M, Magri AS, Agostini T. Full facial feminization surgery: patient satisfaction assessment based on 180 procedures involving 33 consecutive patients. *Plast Reconstr Surg.* 2016;137 (2):438–448.

21. Morrison SD, Vyas KS, Motakef S, et al. Facial feminization: systematic review of the literature. *Plast Reconstr Surg.* 2016;137(6):1759–1770.

22. Wolfort FG, Parry RG. Laryngeal chondroplasty for appearance. *Plast Reconstr Surg.* 1975;56 (4):371–374.

23. Wolfort FG, Dejerine ES, Ramos DJ, Parry RG. Chondrolaryngoplasty for appearance. *Plast Reconstr Surg.* 1990;86(3):464–469.

24. Irwig MS. Testosterone therapy for transgender men. *Lancet Diabetes Endocrinol.* 2017;5 (4):301–311.

25. Dahl M, Feldman J, Goldberg J, Jaberi A. Physical aspects of transgender endocrine therapy. *Int J Transgend.* 2006;9(3–4):111–134.

26. Wilson SC, Morrison SD, Anzai L, et al. Masculinizing top surgery: a systematic review of techniques and outcomes. *Ann Plast Surg.* 2018;80 (6):679–683.

27. Hage JJ, van Kesteren PJ. Chest-wall contouring in female-to-male transsexuals: basic considerations and review of the literature. *Plast Reconstr Surg.* 1995;96(2):386–391.

28. Monstrey S, Selvaggi G, Ceulemans P, et al. Chest-wall contouring surgery in female-to-male transsexuals: a new algorithm. *Plast Reconstr Surg.* 2008;121(3):849–859.

29. Wierckx K, Gooren L, T'Sjoen G. Clinical review: breast development in trans women receiving cross-sex hormones. *J Sex Med.* 2014;11(5):1240–1247.

30. Gooren L. Hormone treatment of the adult transsexual patient. *Horm Res.* 2005;64:31–36.

31. Kanhai RC, Hage JJ, Asscheman H, Mulder JW. Augmentation mammaplasty in male-to-female transsexuals. *Plast Reconstr Surg.* 1999;104 (2):542–549.

32. Adams Jr WP, Mallucci P. Breast augmentation. *Plast Reconstr Surg.* 2012;130(4):597e–611e.

33. Forster NA, Kunzi W, Giovanoli P. The reoperation cascade after breast augmentation with implants: what the patient needs to know. *J Plast Reconstr Aesthet Surg.* 2013;66 (3):313–322.

34. Hage JJ, De Graaf FH. Addressing the ideal requirements by free flap phalloplasty: some reflections on refinements of technique. *Microsurgery.* 1993;14(9):592–598.

35. Hage JJ. Metaidoioplasty: an alternative phalloplasty technique in transsexuals. *Plast Reconstr Surg.* 1996;97:161–167.

36. Frey JD, Poudrier G, Chiodo MV, Hazen A. An update on genital reconstruction options for the female-to-male transgender patient: a review of the literature. *Plast Reconstr Surg.* 2017;139 (3):728–737.

37. Hage JJ, van Turnhout AA. Long-term outcome of metaidoioplasty in 70 female-to-male transsexuals. *Ann Plast Surg.* 2006;57 (3):312–316.

38. Monstrey S, Ceulemans P, Roche N, Houtmeyers P, Lumen N, Hoebeke P. Reconstruction of male genital defects. In: Song D, Neligan P, eds. *Plastic Surgery: Volume 4: Lower Extremity, Trunk, and Burns.* 4th ed. Elsevier; 2018:297–325 e3 (eBook version).

39. Monstrey S, Hoebeke P, Selvaggi G, et al. Penile reconstruction: is the radial forearm flap really the standard technique? *Plast Reconstr Surg.* 2009;124(2):510–518.

40. Karim RB, Hage JJ, Mulder JW. Neovaginoplasty in male transsexuals: review of surgical techniques and recommendations regarding eligibility. *Ann Plast Surg.* 1996;37(6):669–675.

41. Horbach SE, Bouman MB, Smit JM, Özer M, Buncamper ME, Mullender MG. Outcome of vaginoplasty in male-to-female transgenders: a systematic review of surgical techniques. *J Sex Med.* 2015;12(6):1499–1512.

42. Unger CA. Gynecologic care for transgender youth. *Curr Opin Obstet Gynecol.* 2014;26 (5):347–354.

43. Bouman MB, van der Sluis WB, Buncamper ME, Ozer M, Mullender MG, Meijerink WJ. Primary total laparoscopic sigmoid vaginoplasty in transgender women with penoscrotal hypoplasia: a prospective cohort study of surgical outcomes and follow-up of 42 patients. *Plast Reconstr Surg.* 2016;138(4):614e–623e.

44. Bouman M, van Zeijl MCT, Buncamper ME, Meijerink WJHJ, van Bodegraven AA, Mullender MG. Intestinal vaginoplasty revisited: a review of surgical techniques, complications, and sexual function. *J Sex Med.* 2014;11 (7):1835–1847.

45. Elamin MB, Garcia MZ, Murad MH, Erwin PJ, Montori VM. Effect of sex steroid use on cardiovascular risk in transsexual individuals: a systematic review and meta-analyses. *Clin Endocrinol (Oxf).* 2010;72(1):1–10.

46. Bratzler DW, Dellinger EP, Olsen KM, et al. Clinical practice guidelines for antimicrobial prophylaxis in surgery. *Am J Health Syst Pharm.* 2013;70(3):195–283.

Facial Feminization Surgery and Facial Gender Confirmation Surgery

LUIS CAPITÁN | DANIEL SIMON | FERMÍN CAPITÁN-CAÑADAS

Introduction

From a very early age, everyone is able to recognize whether a face is male or female, long before learning about genital differences. The perception of gender through facial features occurs in a single glance, involuntarily, and definitively. While other parts of the body can be hidden, camouflaged, or exaggerated to appear more feminine, it is difficult to create female facial features without the appropriate surgical reassignment of facial gender. It is for this reason that an individual in the process of transitioning from man to woman may want this surgery in order to modify their face and better integrate into society, the workplace, and the family.[1,2] The surgical reassignment of facial gender is generating considerable interest among trans women and trans-health professionals. Modifying facial gender within the transition protocol is without doubt as important as hormone therapy and genital reconstruction.[3]

Definition and Differences

From a technical point of view, Facial Feminization Surgery (FFS) can be defined as the set of surgical procedures associated with different surgical specialties (Oral and Maxillofacial Surgery, Craniofacial Surgery, Plastic and Reconstructive Surgery) designed to soften and modify facial features perceived as masculine, exaggerated, or nonharmonic, and which, therefore, are decisive in the visual identification of facial gender.[4] On a somewhat more philosophical note, a much more specific term would be more appropriate for the type of surgery discussed in this chapter: Facial Gender Confirmation Surgery (FGCS). The popularly known concept of FFS is, in fact, so broad that it can include groups of patients without any gender dysphoria symptoms, for whom the techniques included in FFS are absolutely indicated (e.g., cis females with unusually prominent supraorbital ridge or cis males with especially wide jaws). This chapter focuses exclusively on male-to-female FGCS (MtF FGCS) due to the low incidence of and indication for surgical treatment in female-to-male patients and its near absence in the scientific literature reviewed.

When evaluating, diagnosing, and planning a patient's feminization needs, it is essential to understand the differences between male and female facial features. Generally speaking, the male facial skeleton has some well-defined features that distinguish it from its female counterpart. The basic pillars for the visual identification of facial gender are the frontonasoorbital complex, the nose, and the maxillomandibular complex.[5] Other aspects, structural and not, can also influence this identification, such as thyroid cartilage (Adam's apple), hairline format, cheekbones, the upper lip, facial hair, skin type and quality, and the distribution of facial fat.[6]

GENDER DIFFERENCES: PRIMARY ASPECTS

Genetic sex is determined at conception, but gonadal hormones play a vital role in the differentiation of male and female phenotypes throughout human development. Prenatal and adolescent levels of testosterone, the most abundant androgen, condition the appearance of facial features related to gender identity,[7,8] which can be divided into primary aspects (structural) and secondary aspects (hormone–dependent).

These differentiating features appear in the frontonasoorbital complex, the nose, the malar region, the upper lip, the jaw and chin complex, and the thyroid cartilage (Fig. 8.1). The development of these structures under hormonal influence is not reversible, and thus these features, which determine a significant part of an individual's facial gender, can only be approached and modified using surgery, always respecting the intrinsic architecture and anatomy of the craniofacial skeleton.

Frontonasoorbital Complex

This area is quite possibly the greatest determinant of facial gender.[4,5,9–11] The region encompasses the forehead surface, the supraorbital ridge (frontal bossing), the eye sockets, the frontomalar buttresses, the temporal ridges, and the frontonasal transition (Fig. 8.2). The supraorbital ridge is almost invariably much more strongly developed in the male than in the female, although, typically, all of these areas are more pronounced and have greater bone volume in the male skeleton than in the female skeleton. The forehead contour in the female is higher, smoother, more vertical, and may be rounded to the point of forward protrusion. It determines the position of the eyebrows and the positioning of the periorbital soft tissues like the eyelids.

Nose

From the perspective of gender difference, the male nose is usually larger than the female because it has a greater component of bone and cartilage. The male nasal bones are larger and tend to meet in the midline at a sharper angle. Female noses tend to be narrower, the tip is often sharper, and the nostrils may be smaller.[12] The frontonasal transition can be another important area with regard to facial gender differences. In males, the angle formed by the transition between forehead and nose tends to be more acute.[13,14] However, the nose has characteristics conditioned by ethnicity and age that are almost as important as gender-based differences.

Malar Region

The cheek area (zygomatic-malar region of the facial skeleton) usually has some structural differences that must be defined, since it can readily lead to confusion with regard to facial feminization. As a general rule, the malar bone volume is greater in

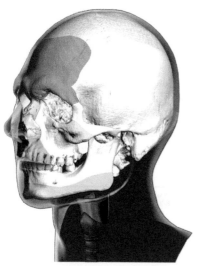

Fig. 8.1 Primary facial features related to gender identity. *From top to bottom:* frontonasoorbital complex, frontonasal transition, nose, malar region, upper lip, lower jaw and chin complex, and thyroid cartilage.

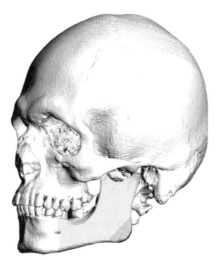

Fig. 8.3 Jaw and chin complex, color coded. *Blue:* mandibular body; *pink:* mandibular angle; *green:* ascending ramus.

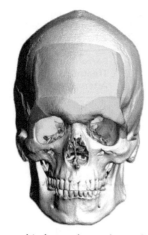

Fig. 8.2 Frontonasoorbital complex, color coded. *Green:* forehead surface; *purple:* temporal ridges; *light orange:* supraorbital ridge (frontal bossing); *dark orange:* frontomalar buttresses; *blue:* eye sockets; *yellow:* frontonasal transition.

men, which can result in well-defined cheeks. However, prominent round cheeks in the middle third of the face are compatible with femininity, due to a greater concentration of fat in this area in women (e.g., the greater volume is due not to the bone but to the soft tissues). This has specific implications when it comes to deciding the best treatment in this region.

Upper Lip

On the whole, the distance between the upper lip and the nose (cutaneous portion) is greater in men than in women.[15] Additionally, a recent study done by Penna et al. found that the ratio of the upper vermillion height/mouth-nose distance of the female lip is significantly higher in the attractive than in the unattractive group, which shows that a full upper lip is clearly an important feature of feminine attractiveness.[16]

Jaw and Chin Complex

To better understand the jaw, it needs to be divided into the mandibular body, the mandibular angle and the ascending ramus (Fig. 8.3). Generally speaking, the male jaw is larger, with greater body height and a broader ascending ramus. The mandibular angle formed by the body and ramus tends to be more acute in males, at times with everted gonial angles. The greater bone volume and vertical height are important factors when planning mandibular reshaping techniques in FGCS.

The male chin tends to be more square-shaped, with more pronounced and defined transitions between the chin and mandibular body, greater bone volume, and a more significant vertical dimension. Gender does not necessarily determine the position of the chin; that is, it is possible to find retro-positioned or over-projected chins in both men and women. However, a well-defined and projected chin may improve the overall aesthetics of the jaw-chin region.

Thyroid Cartilage (Adam's Apple)

The larynx structure, which plays a key role in basic life processes like breathing and phonation, has a greater volume and is larger (greater in diameter and longer) in males. This structure should never be approached with the idea of feminizing it, since this would pose the unacceptable and unnecessary risk of damaging the vocal cords or even causing respiratory problems. Only the most prominent part of the thyroid cartilage should be modified. This allows for a significant reduction in the Adam's apple without compromising its structural integrity.

GENDER DIFFERENCES: SECONDARY ASPECTS

In addition to structural facial features, a series of secondary traits are equally important in the identification of facial gender. These include, most notably, the hair and hairline, facial hair, skin texture, and the distribution and volume of facial fat.

Male hair may be conditioned by androgenic alopecia (loss of hair due to hormonal influence) and tends to have an M-shaped primary hairline with recessions at the temples.[17] The hairline of women usually has a rounded shape, their hair is not normally affected by alopecia, and, proportionally, the hairline implantation is higher in the center than in men.[18,19] Although MtF transgender hairlines are comparable to male hairlines, they are distinctive in that alopecia stabilizes as a consequence of hormone treatment.[20] The most common patterns found in MtF transgender patients are rounded (without recessions), M-shaped (receding hairline at the temples), and undefined (marked front line and temple recessions due to advanced alopecia).[21] Hair density refers to the number of follicular units (FU) per square centimeter (FU/cm²) on the scalp. Density and the composition of the FU can be easily measured with a simple handheld device called a densitometer.[22,23] Additionally, the presence or absence of miniaturization can be assessed with a dermatoscope.[24]

When approaching the upper facial third in MtF transgender patients, both the anatomy of the frontonasoorbital region and the overall condition of the hairline—format, height, and hair density—should be considered as a unit. For a better clinical analysis and broader understanding we have established an MtF hairline classification based on the observation and analysis of the hairlines of every transgender patient treated by our team through December 2015, a total of 492 patients.[21] The analysis establishes five possible hairline height and format types: type I, hairline with normal height and rounded format; type II, hairline with normal height and receding hairline at the temples, often called an M-shaped hairline; type III, naturally high hairline; type IV, high hairline due to alopecia, which is usually associated with a receding hairline at the temples; and type V, undefined hairline due to advanced alopecia (Table 8.1).

Almost all men have facial hair, which to a large extent conditions their skin type and quality, making it thicker and rougher. For many patients, facial hair is an important determining factor in their transition process.

The distribution and volume of facial fat is equally influenced by hormones. Women have a greater volume of facial fat with the distribution more concentrated in the middle third of the face (cheek area).[25]

Since all of these features can be heavily determined by hormones, they generally respond well to hormone therapy.[26] Conceptually, secondary features play an important role in determining facial gender and it is therefore preferable to treat them before beginning structural FGCS (at least 6 months before surgery) (Fig. 8.4). Prior hormone therapy and FGCS is a combination that improves the results obtained with surgery.

Facial Feminization Procedures: Techniques, Goals, and Considerations

This section describes the main procedures that comprise FGCS. For a better understanding, the face is divided into four key areas and the most important procedures for each area are discussed (Table 8.2).

THE UPPER THIRD: FOREHEAD AND HAIRLINE

Despite the fact that the frontonasoorbital complex is one of the main areas that determines the identification of facial gender, the hairline also plays a crucial role in the upper third of the face. The combined evaluation of these two features should be a basic premise of FGCS.

TABLE 8.1	Hairline Variations, Possible Treatments, and Transplant Design in Male-to-Female Transgender Patients[a,b]		
	Hairline	**Description**	**Transplant Design[c]**
Type I Rounded format Normal height		Ideal condition **Percentage:** 22% **Treatment:** none required	
Type II M-shaped format Normal height		Receding hairline at temples **Percentage:** 43% **Treatment:** SHT **Contraindication:** HLS[d]	
Type III Rounded format High height		Naturally high **Percentage:** 4% **Treatment:** HLS or SHT[e]	
Type IV M-shaped format High height		Naturally high or due to alopecia. Receding hairline at temples **Percentage:** 21% **Treatment:** SHT[e] **Alternative:** HLS + DHT	
Type V Undefined		Advanced alopecia **Percentage:** 10% **Treatment:** SHT + DHT or untreated	

[a]Based on the hairline analysis of transgender patients treated until December 2015 (n = 492) for any facial feminization procedure by our team.

[b]Both treatments, SHT (FUSS technique) and HLS, are performed in combination with an FR during the same surgery. A DHT treatment (FUSS or FUE technique) is performed alone in a second session.

[c]The blue indicates the surface area to cover with the SHT. The yellow indicates a surface that could benefit from a second hair transplant session (unassociated with the FR), when necessary.

[d]This does not improve or correct recessions.

[e]SHT: only if a small advancement (up to 1 cm) of the hairline is desired.

DHT, Deferred hair transplant; *FR,* forehead reconstruction; *FUE,* follicular unit extraction; *FUSS,* follicular unit strip surgery; *HLS,* hairline lowering surgery; *SHT,* simultaneous hair transplant.

Forehead Reconstruction

This is one of the basic procedures in facial feminization. It completely modifies the frontonasoorbital region and softens and feminizes the patient's expression. The surgical plan is devised to open the frontonasal angle, retroposition the anterior wall of the frontal sinus, open the orbital areas, soften the entire forehead surface, and reposition the eyebrows above the new supraorbital ridge, while always maintaining the anatomical integrity of the entire area (Figs. 8.5 and 8.6).[4] The sequence in Fig. 8.7 provides a step-by-step description of the reconstruction technique proposed by our team. Despite the fact that other

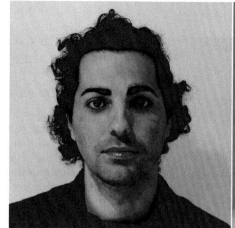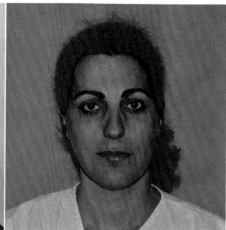

Fig. 8.4 Patient before and after (1 year) hormone treatment. Note the change in secondary aspects (hair, facial hair, skin texture, facial fat) before any type of surgical procedure.

TABLE 8.2	Facial Feminization Procedures			

Area	Feature	Procedure		Description
Upper third	Hairline	**Hair transplant**	FUSS	Follicular unit strip surgery: follicles obtained from a strip of scalp
			FUE	Follicular unit extraction: follicles obtained directly one by one
		Hairline lowering surgery		Decrease the overall height of the forehead and serve as an access point to reconstruct the frontonasoorbital complex (if required)
	Forehead	Forehead reconstruction and simultaneous hair transplant		Take advantage of the strip of scalp obtained in the coronal approach used to access the frontal region (to perform the forehead reconstruction) in order to harvest the hair follicles in the same way that they are obtained with conventional FUSS
		Forehead reconstruction		Retroposition the anterior wall of the frontal sinus, orbital opening, smooth the forehead surface, and reposition the eyebrows above the new supraorbital ridge
Middle third		Forehead reconstruction and rhinoplasty (frontonasal transition)		During forehead reconstruction, a rounded or conical burr can be used to lower the frontonasal transition, marking the level of the osteotomy or point of rasping of the new bony nasal dorsum during the subsequent rhinoplasty
	Nose	Rhinoplasty		Depending on individual needs: refinement of the tip, feminization of the profile, shortening the nose or narrowing of the nasal bone, always considering the harmonization of the nose with regard to the other modified structures
	Upper lip	Rhinoplasty and lip-lift		When a rhinoplasty is performed together with a lip-lift, the open rhinoplasty is carried out at the level of the superior incision of the lip-lift and the columellar skin flap is raised without any other higher incision
		Lip-lift		Reduce vertical excess of the upper lip and change the profile of the lip from flat to curved
	Cheeks	**Malar augmentation**	Implants	Rigid implants fixed to the bone using osteosynthesis
			Fat transfer	Autologous fat graft
Lower third	Chin	Chin contouring		Modify the format, volume (vertical reduction of the chin), and position of the chin (advancement, recession, lowering)
	Lower jaw	Lower jaw and chin contouring (triple approach technique)		When it is necessary to approach the entire mandibular surface as a unit. This is characterized by a triple approach with submucosal tunneling to protect the mental nerves and avoid an excessively large incision (mandibular degloving)
		Lower jaw contouring		Reduce the volume of the jaw and soften the mandibular angles
Neck	Thyroid cartilage	Thyroid cartilage contouring		Only the most prominent part of the thyroid cartilage should be modified, making it possible to significantly reduce the Adam's apple without compromising its structural integrity

FUE, Follicular unit extraction; *FUSS,* follicular unit strip surgery.

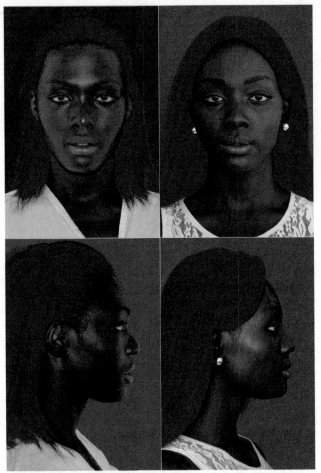

Fig. 8.5 Patient before and after forehead reconstruction. Procedures done: forehead reconstruction and chin contouring.

authors defend different techniques (isolated burring, the use of filling materials),[5,9,11,27] in our experience, the proposed reconstruction technique offers satisfactory and safe results regardless of the anatomy of the frontal region (Fig. 8.8).[28]

Finally, it is important to discuss the best access (approach route) to reach the frontal bone region: modified coronal approach (anterior or posterior) or hairline approach. In our opinion, this access should be based on the characteristics of the patient's hairline and its implantation (the distance from the nasal root to the beginning of the hairline).

Hairline Treatment

The hairline is a basic element in the identification of facial gender and, therefore, must be addressed to obtain a satisfactory and natural result in the upper third of the face. There are two options for treatment of the hairline. First, the hairline can be redefined using a hair transplant technique. The main areas to treat with a hair transplant are the receding hairline at the temples; however, the central section can also be addressed if the density is poor or if a small advancement (up to 1 cm) of the hairline is desired. This is recommended for patients with an M-shaped hairline, with sufficient hair density, and without active androgenetic alopecia (or with stabilized alopecia due to hormone treatment—type II MtF hairline). Depending on how the hair follicles are obtained, either follicular unit strip surgery (FUSS) or follicular unit extraction (FUE) can be used.[29,30] In the FUSS technique the follicles are obtained from a strip of scalp removed in a surgical procedure, while in the FUE technique the follicles are obtained one by one, without any need for an invasive surgical process. This latter technique usually requires more experience given its technical complexity and it generally takes longer. The new hairline is designed to look natural, paying attention to parameters such as density and unevenness.

An alternative treatment to hair transplantation involves a hairline lowering surgery (HLS). The objective of HLS is twofold: to decrease the overall height of the forehead and to serve as an access point to reconstruct the frontonasoorbital complex (if required). This is only recommended for patients with a significantly and disproportionately high hairline (type III MtF hairline).[31] A maximum of 2.5 cm of skin is removed and a 2 mm incision (future scar) is made above the hairline. Resorbable anchors (Endotine Forehead-mini device, Coapt Systems Inc., Palo Alto, CA, USA) can be placed to facilitate the advancement and eliminate the tension between the edges of the wound, helping to improve scarring. The lateral extension of the incision is hidden in the hair, since advancement in this area is not an objective of the surgery.

In most cases, there are a number of disadvantages to this technique: (1) the possibility of leaving a visible scar in a highly exposed part of the face; (2) the possibility of leaving an

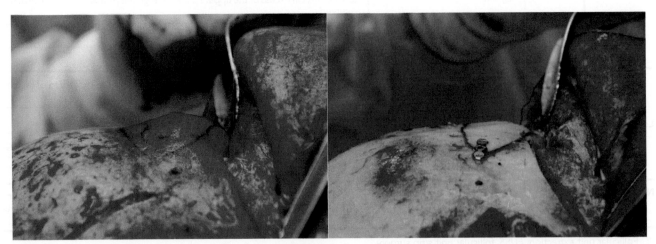

Fig. 8.6 Before and after surgical photos of forehead reconstruction. Note the fixation mechanism used (osteosynthesis with titanium micro screws).

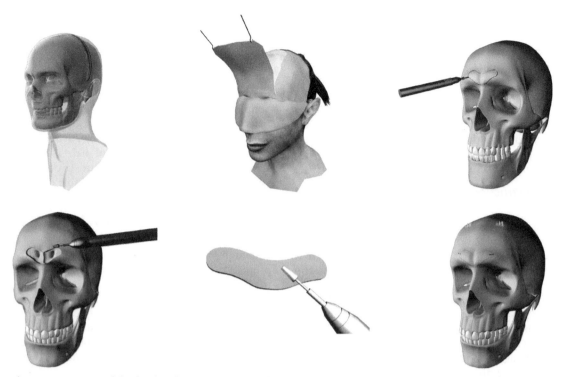

Fig. 8.7 Step-by-step sequence of the forehead reconstruction technique in facial gender confirmation surgery. *(Above, left)* Modified coronal approach, with elimination of the scalp strip. *(Above, center)* Pericranial flap until supraorbital ridge and both frontomalar buttresses are reached. *(Above, right)* Osteotomy of the anterior wall of the frontal sinus using a saw. Access to the frontal sinus. The anterior wall is preserved in saline solution during skull contouring. *(Below, left)* Sculpture of the entire frontonasoorbital complex, paying special attention to the frontonasal transition. *(Below, center)* Elimination of bony interferences of the anterior wall of the frontal sinus. *(Below, right)* Stable fixation of the anterior wall of the frontal sinus with osteosynthesis and placement of resorbable anchors (Endotine Forehead-mini device, Coapt Systems Inc., Palo Alto, CA, USA) to correctly reposition the eyebrows over the new bone structure.

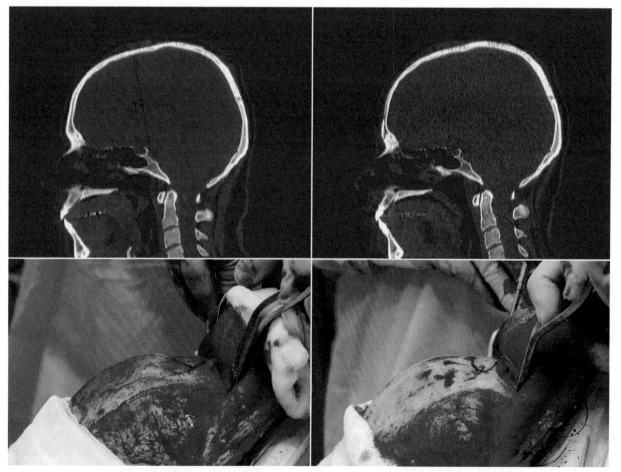

Fig. 8.8 Forehead reconstruction in a patient with complete agenesis of the frontal sinus. *(Above)* Pre- and postoperative sequence with sagittal computerized tomography (CT) images. *(Below)* Surgical before and after images of forehead reconstruction with osteotomy of the frontal sinus area; note the bone fixation method.

excessively short forehead in the center region, which could produce unnatural results; and (3) potentially limited results if surgical closure of the side temples is attempted due to excessive tension in the scarring area. In our experience, only 1 out of every 20 patients is a candidate for this type of approach and treatment. However, and despite the almost total lack of relevant bibliographic references,[32] our professional experience suggests that this is the approach most commonly used around the world to treat the hairline in FGCS.

Forehead Reconstruction and Simultaneous Hair Transplant

If the patient is a candidate for hairline treatment via hair transplant and also a candidate for forehead reconstruction, our team has developed a simultaneous hair transplant (SHT) technique.[21] This technique consists of taking advantage of the strip of scalp obtained in the modified coronal approach, which we have used to access the frontal region. This allows us to harvest the hair follicles on this strip in the same way that they are obtained with the conventional FUSS transplant technique described above. Once the forehead reconstruction is done, a new hairline is designed and the hair follicles obtained are grafted in place (there are an average of 2000 FU per strip, meaning some 3900 hairs). To reduce the risks associated with prolonged general anesthesia, the patient is woken up and kept under light sedation for the duration of the SHT procedure. Thanks to this technique, the entire upper third can be treated as part of the same surgical process, which is highly advantageous for many patients (Figs. 8.9 and 8.10). Androgenic alopecia

must be completely stabilized before this technique can be used. In cases where there has been notable hair loss from the area where the strip of scalp would normally be obtained, we can simply position the coronal incision further back, even in the occipital region if necessary (posterior). The number of follicles that can be obtained from the strip is limited, so if the result of the SHT does not fully meet the objective of closing the temple recession, or if more density of hair is required, a second standard hair transplant procedure (FUSS or FUE) can be performed some months later (see Table 8.1).

THE MIDDLE THIRD: CHEEKS, NOSE, AND UPPER LIP
Malar Augmentation

Although various cheek augmentation alternatives exist,[33] we propose two options based on our experience. The first involves the use of rigid implants that are fixed to the bone using osteosynthesis material (positioning screws) to ensure stability (Fig. 8.11).[34] When necessary, they can be customized to the patient's specific needs. They must be placed via an intraoral approach. The results are quite stable over time. If the volume of the implant is not carefully considered, the results may be artificial.

The second option for cheek augmentation involves fat transfer. An autologous fat graft is obtained, usually from the abdominal region, inner thigh, or hips, and after a purifying process, the fat is deposited in the supraperiosteal zone avoiding excessively superficial areas.[35] Quite satisfactory, natural results can be obtained, but this technique requires extensive

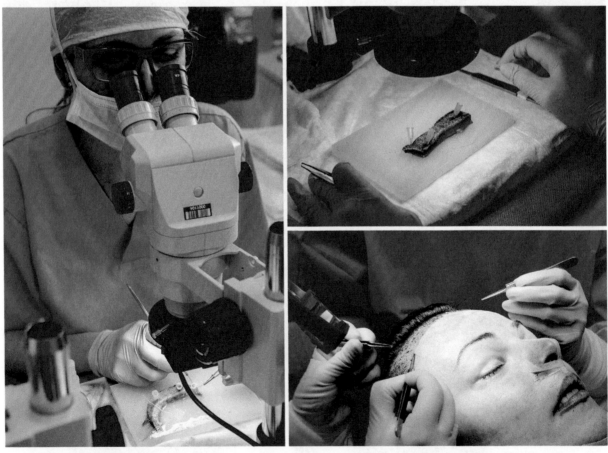

Fig. 8.9 Obtaining follicular units from the strip taken during a modified coronal approach and surgical implantation.

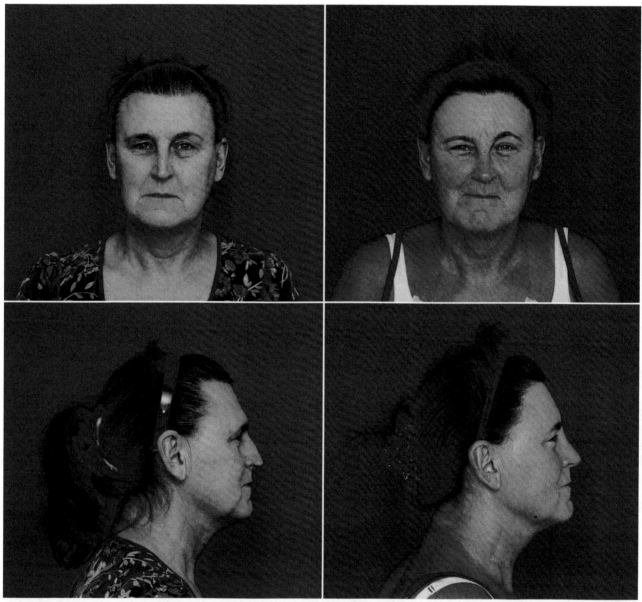

Fig. 8.10 Patient before and after forehead reconstruction and simultaneous hair transplant. Procedures done: forehead reconstruction and simultaneous hair transplant, rhinoplasty, and lower and upper blepharoplasty.

experience on the part of the specialist to collect and manipulate the graft and meticulously place it in the key areas. Fat transfer has two different objectives: to increase the volume of the cheekbones and to improve the quality of the skin thanks to the nourishing and restorative effect that fat transfer has on the skin. Much of the fat may be reabsorbed (up to 65%) so the technique typically requires multiple sessions to build permanent volume.[36] The main advantages of the fat transfer are the amount of fat that can be harvested and the absence of rejection, since the tissue comes from the patient.

Rhinoplasty

The size, shape, age, and ethnicity of the nose all must be evaluated when planning a rhinoplasty in the context of FGCS in order to achieve a threefold objective: (1) feminization of the nose, (2) harmonization with regard to the other modified structures

(primarily the forehead and maxillomandibular complex), and (3) achieving an aesthetic result beyond gender differences.[37]

Rhinoplasty is a highly individualized procedure, which requires an exhaustive evaluation of the bone and cartilaginous structures that form the nose (Fig. 8.12). Depending on the individual needs of the patient, the following procedures are possible: refinement of the tip, feminization of the profile (any excess bridge composed of bone and cartilage is removed to lower the profile), shortening the nose, and narrowing the nasal bone.

The frontonasal transition can be another important area with regard to facial gender differences. Correction of the supraorbital ridge and frontal bossing softens this angle. During forehead reconstruction, when the root of the nose is too high or projected, a rounded or conical burr can be used to lower the frontonasal transition to the optimal and desired position, which will mark

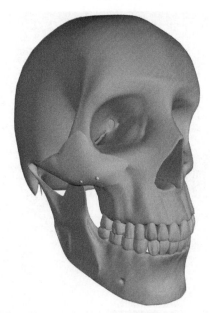

Fig. 8.11 Malar augmentation with rigid implant fixed to the bone using osteosynthesis (positioning screws) to ensure stability.

the level of the osteotomy or rasping of the new bony nasal dorsum during the subsequent rhinoplasty (Fig. 8.13).

Lip-Lift

Lifting the upper lip is proposed to reduce its vertical excess, obtaining partial exposure of the central incisor teeth at rest. Additionally, the lip profile is altered from flat to curved (Fig. 8.14).[38]

Our lip-lift technique is a modification of the bullhorn technique.[39] First the key points are tattooed with a needle and methylene blue and then the incisions are made with a No. 11 blade. These incisions are straight and join the points, removing a strip of skin and subcutaneous tissue without violating the *orbicularis oris* muscle. When a rhinoplasty is performed together with a lip-lift, the open rhinoplasty is carried out at the level of the superior incision of the lip-lift and the columellar skin flap is raised without any other higher incision (Fig. 8.15).[37] In this way, there is no potential risk of skin necrosis and the scar is perfectly hidden.

THE LOWER THIRD: LOWER JAW AND CHIN

The procedures used on the jaw and chin are fundamental to achieving adequate feminization of the lower third of the face. The possible goals of this treatment include: modifying the width and height of the jaw; softening the jawline (including the transition between the jaw and chin); and modifying the size, shape, and position of the chin.

The choice of treatment must be based on image diagnosis and the clinical evaluation of the patient. In this context, it is important to note that a strong jawline or one with pronounced angles is not necessarily synonymous with masculinity, since these features fit some female facial profiles quite well; hence the importance of a personalized evaluation that meets the particular patient's needs.

Lower Jaw and Chin Contouring

Access to the jaw and chin should always be via intraoral approaches to prevent visible external scars. With the jaw, two small incisions are made at the base of the vestibule parallel to the end molars. To access the chin, an incision is made in the lip mucosal area (far from the teeth and dental gums), which provides an excellent view and access to the area to be treated, and a scar that is imperceptible after the scarring period. On many occasions, it is necessary to treat the jaw

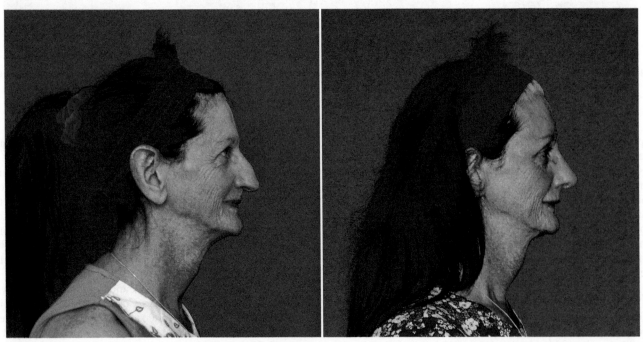

Fig. 8.12 Patient before and after feminization rhinoplasty. Procedures done: forehead reconstruction, rhinoplasty, thyroid cartilage contouring, otoplasty, lower blepharoplasty, and upper lip fill with hyaluronic acid.

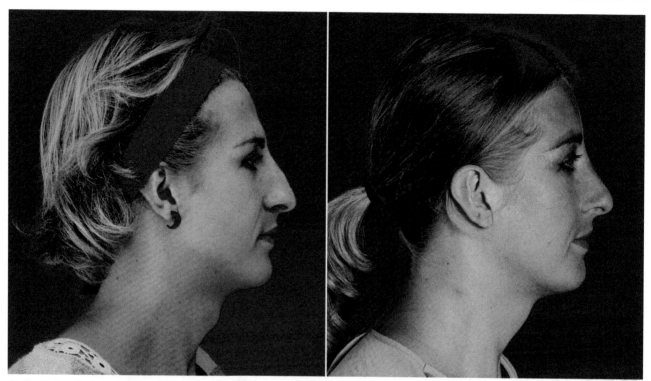

Fig. 8.13 **Patient before and after lowering the frontonasal transition during a forehead reconstruction.** Procedures done: forehead reconstruction, rhinoplasty, lower jaw contouring, thyroid cartilage contouring, and otoplasty.

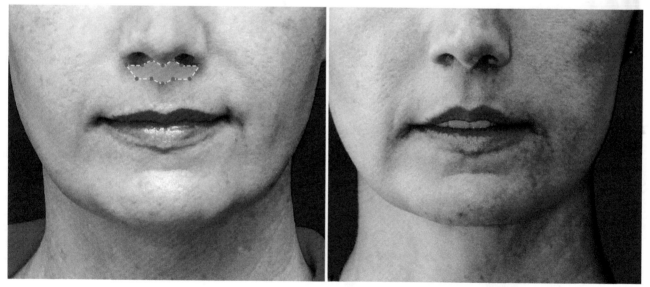

Fig. 8.14 Lip-lift design and postoperative result.

and chin as a whole (Fig. 8.16). In this case, we recommend connecting the described incisions through a subperiosteal tunnel, which creates an excellent working area, avoids an overly large incision (mandibular degloving), and helps to protect the mental nerves by not exposing them. This produces a better postoperative experience with regard to scarring and functional recovery.

Surgical techniques are based on bone sculpture, namely burring, standard osteotomies (bone cutting), and osteotomies with piezosurgery (ultrasonic cutting). Generally speaking, burring techniques make it possible to decrease the bone volume of

the chin, mandibular body, and mandibular angles. A very high degree of control is required with this technique to prevent damage to the surrounding structures (mental nerves, muscles, or vessels), weakening of the jaw, and medulla exposure.

We recommend the use of standard osteotomies in areas where the design and type of cut are highly predictable and where we can completely control instrument access (primarily recommended for the chin). This involves making cuts in the bone with a reciprocating saw or similar that makes it possible to move the bone segments and modify the chin position (e.g., to advance it) (Fig. 8.17).

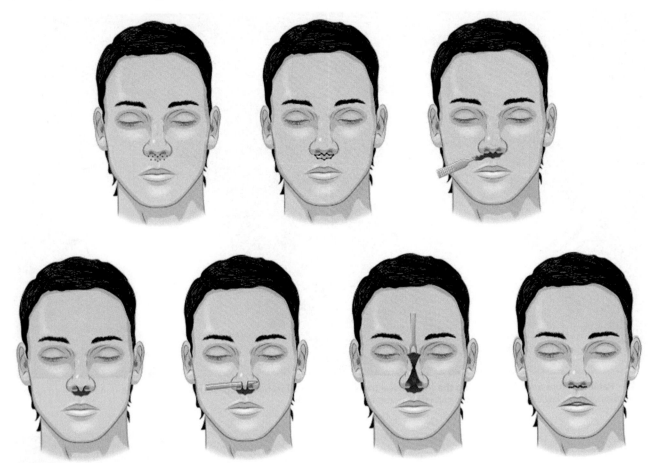

Fig. 8.15   Rhinoplasty and lip-lift sequence. From left to right and top to bottom: (1) Drawing the key points. (2) Skin excision. (3) Skin removed leaving the muscle layer intact. (4) Drawing of the incisions for the external approach. (5) Raising the columellar flap. (6) Elevation of the columellar flap and complete exposure of medial crura and domes. (7) Skin closure.

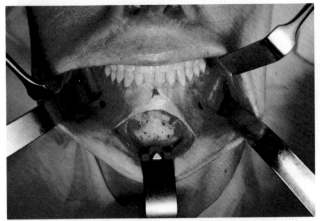

Fig. 8.16   Triple approach to treat the jaw and chin simultaneously. Surgical photo showing jaw and chin exposure without degloving; note the mucosal bridges protecting the mental nerves (marked in *black*).

We recommend the use of ultrasound osteotomies in areas that are difficult to access, for cuts affecting part of the curved section, for localized cuts on the mandibular base, and whenever we wish to avoid damaging the tissues near the osteotomy (e.g., mandibular angle lingual cuts) (Fig. 8.18). With piezoelectric bone surgery, it is possible to make very precise cuts into the mineralized tissue (bone) without affecting other structures,

thus preventing any type of damage to the mucosa, muscle, nerves, or blood vessels.[40]

For every procedure, the use of field magnification is recommended. In areas with low visibility, we also advocate the use of a forehead light. Endoscopic control is highly useful when checking mandibular osteotomies, particularly in the distal part of the angle, a region that is difficult to access and can present great technical complexity (Figs. 8.19 and 8.20). Finally, none of the facial harmonization or feminization techniques described are intended to modify or treat dental occlusion or make dentoskeletal alterations to the patient.

THE NECK: THYROID CARTILAGE (ADAM'S APPLE)

Considered on its own, this feature is one of the most prominent hallmarks of male gender and a true source of stigma for a large number of transgender women.

Thyroid Cartilage Contouring

When approaching the Adam's apple, we recommend making an incision far from the cartilage itself, preferably in the submental zone. This prevents visible scarring and scar adhesions between the thyroid cartilage and the overlying layers. The incision must not be larger than 2 cm. The dissection must be very

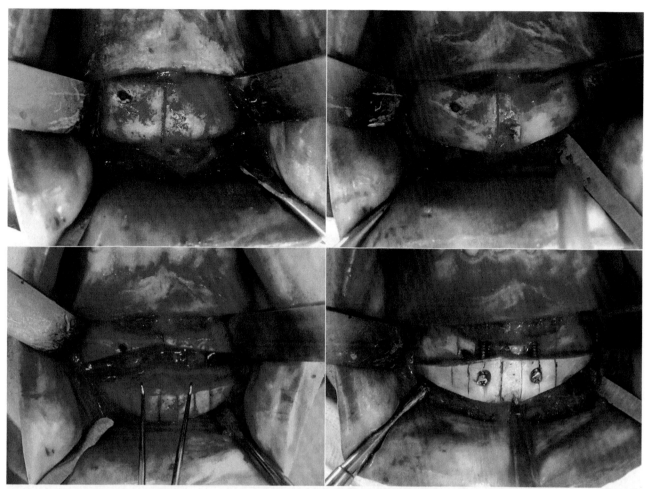

Fig. 8.17 **Surgical technique to contour the chin: modification of the position.** *(Above, left)* High vestibular approach with subsequent dissection of the chin musculature. *(Above, right)* Bone contouring. *(Below, left)* Standard osteotomy. *(Below, right)* Appropriate fixation for the type of movement (advancement).

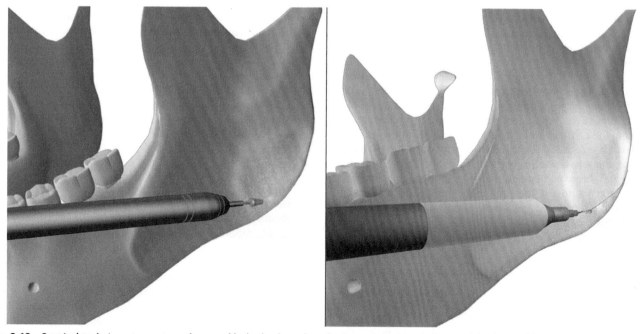

Fig. 8.18 **Surgical technique to contour the mandibular body and angle.** Bone contouring is done with high-speed burring *(left)* and ultrasound osteotomy of the angle *(right)*.

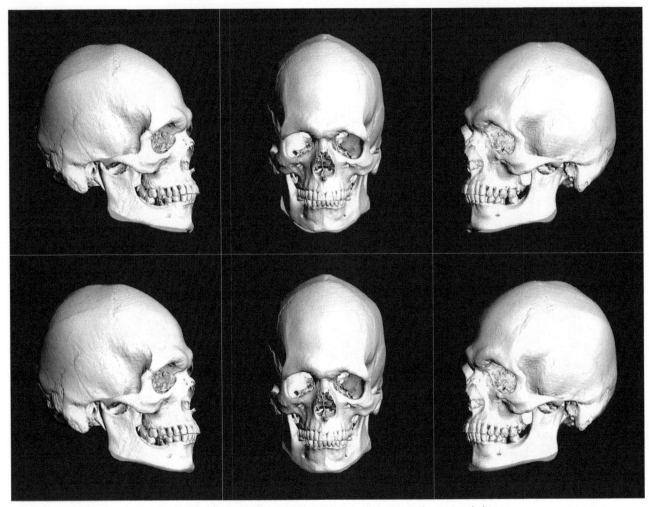

Fig. 8.19 Working areas and possible osteotomies on the jaw and chin.

precise and the different dissection layers must be identified exactly to avoid cutting the musculature, such that the scarring and final result are not affected. Once the thyroid cartilage is completely exposed, the most prominent area is identified. According to the characteristics of the cartilage (hardness, position), the reduction can be performed by burring or with a cold scalpel. When the contouring is done by burring, the use of diamond burrs is recommended, since they are very effective for sculpting the cartilage and not very aggressive with the adjacent soft tissue. Once the cartilage reduction procedure has been carried out, the area is washed with cold saline solution. If the dissection has been meticulous, following the middle line and taking care not to cut the pretracheal musculature, the skin can be directly sutured, positively affecting scarring and the postoperative aesthetic result (Fig. 8.21).

Perioperative Considerations and Postoperative Care

PERIOPERATIVE CONSIDERATIONS

One of the most important preliminary steps in FGCS is a meticulous evaluation and diagnosis of the patient. Each patient has a unique facial structure with specific features responsible for the male identification of the face, so it is important to adapt surgical options to a patient's individual needs rather than taking a standardized approach. The indication for facial feminization procedures must be based on the clinical parameters of the patient as well as on a detailed anatomical study of the craniofacial structure, preferably based on a three-dimensional (3D) computerized tomography (CT) reconstruction that will be used to design the surgical plan.

Clinical Evaluation

The clinical evaluation consists of recognizing the features that contribute to male facial identification in a particular patient, and identifying which of these features can be realistically and predictably modified with surgery. In this process, a distinction must be made between secondary aspects, which can be corrected with nonsurgical treatment (except for the hairline), and the primary aspects that are conditioned by the individual's craniofacial structure. For this reason, it is preferable for the patient to begin her hormonal transition early enough (at least 6 months before surgery) so that the secondary aspects do not obscure the diagnosis. The surgeon's experience is essential when deciding the procedures that can most effectively contribute to the feminization of the face and, therefore, achieve a satisfactory result.

Each of the features in the four key areas into which the face is divided (upper third, middle third, lower third, and neck) must be evaluated not only on an individual basis, but also in the context of the proportionality and symmetry of the face as a whole.

Imaging Tests

Imaging tests are an essential part of a correct diagnosis and proper surgical planning. Today, the combination of CT and 3D reconstruction makes it possible to obtain detailed anatomical information. This is essential when it comes to detecting the facial features that can be modified, providing the patient with precise information, and assisting surgical planning. Moreover, being able to compare these images with postoperative CT results is extremely useful when assessing and explaining the changes made to the bone structure.

Evaluating Requests and Adjusting Expectations

It is critical to listen to, and to understand, the patient's own ideas about her face. She will often provide valid ideas about the features that, from her perspective, determine the recognition of her facial gender. However, patients often have expectations about the results of their feminization surgery that are out of proportion with reality. It is important to explain that the surgery will modify certain features, but that at no time will it modify the core identity of their face or change it completely, since this would go against the principle of naturalness, a basic tenet of facial gender modification surgery. If these factors are correctly addressed by the FGCS specialist using appropriate consultation methods, the facial feminization treatment has the potential to emerge as a crucial step in the complex process of transition.

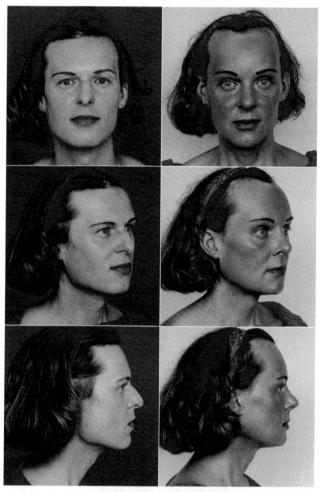

Fig. 8.20 Patient before and after lower jaw and chin contouring. Procedures done: forehead construction, rhinoplasty, lower jaw and chin contouring, and thyroid cartilage contouring.

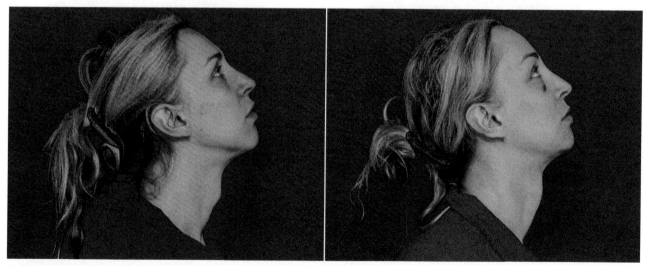

Fig. 8.21 Patient before and after thyroid cartilage contouring. Procedures done: forehead reconstruction, chin contouring, and thyroid cartilage contouring.

Clinical Documentation

The entire process of a patient's facial gender modification must be recorded in photographs, following a clear protocol. These should include clinical photographs, both pre- and postoperative (7 days, 6 months, and 1 year after the operation) and intraoperative photographs of the procedures carried out.

This complete photographic record gives an objective view of the changes obtained with FGCS at different stages in the patient's postoperative evolution.

Virtual Facial Feminization Surgery

Virtual facial feminization surgery (VFFS) is a powerful tool that makes it possible to simulate the potential results of facial feminization procedures on photographs of the patient (Fig. 8.22). It helps to establish the feminization potential for any given procedure or set of procedures, it can help both the patient and surgeon decide whether to go ahead with procedures of marginal benefit, and it helps the patient maintain realistic expectations.

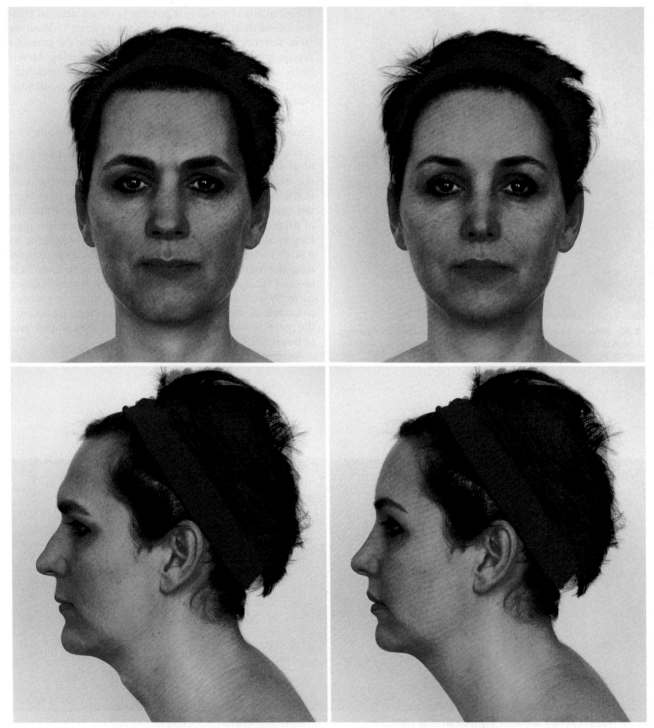

Fig. 8.22 Virtual Facial Feminization Surgery (VFFS). Courtesy of Alexandra Hamer.

VFFS is highly realistic when done by experts in facial gender who can accurately simulate the expected facial changes after the bone structure has been modified. However, the patient should be made aware that, as with all simulations, there is some margin of variability with respect to the results obtained with FGCS, and that the simulations are always of mid- or long-term results, once the postoperative recovery phase has ended.

New Implementations: Three-Dimensional Camera and Three-Dimensional Printing

The introduction of 3D stereophotogrammetry (3D camera technology) provides a practical method for objectively comparing surgical results. Stereophotogrammetry involves estimating the 3D coordinates of points on an object (the face, in our case), employing measurements made in two or more photographic images taken from different positions. The image is calculated from a collection of points obtained along an x, y, and z coordinate system. The data, besides rendering a 3D image, is easily obtained and, thanks to included software, can be utilized to perform anthropometric analyses of facial soft tissue landmarks with a reliability of less than 1 mm.[41]

This technology offers a unique tool in the field of FGCS for visual communication with the patient and makes it possible to enhance the process of clinical documentation. Thanks to 3D simulation and evaluation tools, the patient's own image can be used to explore possible outcomes, educate them about their options, explain limitations, and establish appropriate expectations.

In some cases, we recommend the use of stereolithographic 3D models to improve preoperative planning as the standardized incorporation of 3D printing is an important advance in diagnosis. The 3D printing of CT scans of skulls allows for model surgery to be practiced, which enables surgeons to refine the precise procedures that should be performed on the patient on the day of surgery. The combination of 3D technologies, facial scanning, and skull printing allow for a high standard of surgical planning.

POSTOPERATIVE CARE

One of the most important factors in FGCS entails the appropriate postoperative management of the patient, both immediately after the operation and in the mid- to long-term. Proper recovery has a strong influence on whether the patient returns to her usual routine swiftly. The immediate postoperative period is the most intensely influential phase, both physically and emotionally. It requires a strict protocol to ensure that the patient is given constant care and is made to feel that she is receiving the close support of the professionals involved in her treatment. Finally, the patient should know that definitive and stable results may not appear until up to a year after the operation. The patient must have easy access to the specialists involved in her case at all times, keeping them up to date about her evolution and making them aware of any complications that need to be resolved.

Inflammation Management

While the situation may vary according to the patient, the face usually experiences significant inflammation after surgical manipulation, which is most obvious in the eyelid, nose, jaw, and chin areas. The immediate application of hilotherapy (Hilotherm Clinic device, Hilotherm GmbH, Ludwigsburg, Germany), which is a controlled cooling therapy that does not impede lymphatic drainage, can help to resolve edema and produces a subjective feeling of well-being in the patient.[42] Additionally, the early (2 to 5 days after surgery) application of manual lymphatic drainage by specialists considerably decreases any edema and speeds the recovery and adjustment of the soft tissues.[43] Finally, we recommend using compression therapy for 2 to 3 weeks after jaw and chin contouring surgery to assist in tissue repositioning.

It requires some time, possibly up to 12 months, for the soft tissues to readjust to the new jaw and chin structure, volume, and position. For patients with prior soft tissue drooping or significant laxity postoperatively, we recommend surgical readjustment via lifting in a second surgical session to correct the laxity and highlight the bone work.

Physical Activity

Between six and ten days after surgery, when acute inflammation and other symptoms are under control, the patient enters a 2- to 3-week period of progressive recovery, during which time we recommend that the patient takes it as easy as possible and avoids overexertion. After this period, the patient can return to her usual routine. Moderate physical exercise can begin 3 to 6 months after surgery.

Nutritional Guidance

Before any oral surgery, patients must follow some nutritional guidelines in order to complete the pre- and postoperative recovery process more successfully and rapidly. To ensure proper scarring in the area, the adequate intake of the correct liquid or soft diet, as appropriate, is essential. Moreover, chewing and swallowing may be difficult due to incisions or possible swelling caused by the operation. These problems may interfere with the patient's consumption of necessary nutrients, which is why collaboration with and counseling from a nutritionist is a fundamental complement to an effective and healthy surgery. The tissues require a balanced diet to recover and, as a general rule, food consumption should not be reduced.

Psychological Support

While physical control of inflammation and the maintenance of the patient's well-being are essential, regular counseling from a psychologist who specializes in transgender health should also be provided throughout the entire FGCS process.

During the preoperative period, the patient may present with signs of anxiety about the operation. This might be due to fear of pain, fear of anesthesia, very high expectations, or uncertainty about how family members and friends are going to react to the surgery. In the postoperative phase, anxiety can result from a variety of factors, including slow recovery, dissatisfaction with some results, concerns about recovering their social and/or work lives, or not feeling supported by loved ones.

The psychologist's primary role is to help the patient feel supported during the pre- and postoperative period by providing the necessary counsel required.

Management of Complications

The management of complications is of extreme importance in FGCS. While the surgeries are highly predictable, they are not without complications, which can prolong the postoperative period and compromise the final result. Below are the primary complications associated with basic feminization procedures (forehead reconstruction, HLS, lower jaw and chin contouring, and thyroid cartilage contouring), as well as the different management and treatment alternatives.

COMPLICATIONS ASSOCIATED WITH FOREHEAD RECONSTRUCTION

Complications Associated With the Coronal Approach (Anterior or Posterior)

Hematoma usually occurs in the immediate postoperative period. The bleeding usually comes from the scalp or subgaleal vessels. As a rule, these bleeds do not compromise the patient's hemodynamic stability, but can produce a significant accumulation of blood, capable of dissecting the different surgical layers and reaching the orbital region. To prevent this, we recommend exhaustive control of the hemostasis during surgery, placing drainage devices during the first 24 to 48 hours after surgery, and applying moderate compression in the region. If the patient develops a hematoma, according to the accumulation, type of bleeding, and the areas affected, we recommend surgical drainage, control of the hemostasis, and close monitoring after drainage.

Suture dehiscence is usually associated with sutures placed on excess tension. Although it is not a serious complication, it may delay scarring, leave low quality scar tissue in the incision area, or produce alopecic areas resulting from damaged hair follicles. These complications must and can be avoided by guaranteeing a tension-free closure along the coronal incision.

At times during the intermediate postoperative period (beginning one month after surgery), irregularly distributed **alopecic areas** may appear on the scalp, especially in the approach zone. These are usually secondary to postoperative hormonal phenomena due to surgical stress and tend to stabilize and disappear over time. Occasionally, administration of vitamin complexes may be beneficial to the recovery process.

Complications Associated With the Reconstruction Technique

Perforation of the posterior wall of the frontal sinus is an intraoperative complication that can occur during the osteotomy of the anterior wall of the frontal sinus or during bone burring. At times, it can be associated with the visible leak of cerebrospinal fluid. It is extremely important to seal the perforation during surgery to avoid subsequent clinically important complications like cerebrospinal fluid fistulas and infectious problems (meningitis, empyema, etc.).

Postoperative **sinus dysfunction** is a rare complication, but can occur and may have serious implications for the patient's quality of life. The most likely sinus alteration is sinusopathy due to obstruction of the frontonasal duct with or without associated signs of infection. This complication usually appears during the intermediate or late postoperative period (after 6 months) and can manifest itself in various ways on the clinical spectrum: pain in the area, a feeling of sinus pressure, increased mucus, etc. In the case of infection, symptoms can range from fever and possible sinus abscess (presence of pus) to bone reabsorption. The diagnosis of this complication is clinical and radiological. Initially, medical treatment can be done in an outpatient setting, although surgical interventions may be required, ranging from a sinus cleaning and repermeabilization of the drainage duct using an endoscopic approach to open surgery for a sinus cleaning, obliteration, and sealing or to correct bone defects.

Reabsorption of the anterior wall of the frontal sinus can also occur. This complication usually appears in the late postoperative period and can be due to various factors: bad osteotomy design, inadequate fixation technique with the anterior wall of the frontal sinus, a lack of reconstruction of the anterior wall areas of the sinus perforated during surgery, or poor covering of the soft tissues over the area. This type of complication may not have associated clinical signs and at times it can be diagnosed using imaging tests alone. If symptoms appear, they may be associated with functional alterations of the sinus or aesthetic problems in the frontal region secondary to a lack of bone support. Treatment is surgical in order to achieve the anatomical and functional restoration of the entire affected region (Fig. 8.23).

COMPLICATIONS ASSOCIATED WITH HAIRLINE LOWERING SURGERY

Although this procedure is very rarely indicated, many facial feminization specialists use it as an alternative to hairline treatment. One of the main complications associated with this technique is **poor scarring** in a very visible and exposed area, the forehead. The scar quality depends on the patient's type of hair, the scarring itself, the type of suture, and the tension applied during the closure. This complication may appear at any point in the postoperative period and could be very difficult to manage (Fig. 8.24).

COMPLICATIONS ASSOCIATED WITH LOWER JAW AND CHIN CONTOURING

The complications associated with jaw and chin procedures are usually intraoperative or appear in the immediate postoperative period.

Bleeding and/or hematoma formation are known complications and are usually acute, complex, and require fast action. The accumulation of blood in the floor of the mouth after a mentoplasty is extremely urgent since it may compromise the patient's airway, meaning that it is vitally important to take immediate action. Treatment consists of surgically draining the hematoma (preferably under local anesthetic) and hemostatic control.

Infection is an uncommon complication. It may occur during the immediate or mid-term postoperative period. At times, it has a dental etiology, given the closeness of the dentoalveolar region to the surgical area. It may require medical treatment (antibiotic therapy) or surgical treatment depending on the progression and severity of the infection.

Fractures are very uncommon complications. A fracture may occur during the surgical procedure or in the short-term postoperative period. It usually appears in high-risk mandibular areas (symphysis, mandibular body near the mental nerve exit, the mandibular angle), which have become excessively weakened during bone burring or during the osteotomy manipulation, either because of a bad split or a fracture with an axis different from that of the osteotomy. This complication must be resolved immediately by reducing the fracture site followed by fixation with osteosynthesis material. If the dental occlusion

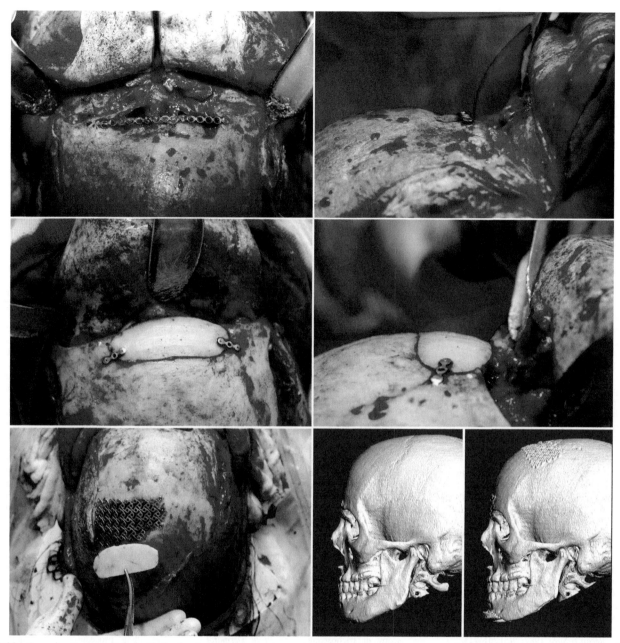

Fig. 8.23 Complication associated with the forehead reconstruction technique and secondary surgery: reabsorption of the anterior wall of the frontal sinus. *(Above)* Presurgical photos showing the complete exposure of the frontal sinus. *(Below)* Postsurgical photos. After removing the osteosynthesis material and frontal setback, the cranial vault graft is placed. *(Below, left)* Obtaining the graft from the cranial vault using ultrasounds to create the new anterior wall of the frontal sinus. *(Below, right)* Computerized tomography (CT) images before and after secondary surgery.

Fig. 8.24 Complication associated with the hairline lowering surgery.

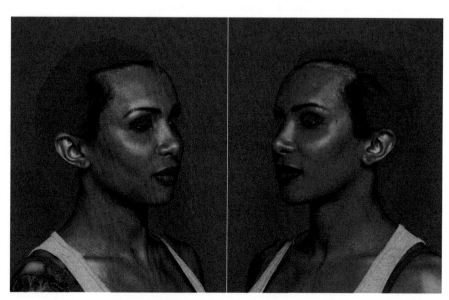

is altered, this must be reestablished to avoid functional repercussions for the patient.

COMPLICATIONS ASSOCIATED WITH THYROID CARTILAGE CONTOURING

The main complications associated with this procedure are linked to the surgical lesioning of anatomical structures near the contouring area.

It is difficult to directly **damage the vocal cords**, but if damage does occur, it is usually located at the insertion area anterior to the cord, which can cause phonatory problems that are difficult to manage, which may be of great clinical importance to the patient.

Airway impairment can occur as a result of excessive burring of the cartilage or from damage to the cricothyroid membrane, which may expose the larynx and lead to difficulties managing the patient's airway, affecting postoperative recovery.

ACKNOWLEDGMENTS

To our team, our families, and our patients.

REFERENCES

1. Tugnet N, Goddard JC, Vickery RM, Khoosal D, Terry TR. Current management of male-to-female gender identity disorder in the UK. *Postgrad Med J.* 2007;83(984):638–642.
2. Ainsworth TA, Spiegel JH. Quality of life of individuals with and without facial feminization surgery or gender reassignment surgery. *Qual Life Res.* 2010;19(7):1019–1024.
3. Ettner R, Monstrey S, Coleman E, eds. *Principles of Transgender Medicine and Surgery.* 2nd ed. New York: Routledge (Taylor & Francis); 2016.
4. Capitán L, Simon D, Kaye K, Tenório T. Facial feminization surgery: the forehead. Surgical techniques and analysis of results. *Plast Reconstr Surg.* 2014;134(4):609–619.
5. Spiegel JH. Facial determinants of female gender and feminizing forehead cranioplasty. *Laryngoscope.* 2011;121(2):250–261.
6. Brown E, Perrett DI. What gives a face its gender? *Perception.* 1993;22(7):829–840.
7. Mareckova K, Weinbrand Z, Chakravarty MM, et al. Testosterone-mediated sex differences in the face shape during adolescence: subjective impressions and objective features. *Horm Behav.* 2011;60(5):681–690.
8. Whitehouse AJ, Gilani SZ, Shafait F, et al. Prenatal testosterone exposure is related to sexually dimorphic facial morphology in adulthood. *Proc Biol Sci.* 2015;282(1816):20151351. https://doi.org/10.1098/rspb.2015.1351.
9. Ousterhout DK. Feminization of the forehead: contour changing to improve female aesthetics. *Plast Reconstr Surg.* 1987;79(5):701–713.
10. Becking AG, Tuinzing DB, Hage JJ, Gooren LJ. Transgender feminization of the facial skeleton. *Clin Plast Surg.* 2007;34(3):557–564.
11. Hoenig JF. Frontal bone remodeling for gender reassignment of the male forehead: a gender-reassignment surgery. *Aesthetic Plast Surg.* 2011; 35(6):1043–1049.
12. Springer IN, Zernial O, Nolke F, et al. Gender and nasal shape: measures for rhinoplasty. *Plast Reconstr Surg.* 2008;121(2):629–637.
13. Farkas LG, Kolar JC. Anthropometric guidelines in cranio-orbital surgery. *Clin Plast Surg.* 1987;14 (1):1–16.
14. Hwang HS, Kim WS, McNamara Jr JA. Ethnic differences in the soft tissue profile of Korean and European-American adults with normal occlusions and well-balanced faces. *Angle Orthod.* 2002;72(1):72–80.
15. Farkas LG, Katic MJ, Hreczko TA, Deutsch C, Munro IR. Anthropometric proportions in the upper lip-lower lip-chin area of the lower face in young white adults. *Am J Orthod.* 1984;86 (1):52–60.
16. Penna V, Fricke A, Iblher N, Eisenhardt SU, Stark GB. The attractive lip: a photomorphometric analysis. *J Plast Reconstr Aesthet Surg.* 2015;68(7):920–929.
17. Norwood OT. Male pattern baldness: classification and incidence. *South Med J.* 1975;68 (11):1359–1365.
18. Nusbaum BP, Fuentefria S. Naturally occurring female hairline patterns. *Dermatol Surg.* 2009;35(6):907–913.
19. Hamer A. Hair and Hairline. Accessed September 3, 2012. <http://www.virtualffs. co.uk>.
20. Giltay EJ, Gooren LJ. Effects of sex steroid deprivation/administration on hair growth and skin sebum production in transsexual males and females. *J Clin Endocrinol Metab.* 2000;85(8): 2913–2921.
21. Capitán L, Simon D, Meyer T, et al. Facial feminization surgery: simultaneous hair transplant during forehead reconstruction. *Plast Reconstr Surg.* 2017;139(3):573–584.
22. Rassman WR. The measurement of hair density in the diagnosis and treatment of hair loss. *J Dermatol Surg Oncol.* 1994;20(11):773.
23. Berg D, Cotterill P. Hair transplantation. In: Alam M, Gladstone H, Tung R, eds. *Cosmetic Dermatology.* Toronto: Saunders; 2009: 187–232.
24. Lacarrubba F, Micali G, Tosti A. Scalp dermoscopy or trichoscopy. *Curr Probl Dermatol.* 2015;47:21–32.
25. Wan D, Amirlak B, Rohrich R, Davis K. The clinical importance of the fat compartments in midfacial aging. *Plast Reconstr Surg Glob Open.* 2013;1(9). e92.
26. Hembree WC, Cohen-Kettenis P. Delemarre-van de Waal HA, et al. Endocrine treatment of transsexual persons: an Endocrine Society clinical practice guideline. *J Clin Endocrinol Metab.* 2009;94(9):3132–3154.
27. Ousterhout DK, Zlotolow IM. Aesthetic improvement of the forehead utilizing methylmethacrylate onlay implants. *Aesthetic Plast Surg.* 1990;14(4):281–285.
28. Capitán L, Simon D, Kaye K, Tenório T. Reply: facial feminization surgery: the forehead. Surgical techniques and analysis of results. *Plast Reconstr Surg.* 2015;136(4):561e–563e.
29. Rogers NE. Hair transplantation update. *Semin Cutan Med Surg.* 2015;34(2):89–94.
30. Gupta AK, Lyons DC, Daigle D. Progression of surgical hair restoration techniques. *J Cutan Med Surg.* 2015;19(1):17–21.
31. Kabaker SS, Champagne JP. Hairline lowering. *Facial Plast Surg Clin North Am.* 2013;21 (3):479–486.
32. Cho SW, Jin HR. Feminization of the forehead in a transgender: frontal sinus reshaping combined with brow lift and hairline lowering. *Aesthetic Plast Surg.* 2012;36(5):1207–1210.
33. Binder WJ, Azizzadeh B. Malar and submalar augmentation. *Facial Plast Surg Clin North Am.* 2008;16(1):11–32.
34. Matros E, Momoh A, Yaremchuk MJ. The aging midfacial skeleton: implications for rejuvenation and reconstruction using implants. *Facial Plast Surg.* 2009;25(4):252–259.
35. Marten TJ, Elyassnia D. Fat grafting in facial rejuvenation. *Clin Plast Surg.* 2015;42(2): 219–252.
36. Clauser LC, Consorti G, Elia G, Galie M, Tieghi R. Three-dimensional volumetric restoration by structural fat grafting. *Craniomaxillofac Trauma Reconstr.* 2014;7(1):63–70.
37. Bellinga RJ, Capitán L, Simon D, Tenório T. Technical and clinical considerations for facial feminization surgery with rhinoplasty and related procedures. *JAMA Facial Plast Surg.* 2017;19(3):1–7.
38. Altman K. Facial feminization surgery: current state of the art. *Int J Oral Maxillofac Surg.* 2012;41(8):885–894.
39. Moragas JS, Vercruysse HJ, Mommaerts MY. "Non-filling" procedures for lip augmentation: a systematic review of contemporary techniques and their outcomes. *J Craniomaxillofac Surg.* 2014;42(6):943–952.
40. Pavlikova G, Foltan R, Horka M, Hanzelka T, Borunska H, Sedy J. Piezosurgery in oral and maxillofacial surgery. *Int J Oral Maxillofac Surg.* 2011;40(5):451–457.
41. Mailey B, Baker JL, Hosseini A, et al. Evaluation of facial volume changes after rejuvenation surgery using a 3-dimensional camera. *Aesthet Surg J.* 2016;36(4):379–387.
42. Rana M, Gellrich NC, Joos U, Piffko J, Kater W. 3D evaluation of postoperative swelling using two different cooling methods following orthognathic surgery: a randomised observer blind prospective pilot study. *Int J Oral Maxillofac Surg.* 2011;40(7):690–696.
43. Leduc A, Leduc O. Drenaje linfático. Teoría y práctica. In: *Issy les Moulineaux.* 1st ed. Elsevier Masson: France; 2003.

9

Breast and Chest Surgery for Transgender Patients

LOREN S. SCHECHTER | REBECCA B. SCHECHTER

Introduction

Breast or chest surgery, specifically either augmentation mammaplasty or mastectomy/chest reconstruction, are commonly requested procedures in the transgender and gender diverse population. The overarching goal of such surgeries is to alleviate symptoms of gender dysphoria and to allow individuals to live as their true selves. Individual goals vary between patients. In some individuals, breast or chest surgery is the only desired procedure, while in others, such surgery is one of many steps in their transition. From a technical perspective, the goals of surgery include a successful cosmetic and functional result with minimal complications.

In caring for the transgender individual, the surgeon functions as part of the multidisciplinary health-care team that may include mental health professionals, primary care providers, endocrinologists, and midlevel practitioners. It is the responsibility of the operating surgeon to understand the diagnosis that has led to the recommendation for surgery, medical comorbidities that may impact the surgical outcome, the effects of hormonal therapy (when applicable) on the patient's health, and the patient's ultimate satisfaction with the surgical result.[1] Furthermore, the surgeon should assist with the coordination of the patient's postoperative care in order to assure continuity.

Surgeons performing breast and chest surgery should also be familiar with the World Professional Association for Transgender Health's (WPATH) Standards of Care (SOC).[2] As previously mentioned, these guidelines offer a flexible framework to aid with providing care to transgender and gender diverse individuals. While procedures such as augmentation mammaplasty and chest surgery are not as invasive as genital surgery, care should nonetheless be taken to assure that individuals pursuing such surgery are appropriate candidates.

The SOC recommend that individuals who request breast or chest surgery have one referral letter from a mental health provider. In addition, input from a patient's primary care doctor, or in some cases, endocrinologist, is useful in confirming that an individual is medically fit for surgery. The surgeon should, when needed, communicate directly with members of the health-care team, especially if there are any questions regarding a patient's appropriateness for surgery. The SOC recommend the following criterion for individuals who desire breast or chest surgery[2]:

1. Persistent, well-documented gender dysphoria;
2. Capacity to make a fully informed decision and to consent for treatment;
3. Age of majority in a given country (if younger, additional recommendations apply);
4. If significant medical or mental health concerns are present, they must be reasonably well-controlled.

Hormone therapy is not required for mastectomy/chest reconstruction surgery. Although hormone therapy is not specifically required for augmentation mammaplasty, it is recommended that individuals requesting such surgery undergo at least 12 months of feminizing hormone therapy prior to surgery in order to maximize breast growth to improve the aesthetic results of surgery.

If an individual is an appropriate candidate for surgery, a surgical consultation should be obtained. During the consultation, the surgeon should discuss the available surgical techniques, the advantages and disadvantages of each technique, the limitations of the procedure, and the risks and possible complications of various techniques.[2] Furthermore, the surgeon should review the postoperative course and discuss the individual's expectations from surgery. Patients who have unrealistic expectations risk disappointment with their final results.

If an individual decides to proceed with surgery, written documentation of informed consent should be included in the patient's chart.

Augmentation Mammaplasty, Techniques, and Considerations

BREAST DEVELOPMENT AND HORMONE THERAPY

Development of the breasts during the prenatal stage of life is independent of sex hormones and is, therefore, the same in males and females.[3] During embryonic development, breast buds composed of networks of tubules develop from the ectoderm. In females, these tubules will eventually become the matured milk ducts. Until puberty, the tubule networks of the breast buds remain quiet. At puberty, male and female breast development diverges. In females, high levels of estrogen and progestins, in conjunction with growth hormone and insulin-like growth factor-1, result in growth and maturation of the tubules into the ductal system of the breasts. Estrogens are generally believed to induce breast proliferation whereas progestins result in differentiation.[4] Progestins are not thought to have a significant role in breast volume.[5] In contrast, in puberty of males, androgens (testosterone and dihydrotestosterone) increase about 10-fold higher compared to females, and estrogen is approximately 10-fold lower compared to females. The high levels of androgens strongly suppress the action of estrogen in the breast at puberty, resulting in lack of breast development in men.

The suppression of androgens and supplementation with estrogens can lead to breast growth in transwomen. Androgen blockade can be achieved with antiandrogens. Spironolactone is most commonly used in the United States, whereas cyproterone acetate is widely used in Europe. A major difference between the agents is that cyproterone also has progestogenic properties. As previously mentioned, it is not approved for use in the United States due to concerns of hepatotoxicity. Some centers use gonadotropin-releasing hormone analogs to suppress androgen production, but cost limits the use of these agents. Alternatively, orchiectomy is an effective means to decrease androgen levels.

Breast size typically begins to increase 2 to 3 months after the initiation of hormone therapy. Initially, tender breast buds begin to form and breast growth progresses over 2 years.[4,6] For this reason, the SOC recommend hormone therapy for at least 1 year prior to breast augmentation.[2] Response to therapy varies among individuals, but breast and nipple development in transwomen is rarely as complete as it is in cisgender women. Few studies have addressed the optimal hormone regimen to maximize breast growth in transwomen. While studies have demonstrated the efficacy of various hormone therapies, reported data are observational and subjective.[7–10] The majority of available literature does not suggest that estrogen type or dose affects the final breast size in transwomen.[4] In addition, current data do not provide evidence that progestins enhance breast growth.[4] Some, but not all authors suggest that younger age, tissue sensitivity, and body weight may impact breast size.[11–15] Furthermore, shoulder width may play a role in perceived breast size and adequacy of growth.[16] Overall, data do suggest that final breast size with hormone therapy is unsatisfactory in many transwomen; 60% to 70% seek surgical breast augmentation.[4]

Patients should be counseled on the degree of breast growth they may expect from hormone therapy and the appropriate options should they desire larger breasts. Some transwomen have unfortunately resorted to "pumping," an illegal and dangerous practice of injecting liquid silicone into breast tissue to enhance breast size. Serious complications of pumping range from local inflammatory reactions to pulmonary embolism and death.[17] Still, because it is a cheap alternative compared to approved treatments, this potential deadly practice continues.[18]

AUGMENTATION MAMMAPLASTY

Many transwomen who report inadequate breast growth with hormone therapy continue to wear external prostheses or padded bras. As such, augmentation mammaplasty may be requested. Breast augmentation can be performed at the same time as vaginoplasty; this can help decrease surgery time and cost in individuals who desire both procedures. In a retrospective survey of 107 transwomen, Kanhai et al. reported that 80% of participants had mammaplasty and vaginoplasty simultaneously.[19] The percentage of patients undergoing both procedures at the same time is likely far lower and variable between clinical practices.

Anatomic differences between the male and female chest are relevant to implant selection, incision choice, and pocket location.[20] The cis male chest is not only wider than the cis female chest, but the pectoralis major muscle is usually more developed. Furthermore, the cis male areola is smaller than the cis female areola, the distance between the nipple and inframammary crease is less, and there is less ptosis in the breasts of transmen, even after hormonal therapy (Figs. 9.1A, B and 9.2A, B).[21]

While the principles of augmentation mammaplasty in transwomen are similar to that of cis women, the broader chest, larger pectoralis muscle, and shorter distance between the nipple and inframammary crease warrant additional consideration. These anatomic characteristics may require lowering the inframammary crease and releasing the lower sternal attachments of the pectoralis major muscle (Fig. 9.3). When releasing the sternal attachments of the pectoralis muscle, the overlying pectoralis fascia is left intact. These maneuvers may assist with implant positioning relative to the position of the nipple-areola complex, and help to prevent lateral implant displacement. Due to the wider chest wall diameter in transmen, a wide interbreast width is common, even with the selection of larger implants.

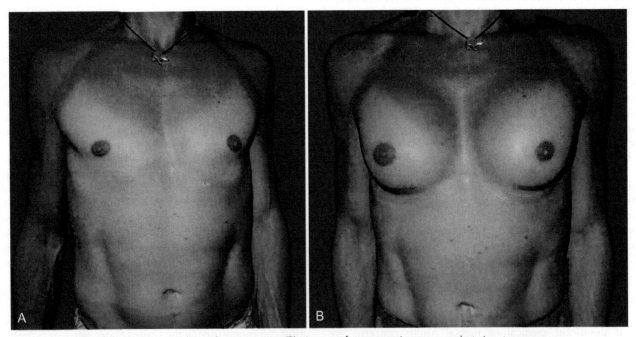

Fig. 9.1   Preoperative (A) and postoperative (B) pictures of augmentation mammaplasty in a transwoman.

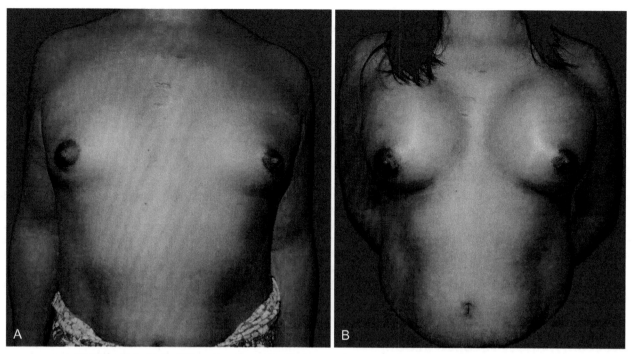

Fig. 9.2 Preoperative (A) and postoperative (B) pictures of augmentation mammaplasty in a transwoman.

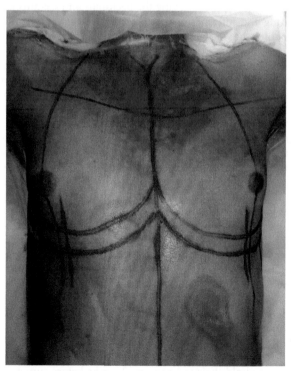

Fig. 9.3 Preoperative markings for augmentation mammoplasty in a transwoman. The lower lines denote the proposed position of inframammary crease.

The implants may be placed in either a subglandular or subpectoral pocket. This decision depends upon the degree of breast growth in response to hormonal therapy. Subglandular implants may be more palpable and may have higher rates of capsular contracture due to less soft tissue coverage overlying the implant. However, subpectoral implants may be more prone to displacement due to the activity of the overlying pectoralis major muscle. Overall, the subpectoral position remains the most common pocket location.

In terms of incisions, transaxillary, periareolar, or inframammary crease approaches may be used. The choice of incision is tailored to the requests and the anatomy of the individual. Due to the smaller size of the male areola and the use of larger implants, an inframammary crease approach is most commonly chosen. Trans axillary incisions are sometimes used, whereas periareolar incisions are infrequently utilized. With the increased use of form-stable implants, larger incisions are often required, which also favor an inframammary crease approach.

While both saline and silicone implants are available, recently, the authors have favored form-stable implants placed in a subpectoral pocket through an inframammary crease incision. In the authors' opinion, this approach allows the surgeon to most effectively lower the inframammary crease, centralize the implant underneath the nipple-areola complex, and release the pectoralis major muscle.

Many transwomen prefer larger implants. Kanhai et al. reported that the average size of implants in transwomen nearly doubled in their practice from 165 mL in 1979 to 287 mL in 1996.[20] In a long-term follow-up study of 107 patients, the authors reported that 25% of patients were unhappy with their mammaplasty.[19] The most common reason for dissatisfaction was that that the breasts were too small. Further augmentation was reported in 19% of these patients.

In order to decrease the risk of venous thromboembolism (VTE), hormones are discontinued prior to surgery, and either fractionated or unfractionated heparin is administered subcutaneously upon induction of anesthesia. In our practice, estrogens are discontinued 2 weeks prior to surgery. Following surgery, a compression bra is worn for 3 weeks. The individual is also instructed to limit upper body exercise for the first several weeks following surgery to decrease the risk of implant displacement. Gentle breast massage is instituted approximately 7 to 10 days following surgery.

THIRD-PARTY PAYER COVERAGE

While there has been significant progress in third-party coverage for gender confirming procedures, many insurance providers continue to consider breast augmentation a "cosmetic" procedure and, therefore, do not provide benefits. However, the SOC point out that in some individuals, a "cosmetic" procedure can have a radical and permanent effect on their quality of life.[2] In fact, research has suggested that gains in breast satisfaction, psychosocial well-being, and sexual well-being after breast augmentation in transgender individuals are statistically significant and clinically meaningful.[22] Because insurance benefits vary, it is worthwhile to review benefits on a case-by-case basis to determine if augmentation mammaplasty is covered.

Mastectomy/Chest reconstruction, Techniques, and Considerations

HORMONE THERAPY

Many transgender men desire masculinization with testosterone therapy. However, testosterone therapy is not a prerequisite for mastectomy/chest reconstruction surgery. Several formulations of testosterone are available and it is most commonly administered intramuscularly or topically. Dosage should be titrated to reach plasma concentrations of an adult man. Testosterone binds to androgen receptors throughout the body and can suppress ovarian production of estrogen and progesterone. Because testosterone is converted peripherally to estradiol by the aromatase enzyme, estradiol will often remain measurable in transmen.

Aside from growth of chest hair, testosterone therapy does not cause significant change in breast appearance. On a microscopic level, some changes have been observed. Evaluation of surgically removed breast tissue from 100 transmen who had received testosterone therapy for at least 6 months showed decreased glandular tissue and increased fibrous connective tissue in 93% of the pathologic samples.[23] In addition, there was mild lobular atrophy and severe lobular atrophy in 86% and 7% of the tissue samples, respectively. Two fibroadenomas, 34 fibrocystic lesions, and no carcinomas were reported in this series.

BREAST BINDING

Transgender individuals often use breast binding as a means to hide breast tissue. Breast binding involves using tight material to hold the breasts flat against the torso to allow them to be more easily hidden beneath clothing. Little is known about the long-term health effects, if any, of breast binding. However, breast binding over several years can decrease skin elasticity and quality, and, as a result, can affect the surgical technique and aesthetic results from mastectomy and chest reconstruction.

MASTECTOMY/CHEST RECONSTRUCTION

Chest-wall contouring is an important surgical step for many transmen. For some transgender and gender diverse individuals, chest surgery is the only desired surgery to alleviate gender dysphoria while in others, chest surgery is one of many steps in transitioning. The goals of chest surgery include the aesthetic contouring of the chest by removing breast tissue and excess skin, reducing and repositioning the nipple-areola complex when necessary, releasing the inframammary crease, performing liposuction of the chest, and, when possible, minimizing chest scars and preserving nipple sensitivity.[24]

Before chest surgery is performed, preoperative breast imaging (i.e., mammogram or ultrasound) may be considered depending upon patient age, personal and family history, and physical examination. The American Congress of Obstetricians and Gynecologists recommends annual mammograms beginning at age 40. Earlier and additional testing may be warranted in high-risk individuals.

Chest surgery in transmen may present an aesthetic challenge due to breast volume, breast ptosis, nipple-areola size and position, degree of skin excess, and potential loss of skin elasticity. Breast binding may necessitate significant amounts of skin removal. Several surgical methods are utilized, and the choice of technique depends upon the skin quality and elasticity, the degree of breast ptosis, and the position of the nipple-areola complex.[24] In addition, preserving subcutaneous fat on the mastectomy skin flaps, preserving the pectoralis and serratus fascia, releasing the inframammary crease and sternal attachments, and contouring the lateral chest wall are also important components of chest surgery and chest wall contouring.

Small, nonptotic breasts can often be treated with periareolar incisions ("limited incision"). In these cases, the nipple may be reduced by a wedge resection of the lower pole, but the areola is not repositioned. A small amount of tissue is left beneath the nipple-areola to preserve viability (Fig. 9.4). Circumareolar ("pursestring") or vertical incisions with free nipple-areola grafts can be used for larger breasts with mild ptosis requiring smaller amounts of skin removal (Fig. 9.5). Finally, traditional transverse inframammary crease incisions ("double incision") with free nipple-areola grafts may better serve individuals with larger breast volumes and increased breast ptosis requiring large amounts of skin removal (Fig. 9.6A and B). Nipple reduction is commonly employed, and often in conjunction with free nipple-areola grafts. In addition, liposuction is frequently used for discontiguous undermining of the inframammary crease and lateral chest wall. Generally, free nipple-areola grafts, as opposed to maintenance of the nipple-areola complex on a dermoglandular pedicle, are the preferred techniques for nipple transposition to prevent residual breast fullness.

For patients on hormone therapy, testosterone is discontinued prior to surgery. Similar to our transfemale patients, we ask patients to hold their testosterone 2 weeks before surgery. The patient is marked in the upright position. The relevant reference points include the inframammary crease, the midbreast meridian, the lateral border of the pectoralis major muscle, the axillary tail of the breast, midline, and the anticipated position of the nipple-areola complex (Fig. 9.7).

Prior to surgery, sequential compression devices are placed and intravenous antibiotics are administered. Following induction of general anesthesia, chemoprophylaxis for VTE is administered subcutaneously (either fractionated or unfractionated

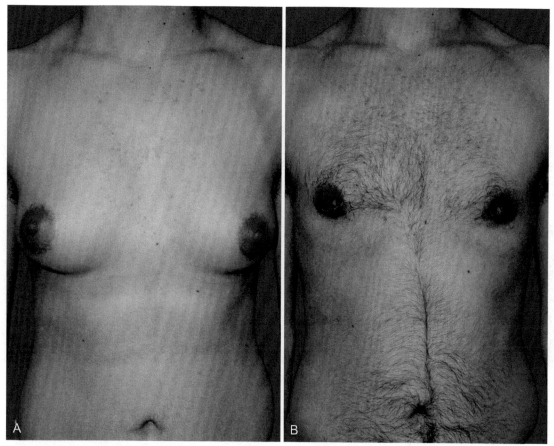

Fig. 9.4   Preoperative (A) and postoperative (B) pictures of a limited incision mastectomy in a transman.

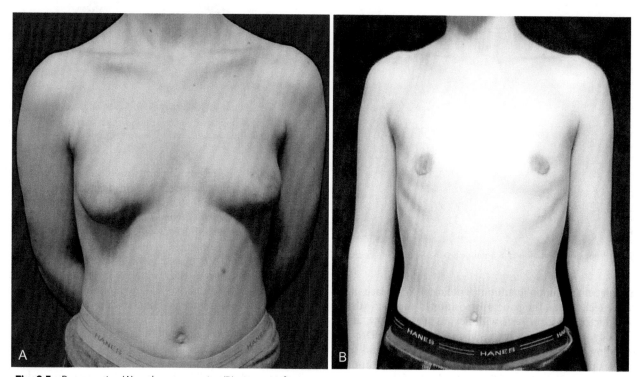

Fig. 9.5   Preoperative (A) and postoperative (B) pictures of a mastectomy using circumareolar ("pursestring") technique in a transman.

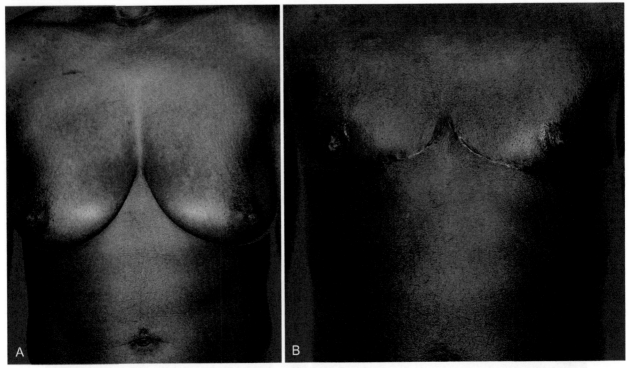

Fig. 9.6 Preoperative (A) and postoperative (B) pictures of a double incision mastectomy in a transman.

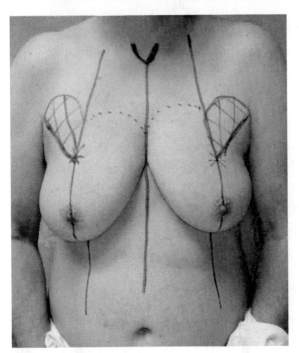

Fig. 9.7 Preoperative markings in a transman undergoing mastectomy.

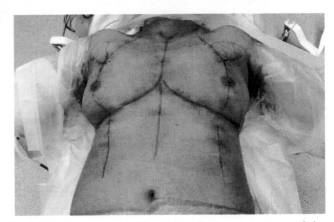

Fig. 9.8 Intraoperative markings during chest surgery using methylene blue to aid in the identification of reference points.

heparin depending upon institutional policies). With each of the operative techniques, the patient is positioned supine, with the arms abducted on foam rests with flexion at the elbow, and a lower body forced-air warming blanket is placed. Draping should allow access to the surgical field from above and from below the upper extremity. In addition, the patient is positioned and secured in anticipation of flexing the back of the operating table to assess symmetry and to guide placement of the nipple-

areola grafts. The reference points are tattooed with methylene blue to aid with intraoperative identification (Fig. 9.8). If free nipple-areola grafts are to be performed, the nipple-areola complex is resized to a diameter of 2.5 to 3.0 cm. In addition, if a nipple reduction is required, a wedge resection of the lower pole of the nipple is performed. The nipple-areola grafts are harvested, defatted, and placed in moist gauze sponges for later use. When a skin resection is planned, regardless of the technique, the anticipated area of skin resection is incised in order to facilitate breast removal. The skin flaps are developed at the junction between the breast tissue and the subcutaneous fat. The inframammary crease is undermined approximately 1 to 2 cm. The medial dissection of the breast stops at the sternal border, and the perforating branches of the internal mammary artery are preserved, if possible. The lateral dissection proceeds subcutaneously over the serratus muscle, with preservation of the

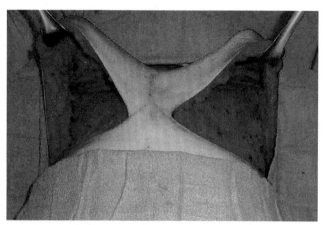

Fig. 9.9 Completion of a bilateral mastectomy with preservation of the pectoralis and serratus fascia.

serratus fascia, and the breast is reflected off of the chest wall, with preservation of the pectoralis fascia (Fig. 9.9). Liposuction of the inframammary crease, the lateral chest, and the axillary tail is performed. Fibrin sealant is placed in the cavity, the patient is sat upright, and the skin flaps are tailored and inset in a layered fashion over a 15 French closed suction drain. Following resection, the breast tissue is marked and sent to pathology for routine examination.

There are no universally established guidelines for nipple position and areola diameter in transmen. Some believe there is a tendency to create areolas that are too large and placed too high and medial.[25,26] Atiyeh et al. proposed a mathematical formula for determining the ideal position for nipple placement in men after massive weight loss using the umbilicus-anterior axillary fold apex distance and the umbilicus-suprasternal notch distance.[27] In addition, McGregor and Whallett reported on their technique for nipple-areola placement.[28] The authors suggest suturing threads at key points: the midclavicular position as the vertical axis, the midline axis of the sternum as the horizontal axis, and the suprasternal notch. The midline axis of the sternum is determined from a point on the upper arm midway between the elbow crease and the apex of the anterior axillary fold. The sutures are pulled along their axes. The point at which the sutures intersect is chosen for the nipple site. A 2 cm disc at this site is de-epithelialized for reception of the nipple-areola graft. However, according to Monstrey et al., "absolute measurements can be misleading."[24] In our experience, clinical judgment is best in positioning the nipple-areola complex in transmen. In general, the nipple-areola is positioned medial to the lateral border of the pectoralis major muscle, approximately 1 to 2 cm above the inferior insertion of the pectoralis major muscle. The nipple-areola is inset on a dermal bed, and a bolster dressing is placed.

Chest surgery is generally performed as an outpatient procedure, unless the patient is travelling or has other medical comorbidities. Following surgery, an elastic compression wrap remains in place for 4 to 5 days. In addition, closed suction drains are placed bilaterally, and patients are instructed to monitor and record output. Discharge medications include an oral narcotic, an antibiotic, a stool softener, and an antinausea medication. Patients can bathe, but not shower, until dressings are removed. Lifting is limited to 10 to 15 pounds for several weeks, and patients sleep with their back elevated for 1 week after surgery. At an office visit 4 to 6 days after surgery, dressings are changed, bolster dressings are removed from the nipple-areola complexes, and local care with a topical antimicrobial ointment is initiated. The compression wrap is continued for 3 weeks after surgery, followed by a compression shirt for an additional 3 weeks. Drains are removed when output is less than approximately 30 mL per 24-hour period. It is recommended that patients stay locally for approximately 1 week after surgery before travel. For patients on hormone therapy, testosterone can be restarted once they are ambulating.

THIRD-PARTY PAYER COVERAGE

Although far from universal, insurance benefits for mastectomy/chest reconstruction are more common than coverage for augmentation mammaplasty. Many insurance providers follow the WPATH SOC and request referral letters from mental health providers before providing precertification for surgery.

Long-term Postoperative Care

TRANSWOMEN

Transwomen with no known increased risk of breast cancer should follow screening guidelines recommended for cis women.[5] Transwomen at increased risk for breast cancer may need additional testing. There are no large, randomized trials to evaluate the adverse effects of hormone therapy on breast tissue in transwomen.[14] Albeit rare, several cases of breast carcinoma in transwomen have been reported in the literature.[29] Unlike in cis women, the reported cases in transwomen occurred at younger ages, after relatively short spans of estrogen therapy, and shared similarities with breast cancer in cis men.[29] Still, because many breast carcinomas are estrogen receptor positive, it is possible that exogenous hormone therapy may increase cancer risk in transwomen.[10] Studies investigating the risks of estrogen therapy on breast carcinoma in postmenopausal cis women are conflicting.[30,31] Furthermore, these studies are not readily translatable to the transgender population, where individuals often receive higher doses of estrogen and may have higher testosterone levels. Some believe that as the transgender community increases and ages, the incidence of breast carcinoma will increase as well.[32]

The best method for screening transwomen who have undergone augmentation mammaplasty is not yet determined. Options include mammography, ultrasonography, and magnetic resonance imaging. In general, mammography is used for screening and is performed in conjunction with regular self- and clinical breast examinations. However, mammogram screening has been found to be less sensitive for detecting malignancies in cis women with implants compared to those without implants. In a study of 137 augmented and 684 nonaugmented women who had been diagnosed with breast cancer as well as 10,533 augmented women and 974,915 nonaugmented women without breast cancer, breast augmentation was found to decrease the sensitivity of the mammogram (45% vs. 66.8%, $P = .008$).[33] This study did not include transgender women.

TRANSMEN

The incidence of breast cancer following mastectomy in transmen is thought to be low.[34] There are no guidelines as to how, when, or if transmen who have undergone chest surgery should be screened for breast cancer. The American Cancer Society recommends that cis women who have undergone bilateral mastectomies be monitored with yearly clinical examination of the chest wall, skin, and incision.[35] There are no recommendations for radiologic examination for transmen who have undergone surgery.

Bilateral mastectomy does not completely negate the risk of developing breast cancer. Katayama et al., reported on a transman who developed breast cancer 12 years after mastectomy and hysterectomy with bilateral salpingo-oophorectomy.[36] The patient had been receiving testosterone therapy continuously for 15 years. Pathological examination revealed a tumor with androgen and estrogen receptor expression, suggesting that testosterone therapy may have played a role in tumor development. Furthermore, Nikolic et al. described a 43-year-old transman who underwent gender confirmation surgery, including a total abdominal hysterectomy with bilateral salpingo-oophorectomy as well as bilateral nipple-sparing subcutaneous mastectomy.[37] Pathological analysis was unremarkable. Before his genital and chest surgery, breast ultrasound, mammogram, and lung radiology were also unremarkable. He had been on testosterone for approximately 2.5 years. One year after his mastectomy, he presented with a left areolar mass and was diagnosed with invasive ductal carcinoma (estrogen and progesterone receptor negative, Her 2/neu receptor positive) with spread to his left axillary lymph nodes and lung metastases. These cases illustrate that continued surveillance is necessary.

Management of Complications

AUGMENTATION MAMMAPLASTY COMPLICATIONS

Acute complications following augmentation mammaplasty, although uncommon, include hematoma, seroma, and infection. Additionally, some patients experience increased pain based upon placement of the implant in the subpectoral location. Other complications include capsular contracture, breast asymmetry and/or asymmetry of the inframammary crease, implant displacement and/or leak, and an unsatisfactory cosmetic appearance. Patients should be counseled about the need for implant replacement/exchange within 20 years following surgery.

There are several reasons for revision after augmentation mammaplasty. In a 10-year retrospective study, Forster et al. identified 24 transwomen who underwent reoperation (either implant replacement or removal) at the University Hospital Zurich, Switzerland.[38] Aesthetic indications included size ($n = 11$, 45.8%), asymmetry/malposition ($n = 15$, 7.8%), and shape ($n = 1$, 4.1%); and medical indications included capsular contracture ($n = 7$, 29.1%), and capsular contracture and size ($n = 1$, 4.1%).

MASTECTOMY/CHEST RECONSTRUCTION COMPLICATIONS

Complications following mastectomy/chest surgery can be divided into acute complications and secondary revisions. Acute complication rates range from 11% to 33% and include—but are not limited to—hematoma, seroma, infection, delayed healing, and loss of nipple graft.[24,39–41] Reported reoperation rates for acute complications range from 4.3% to 10.4%.[39–41] Hematoma is the most commonly reported reason for reoperation in the acute postoperative period.[39]

Many patients also require later revisions for aesthetic reasons. Rates for aesthetic correction vary between 9.0% and 40.4%[24,39–41] and vary with the technique used; they may be more common in patients who experienced acute complications.[39] The need for correction ranges from 1.4% to 19.6% for scars, 5.5% to 28% for chest contour, and 2.0% to 13.0% for the nipple-areola. In a retrospective review of 404 mastectomies in 202 transmen, Cregten-Escobar et al. found that in general, the larger the breast the larger the incision and scar required; however, on the other hand, the smaller the scars the higher the risk of hematoma.[41] In our experience, obesity is correlated with the need for subsequent revisions. Most often, this relates to secondary excisions of redundant axillary tissue (i.e., "dog ears").

Conclusion

Augmentation mammaplasty and mastectomy/chest surgery can play an important role in alleviating gender dysphoria in some transgender and gender diverse individuals. Care should be taken to ensure that individuals interested in such surgery are appropriate candidates. Surgeons should be familiar with the framework recommended in the WPATH SOC and work closely with the health-care team to assure optimal care. Individuals who decide to pursue surgery must fully understand the risks, benefits, and limitations of surgery before proceeding.

REFERENCES

1. Hage JJ. Medical requirements and consequences of sex reassignment surgery. *Med Sci Law.* 1995;35(1):17–24.
2. World Professional Association for Transgender Health Standards of Care; 2012. https://www.wpath.org/media/cms/Documents/Web%20Transfer/SOC/Standards%20of%20Care%20V7%20-%202011%20WPATH.pdf. Accessed July 1, 2016.
3. Javed A, Lteif A. Development of the human breast. *Semin Plast Surg.* 2013;27(1):5–12.
4. Wierckx K, Gooren L, T'Sjoen G. Clinical review: breast development in trans women receiving cross-sex hormones. *J Sex Med.* 2014;11(5):1240–1247.
5. Hembree WC, Cohen-Kettenis P, Delemarre-van de Waal HA, et al. Endocrine treatment of transsexual persons: an Endocrine Society clinical practice guideline. *J Clin Endocrinol Metab.* 2009;94(9):3132–3154.
6. Dahl M, Feldman J, Goldberg J, Jaberi A. Physial aspects of transgender endocrine therapy. *Int J Transgenderism.* 2006;9(3/4):111–134.
7. Moore E, Wisniewski A, Dobs A. Endocrine treatment of transsexual people: a review of treatment regimens, outcomes, and adverse effects. *J Clin Endocrinol Metab.* 2003;88(8):3467–3473.
8. Tangpricha V, Ducharme SH, Barber TW, Chipkin SR. Endocrinologic treatment of gender identity disorders. *Endocr Pract.* 2003;9(1):12–21.
9. Gooren LJ. Clinical practice. Care of transsexual persons. *N Engl J Med.* 2011;364(13):1251–1257.
10. Gooren LJ, Giltay EJ, Bunck MC. Long-term treatment of transsexuals with cross-sex hormones: extensive personal experience. *J Clin Endocrinol Metab.* 2008;93(1):19–25.
11. Wallace P, Rasmussen S. Analysis of Adulterated Silicone: implications for health promotion. *Int J Transgenderism.* 2010;12:167–175.
12. Orentreich N, Durr NP. Proceedings: mammogenesis in transsexuals. *J Invest Dermatol.* 1974;63(1):142–146.
13. Asscheman H, Gooren L. Hormone treatment in transsexuals. *J Psychol Human Sex.* 1993;5:33–47.
14. Maycock LB, Kennedy HP. Breast care in the transgender individual. *J Midwifery Womens Health.* 2014;59(1):74–81.

15. Levy A, Crown A, Reid R. Endocrine intervention for transsexuals. *Clin Endocrinol (Oxf)*. 2003;59(4):409–418.

16. Seal LJ, Franklin S, Richards C, et al. Predictive markers for mammoplasty and a comparison of side effect profiles in transwomen taking various hormonal regimens. *J Clin Endocrinol Metab*. 2012;97(12):4422–4428.

17. Narins RS, Beer K. Liquid injectable silicone: a review of its history, immunology, technical considerations, complications, and potential. *Plast Reconstr Surg*. 2006;118(3 Suppl):77S–84S.

18. Chasan PE. The history of injectable silicone fluids for soft-tissue augmentation. *Plast Reconstr Surg*. 2007;120(7):2034–2040. discussion 2041–2033.

19. Kanhai RC, Hage JJ, Mulder JW. Long-term outcome of augmentation mammaplasty in male-to-female transsexuals: a questionnaire survey of 107 patients. *Br J Plast Surg*. 2000;53(3):209–211.

20. Kanhai RC, Hage JJ, Asscheman H, Mulder JW. Augmentation mammaplasty in male-to-female transsexuals. *Plast Reconstr Surg*. 1999;104(2):542–549 discussion 550–541.

21. Laub D. Discussion: augmentation mammaplasty in male-to-female transsexuals. *Plast Reconstr Surg*. 1999;104(2):550–551.

22. Weigert R, Frison E, Sessiecq Q, et al. Patient satisfaction with breasts and psychosocial, sexual, and physical well-being after breast augmentation in male-to-female transsexuals. *Plast Reconstr Surg*. 2013;132(6):1421–1429.

23. Grynberg M, Fanchin R, Dubost G, et al. Histology of genital tract and breast tissue after long-term testosterone administration in a female-to-male transsexual population. *Reprod Biomed Online*. 2010;20(4):553–558.

24. Monstrey S, Selvaggi G, Ceulemans P, et al. Chest-wall contouring surgery in female-to-male transsexuals: a new algorithm. *Plast Reconstr Surg*. 2008;121(3):849–859.

25. Beer GM, Budi S, Seifert B, et al. Configuration and localization of the nipple–areola complex in men. *Plast Reconstr Surg*. 2001;108(7):1947–1952. discussion 1953.

26. Lindsay WR. Creation of a male chest in female transsexuals. *Ann Plast Surg*. 1979;3(1):39–46.

27. Atiyeh BS, Dibo SA, El Chafic AH. Vertical and horizontal coordinates of the nipple–areola complex position in males. *Ann Plast Surg*. 2009;63(5):499–502.

28. McGregor JC, Whallett EJ. Some personal suggestions on surgery in large or ptotic breasts for female to male transsexuals. *J Plast Reconstr Aesthet Surg*. 2006;59(8):893–896.

29. Gooren LJ, van Trotsenburg MA, Giltay EJ, van Diest PJ. Breast cancer development in transsexual subjects receiving cross-sex hormone treatment. *J Sex Med*. 2013;10(12):3129–3134.

30. Stefanick ML, Anderson GL, Margolis KL, et al. Effects of conjugated equine estrogens on breast cancer and mammography screening in post-menopausal women with hysterectomy. *JAMA*. 2006;295(14):1647–1657.

31. Rossouw JE, Anderson GL, Prentice RL, et al. Risks and benefits of estrogen plus progestin in healthy postmenopausal women: principal results From the Women's Health Initiative randomized controlled trial. *JAMA*. 2002;288(3):321–333.

32. van Trotsenburg M. Gynecological aspects of transgender healthcare. *Int J Transgenderism*. 2009;11:238–246.

33. Miglioretti DL, Rutter CM, Geller BM, et al. Effect of breast augmentation on the accuracy of mammography and cancer characteristics. *JAMA*. 2004;291(4):442–450.

34. Lawrence A. Transgender Health Concerns. In: Meyer IH, Northridge ME, eds. *The Health of Sexual Minorities: Public Health Perspectives on Lesbian, Gay, Bisexual and Transgender Populations*. New York, NY: Springer; 2007:437–505.

35. American Cancer Society. http://www.cancer.org. Accessed July 1, 2016.

36. Katayama Y, Motoki T, Watanabe S, et al. A very rare case of breast cancer in a female-to-male transsexual. *Breast Cancer*. 2016;23(6):939–944.

37. Nikolic DV, Djordjevic ML, Granic M, et al. Importance of revealing a rare case of breast cancer in a female to male transsexual after bilateral mastectomy. *World J Surg Oncol*. 2012;10:280.

38. Forster NA, Kunzi W, Giovanoli P. The reoperation cascade after breast augmentation with implants: what the patient needs to know. *J Plast Reconstr Aesthet Surg*. 2013;66(3):313–322.

39. Kääriäinen M, Salonen K, Helminen M, Karhunen-Enckell U. Chest-wall contouring surgery in female-to-male transgender patients: a one-center retrospective analysis of applied surgical techniques and results. *Scand J Surg*. 2017;106(1):74–79.

40. Berry MG, Curtis R, Davies D. Female-to-male transgender chest reconstruction: a large consecutive, single-surgeon experience. *J Plast Reconstr Aesthet Surg*. 2012;65(6):711–719.

41. Cregten-Escobar P, Bouman MB, Buncamper ME, Mullender MG. Subcutaneous mastectomy in female-to-male transsexuals: a retrospective cohort-analysis of 202 patients. *J Sex Med*. 2012;9(12):3148–3153.

10

Genital Gender Confirmation Surgery for Patients Assigned Male at Birth

CECILE A. FERRANDO | MARCI L. BOWERS

Introduction

Gender confirmation surgery (GCS) for the male-to-female (MTF) individual fulfills a final, completive step in a process that, for most, has spanned years or decades. Completing this surgical journey is rate-limited historically by cost, by fears of complications, and by uncertainty over the final outcome. When the need to find anatomical wholeness overcomes these reservations, genital reassignment is chosen. Broadening of insurance coverage, reduction in complications, and clearer understanding of the anatomical details and outcomes have led to ever more transgender individuals seeking this major surgical option.

As chronicled in the recent film *The Danish Girl*, the first documented genital reassignment for an MTF individual took place in 1930 in pre-WWII Germany. At this time, the term *transsexual* had been coined by the famous sexologist Magnus Hirschfeld, who cared for and studied transgender individuals. The genital reassignment surgical process was the culmination of 2 decades of research and early scientific interest in the phenomenon of gender incongruence. Although the previously mentioned film's subject, Lili Elbe, died of complications related to her surgical process, the door had been opened, and generations of gradual surgical innovations have followed. Wide publicity and attention was brought to the United States in the 1950s when Christine Jorgensen, a former GI, was the first American to undergo sex reassignment surgery in Europe. Later in the 1950s, the French gynecologic surgeon Georges Burou developed one of the versions of the modern penile inversion vaginoplasty technique. Modifications of this technique are still commonly used today.

Although consensus regarding a definitive surgical approach has not been reached among surgeons, there is broad agreement that hormonal and/or surgical treatment of individuals treated for gender dysphoria is of benefit to the individual in general. Documented cases of true regret are rare and usually are due to the difficulty of the transition process itself.

World Professional Association for Transgender Health Standards of Care

Patients who seek to undergo MTF GAS do so by following a general set of guidelines and recommendations established by the World Professional Association for Transgender Health (WPATH) in its standards of care (SOC). Currently in its seventh edition,[1] the SOC are a series of flexible guidelines for clinical practice set forth by the society, based on evidence and expert consensus, and may be modified to meet the needs of an individual. The guidelines provide a framework for those individuals in the health-care community who provide assessment, mental and physical health care, hormone therapy, and surgery for transgender individuals.

These following criteria are recommended by WPATH for genital surgery: (1) well-documented, persistent gender dysphoria, (2) two letters of referral from mental health professionals well versed in the care of transgender patients, (3) capacity of the patient to engage in informed decision making and consent, (4) well-controlled comorbid medical and mental health conditions, (5) 12 continuous months of hormone therapy, and (6) 12 continuous months of experience living in the gender role consistent with the patient's gender identity. In addition, regular follow-up with a mental health or medical care provider is recommended.

In general, individuals who seek to undergo genital reassignment do so after living at least 1 year in their desired gender role. They are expected to have completed a process of social transition which makes the surgical transition more of a formality than a singular process that defines gender. Instead, it is an affirmation of a role already well adopted.

Preoperative Planning and Care of Patients Undergoing Vaginoplasty

The overall approach to transgender care should be undertaken in a multidisciplinary approach when possible, incorporating input from mental health and medical health-care professionals to ensure that patients are and remain appropriate candidates for surgery. Surgical consultation prior to vaginoplasty should involve an extensive discussion between the surgeon and patient on the individual's history and rationale for surgery, as well as extensive counseling on the types or routes of surgeries available, the risks and benefits related to surgery, and the limitations and expected outcome of the surgery.

Permanent depilatory procedures (e.g., electrolysis or laser hair removal) are recommended (or required by some surgeons) for patients undergoing vaginoplasty via the penile inversion technique, which involves use of a peno-scrotal graft to line the neovaginal cavity. Preoperative depilation optimizes surgical results by preventing future hair growth in the neovagina. Hair removal is recommended on the scrotum, perineum, and proximal penile shaft, all of which are often used to create the graft. Laser hair removal uses a laser light source to target pigmented hair, destroying the follicle with heat while electrolysis destroys the hair follicle through the use of an electric current directed through a needle or probe, and can be used on pigmented or unpigmented hair.[2] These procedures may be uncomfortable, and lidocaine jelly or lidocaine/prilocaine cream may be prescribed to reduce the pain associated with the procedure. For optimal results, several treatments are necessary, and hair removal should be stopped 4 to 6 weeks prior to a scheduled surgery.

Several factors place MTF patients seeking vaginoplasty at risk for venous thromboembolic events (VTE) during the perioperative period. These factors include the use of high-dose exogenous estrogen, a prolonged surgical procedure, and need for postoperative bed rest and decreased mobility.[3] Most surgeons request that patients stop their estrogen regimen 2 to 6 weeks prior to surgery, and allow patients to restart it once they have returned to light activity, generally 1 to 4 weeks after surgery. Some surgeons do not require complete cessation and only ask that their patients modify their estrogen use to a low-dose regimen perioperatively. This may lower the emotional angst and physiologic changes that some patients experience as a result of complete cessation. Patients should receive appropriate VTE prophylaxis in the perioperative and postoperative periods.

Guidelines for prophylactic antibiotic use do not currently exist for vaginoplasty in the transgender population, and therefore appropriate prophylaxis should be administered for urogenital procedures.[4] The specific antibiotic selection and length of administration is based on expert opinion. Many practices use intravenous second-generation cephalosporins such as cefazolin. Some surgeons also choose to provide patients with postoperative prophylaxis to prevent urinary tract infection while an indwelling Foley catheter and vaginal packing are in place.

The use of a mechanical bowel preparation prior to penile inversion vaginoplasty is surgeon dependent. Many experts may choose to perform some degree of modified bowel preparation prior to surgery to avoid fecal contamination in the rare event of a rectal injury, and to delay the immediate return of postoperative bowel movements while a vaginal packing is in place. Modified bowel preparation regimens may involve a combination of clear liquid diet the day prior to surgery and mechanical bowel preparation or enemas. Rectal wash can be performed at the time of surgery with povidone/iodine solution. For intestinal segment vaginoplasty, full mechanical bowel preparation and oral antibiotics are recommended to reduce the risk of surgical site infection and anastomotic leak.[5]

Vaginoplasty: Techniques and Special Considerations

Standardization and consensus among surgeons is rare and, until recently, uncommonly shared. The surgical process itself has remained largely shrouded by proprietary and guarded thinking among surgeons. Patients are wise to compare outcomes between surgeons, communicate with other patients, and in general, act as their own patient advocates in choosing a surgeon.

PENILE INVERSION VAGINOPLASTY

The most commonly performed technique for primary MTF transgender vaginoplasty is the penile inversion vaginoplasty.[6] The technique has been widely researched and described, and modifications have been made over time to improve aesthetic outcome and functional results.[7–9] Penile inversion vaginoplasty is irreversible and generally includes orchiectomy (if not previously performed), penile deconstruction, formation of a sensate neoclitoris from a portion of the glans penis on its dorsal neurovascular pedicle, creation of a neourethral meatus, creation of a vaginal cavity and lining of the neovagina with local

peno-scrotal skin flaps, and labiaplasty to create an aesthetic and feminine external appearance of the genitalia. Surgery may be performed by a variety of surgical specialists including plastic surgery, urology, gynecology, and urogynecology.

The procedure is performed once the patient is positioned in lithotomy, prepped, and draped. To start the procedure, the scrotal flap, which will later be used to line the neovagina, is marked. Surgeons mark out this graft differently. Some refer to it as "butterfly markings," while other graft markings are more oval (Fig. 10.1). It is imperative that the markings be symmetric with the principle of symmetry maintained throughout the surgery. The flap is incised sharply, then excised from the underlying subcutaneous tissue using electrosurgery. To prepare the graft, all excess subcutaneous tissue is removed sharply. If hair removal is suboptimal, remaining hair follicles can be electrosurgically coagulated. The graft is kept moist with saline soaked sponges.

Next, a bilateral orchiectomy is performed by skeletonizing the spermatic cord and isolating the gonadal vessels, which are cross clamped and suture ligated at the level of the external inguinal ring (Fig. 10.2A and B). Excess subcutaneous tissue is then either pinned laterally or removed, depending on how bulky it is, and the penile structures down to the deep fascia (Buck's fascia) are exposed (Fig. 10.3). A circumferential incision is made around the glans of the penis, freeing the epithelium from the underlying tunica albuginea. The penile structures are then sharply de-epithelized, leaving a penile tube

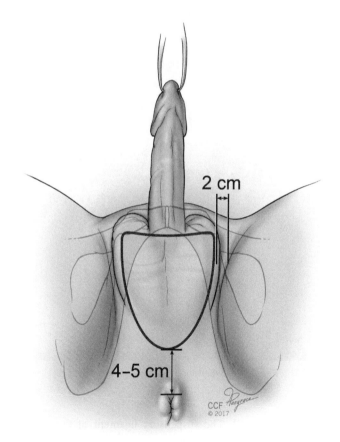

Fig. 10.1 Markings for scrotal flap. The margins of the graft are composed of the ventral base of the penile shaft, the lateral demarcations of the scrotum (approximately 2 cm medial to the groin creases), and the perineum 4–5 cm above the anus.

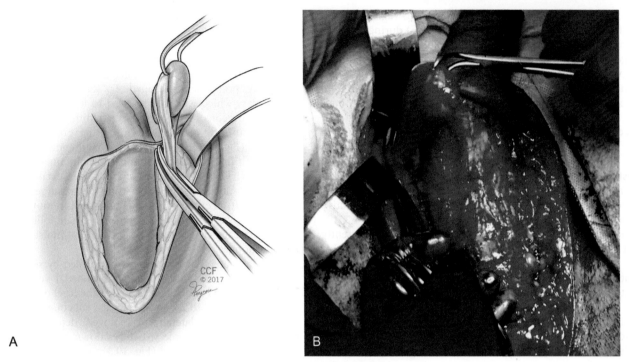

Fig. 10.2 (A and B) Orchiectomy.

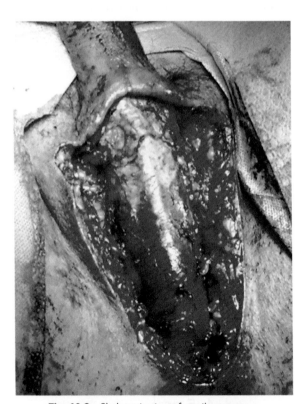

Fig. 10.3 Skeletonization of penile structures.

(Fig. 10.4A and B). The suspensory ligament of the penis is released. A urinary catheter is placed to drain the bladder.

Attention is then turned to creation of the neovagina. In our opinion, the perineal dissection to create the neovaginal cavity is the most technically difficult portion of the procedure. Injuries to the rectum, urethra, or bladder are possible with eventual fistula formation if this step of the surgery is not skillfully performed. Avoiding rectal injury is the most crucial goal. Proper positioning, lighting, and assistance are key to avoiding this. There are three basic landmarks that are traversed in the perineal dissection, and the first 4 cm are the most crucial. Injuries to the rectum in this area are most common, and because of the high-pressure status of the rectum and relative lack of repairable layers in this area, these injuries are the most likely to fistulize. A transverse incision is made in the perineum below the bulbous urethra, transecting the perineal tendon (aponeurosis of the bulbospongiosus muscles) and creating a cavity by separating the levator ani muscles laterally. The midline central tendon is a constant and is a gateway to safety if the dissection remains as anterior as possible once the urethra is safely palpated and protected by retraction. The cathertheterized urethra is palpable and allows progress superiorly until the prostate capsule is entered. Once the prostate capsule has been entered, the risk of rectal injury is markedly lowered. Sharp dissection is then performed through the lower pole of the prostate until Denonvilliers fascia is reached, always with the urethra intermittently palpated behind the retractor. Once the bilateral superior prostatic arteries are encountered near the superior aspect of the prostate capsule, blunt dissection can normally complete the dissection. Dissection can be done with or without a finger in the rectum, depending on the surgeon's preference and choice (Fig. 10.5A and B). Achieving a depth of at least 15 cm is ideal. Once adequate caliber and depth are achieved, meticulous hemostasis is obtained to avoid hematoma formation. A bubble test may be performed to assess for rectal injury by filling the neovagina with irrigation solution and then insufflating the rectum using a large syringe. If bubbles are seen in the neovaginal cavity, further investigation for rectal injury should be performed. Once no injury is confirmed and hemostasis is satisfactory, the neovagina is packed.

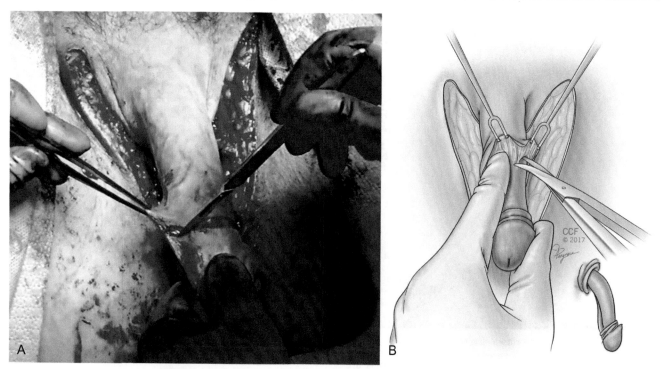

Fig. 10.4 (A and B)   Degloving of the penis and creation of a penile tube.

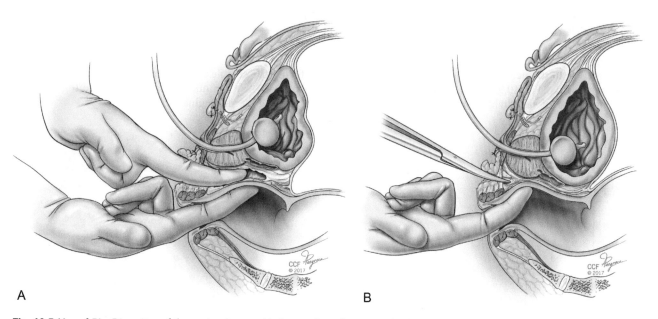

Fig. 10.5 (A and B)   Dissection of the perineal space. Understanding of anatomic landmarks remains key to this portion of the procedure.

Attention is returned to the penile structures. The clitoris is marked in a triangular or heart-shaped fashion on its dorsal tip (Fig. 10.6). A dorsal flap containing the dorsal penile neurovascular blood supply to the neoclitoris (created from a portion of the dorsal glans penis) and a ventral urethral flap are created. The ventral corpora cavernosa are divided with electrocautery from the symphysis to the distal glans, and the ventral portions are discarded (Fig. 10.7). Erectile tissue from the ventral sheath is aggressively removed with scissors or electrocautery and

discarded. Some surgeons dissect the neurovascular structures completely along their length, discarding the tunica—the chief advantage being the lack of bulk and erectile tissue potentially left behind, with perhaps greater risk of clitoral necrosis if there is any compromise to the blood supply.

The clitoral flap is folded on itself to position the neoclitoris approximately 5 cm above the intended location of the neourethral meatus. Additionally, the insertion of the adductor longus tendon in the groin creases bilaterally can also serve as a

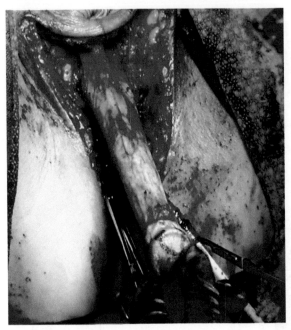

Fig. 10.6 The clitoral flap is marked.

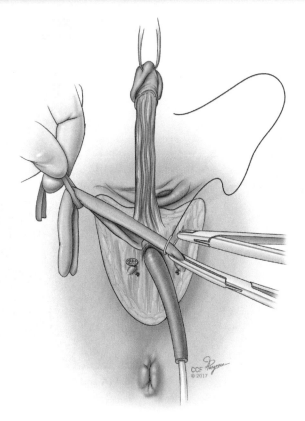

Fig. 10.7 Dismantling of penile structures. The corpora cavernosa have been separated from the overlying clitoral flap and the underlying spongiosum.

landmark for clitoral placement. The edges of the clitoris are folded upon themselves to allow for a conical clitoral shape. The clitoris and folded neurovascular tunica sheath are then sewn bilaterally to the underlying fasica of the symphysis pubis. Care must be taken not to kink the blood supply or place the flap on tension, which could result in necrosis of the neoclitoris (Fig. 10.8A and B).

The spongiosum is then divided down the midline. This allows for creation of the neourethra and the pink mucosa set to line the inner labia (Fig. 10.9A–C). Erectile tissue along the edges of both sides of the divided spongiosum is removed,

reducing the erectile tissue immediately below the neourethral opening—if left behind, arousal will engorge this tissue, often obstructing the neovagina.

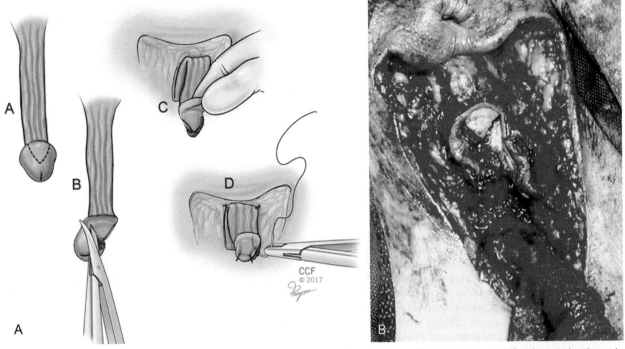

Fig. 10.8 (A and B) Creation of clitoral flap. A portion of the glans penis is removed and the clitoral flap is folded on itself and sutured to the underlying fascia.

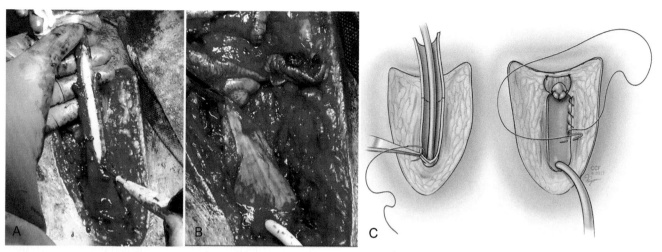

Fig. 10.9 (A–C) Spatulation of the urethra. The underside of the dorsal urethra is used to create the vestibule of the vagina, giving a pink mucosal appearance between the urethra and clitoris.

The prepared graft is sewn onto a large vaginal stent (Fig. 10.10). The stent is then passed through the penile tube and the flaps are sutured together (Fig. 10.11). The vaginal tube and stent are then placed into the neovaginal cavity, and the stent is removed and vaginal packing is placed (Fig. 10.12). An incision is made anteriorly through the penile flap, exposing the underlying clitoris, mucosal urethral flap, and urethral meatus (Fig. 10.13A and B). Labia minora and a clitoral hood are created by imbricating the tissues (Fig. 10.14A–C). Drains are placed to drain the labia majora, and the labia majora incision lines are closed.

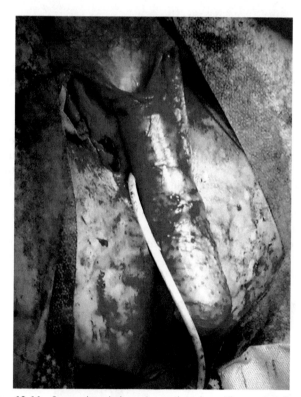

Fig. 10.11 Stent placed through penile tubes. The scrotal flap is anastomosed to the penile tube.

INTESTINAL VAGINOPLASTY

Transgender women with penoscrotal hypoplasia or those who have failed a primary penile inversion vaginoplasty procedure may be candidates for intestinal vaginoplasty.[10,11] Intestinal vaginoplasty involves the use of a segment of small intestine (ileum) or sigmoid colon to create a neovagina, with the advantages of self-lubrication, depth, and reduced risk of stenosis. Disadvantages of the procedure include the risks of abdominal surgery and the creation of a bowel anastomosis, excessive discharge and/or malodor, and prolapse of the neovagina.[12]

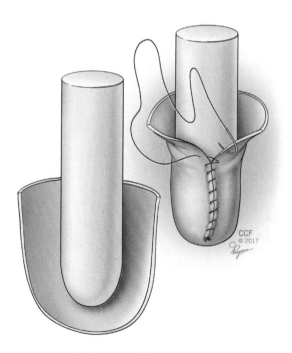

Fig. 10.10 Scrotal flap sewn onto stent.

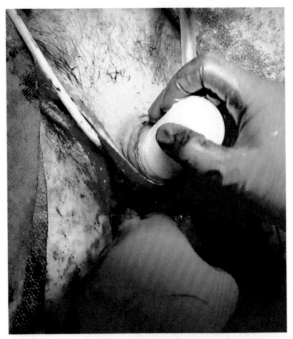

Fig. 10.12   Insertion of stent into neovaginal canal.

Patients with a history of cancer, inflammatory bowel disease, or extensive intra-abdominal adhesions are not candidates for this procedure.

The procedure is performed through a combined abdominal and perineal approach. The perineal portion of the procedure includes perineal dissection of the neovaginal cavity, disassembly of the penile structures, formation of a neoclitoris, neourethreal meatus, labia minora, labia majora, and bowel-perineal anastomosis. The neovaginal dissection, penile disassembly, and creation of vulvar structures are performed similarly to the techniques described previously for penile inversion vaginoplasty. Surgical expertise in bowel surgery is required for the surgeon performing the abdominal portion of the procedure. The abdominal portion may be performed via laparoscopy, laparoscopic-assisted laparotomy, or laparotomy, and includes harvest of an intestinal segment (ileum or sigmoid colon) on its vascular pedicle and bowel anastomosis. Surgeons may also choose to perform a suspension procedure to the sacral promontory to prevent prolapse of the neovagina.[12]

REVISION SURGERY

Data on revision surgery are sparse. One reason for this is that, in general, few large prospective studies have been carried out with this patient population. Second, revision surgeries are not always performed by the surgeon who performed the index procedure, as patients historically have had to travel to have their surgery. Many surgeons may not even be aware of their patients seeking revisions.

In a recent analysis of 330 patients, the authors reported a 9% ($n = 30$) reoperation rate with a median time to reoperation of 10.9 (range 6.2 to 19.6) months.[13] Revision labioplasty was the most commonly performed procedure, with more than half done for cosmetic indications. Other indications for reoperation included excision of granulation tissue (12.5%) and urethral reconstruction for an abnormal urinary stream. Some surgeons report a high anecdotal incidence of urinary stream issues. Often this is related to scarring at the level of the meatus from the penile inversion flap. Revisions for this can be done under sedation or general anesthesia in the outpatient setting and are usually associated with low morbidity. Revision involves release of the scar and creation of an advancement flap of the distal urethral mucosa to open the meatus. In our experience, patients are usually very satisfied with this type of revision surgery (Fig. 10.15).

In another retrospective study of 475 transgender women who underwent penile inversion vaginoplasty, revision vaginoplasty was performed in 14 patients (2.9%), all secondary to neovaginal stenosis.[14] Fig. 10.16 shows an example of neovaginal stenosis. In comparison to primary penile inversion vaginoplasty, revision vaginoplasty caries higher rates of complications, including intraoperative rectal injuries and postoperative complications such as fistula formation.[15] Surgery is more difficult due to the presence of adhesions and contracture

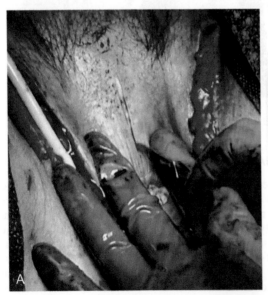

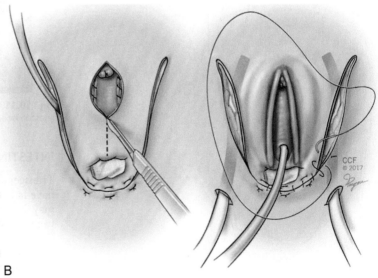

Fig. 10.13 (A and B)   Creation of vulvar structures.

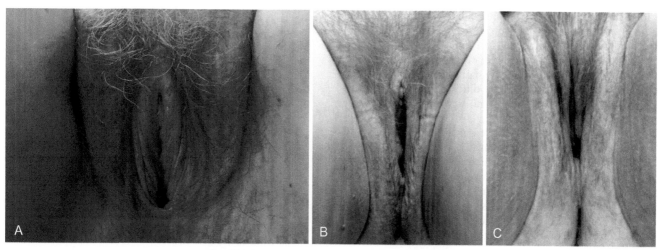

Fig. 10.14 (A–C) Six month postoperative outcomes.

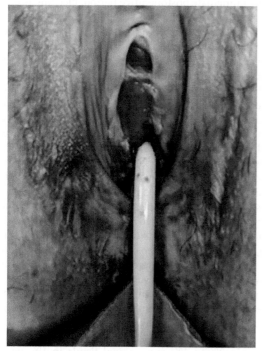

Fig. 10.15 Revision urethroplasty.

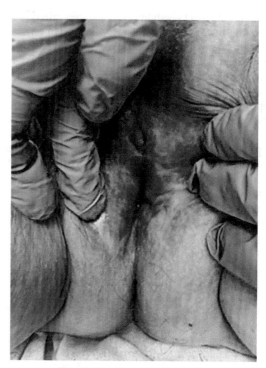

Fig. 10.16 Neovaginal stenosis.

of previous grafts. Options for revision include intestinal vaginoplasty or full-thickness skin grafts from various donor sites. Each technique carries different and specific advantages and disadvantages. Intestinal vaginoplasty provides depth, natural lubrication, and lower risk of stenosis, but confers the risk of bowel-related complications. The use of full-thickness skin grafts is less invasive and avoids abdominal surgery, but carries complications related to skin grafting, including donor site scarring, graft contracture, and poor graft taking.[15] Surgeons are currently studying the use of peritoneal flaps as an option for neovaginal reconstruction. Reported outcomes are preliminary, but this technique is evolving and may be performed more commonly in the future.

USE OF GRAFT MATERIALS

Use of nongenital full-thickness or split-thickness skin grafts is less common, and generally reserved for revision surgery. Few small retrospective studies have described surgical technique, complications, and outcomes.[6] In one report, revision vaginoplasty was performed using abdominal full-thickness skin grafts in six patients with no reported postoperative complications.[16] All patients expressed satisfaction with the results and the ability to have sexual intercourse with vaginal depth reported as 12 cm at 7 (range 3 to 18) months. Others have described the use of an inguinopudendal neurovascular island pedicle flap (*n* = 109).[17] Complications reported included vaginal stenosis urethral meatus stricture, neovaginal hair growth, and flap necrosis. Adequate vaginal depth of 8 to 10 cm was reported.

In a prospective study of transgender women undergoing penile inversion vaginoplasty with ($n = 32$) and without ($n = 68$) an additional full-thickness skin graft, satisfaction, sexual function, and genital self-image were evaluated.[18] Aesthetic outcome as reported by both patients and physicians improved over time, and satisfaction scores did not differ significantly between groups. Preoperative penile skin length was significantly shorter in the full-thickness skin graft group (14.6 ± 1.8 cm vs. 11.5 ± 2.3 cm, $P < .001$), but postoperative mean neovaginal depth at 1 year did not differ between groups (11.3 ± 2.7 cm vs. 11.6 ± 2.1 cm, $P = .65$). Sexual function as assessed by the Female Sexual Function Index was not different between groups, but scores were below levels consistent with sexual dysfunction in cisgender women. Genital self-image as assessed by the Female Genital Self-Image Scale was not different between groups, and scores were indicative of positive self-image.

PATIENTS ON PUBERTY BLOCKERS

Adolescents who meet eligibility and readiness criteria may initiate hormone therapy beginning with GnRH puberty hormone suppression, later incorporating cross-sex steroids for the development of secondary sexual characteristics congruent with the individual's gender identity.[19] Young adult transgender women who have been treated with puberty suppression therapy may develop penoscrotal hypoplasia, resulting in less genital skin availability for reconstructive surgery.[20] In this setting, alternatives to penile inversion vaginoplasty including primary intestinal vaginoplasty or the use of grafts must be considered, as described previously. When considering surgery in the young adult transgender population, the individual patient's maturity and risk of regret must be carefully considered. The WPATH recommends that candidates be of the age of majority (18 in most countries) and have the capacity to make an informed decision and consent for surgery.[1] These guidelines may change over time as younger patients are transitioning and seeking surgical affirmation.

Postoperative Care

Leaving the operating room, patients are dressed with pressure dressings for 36 to 48 hours.

Postoperatively, pain is controlled with intravenous patient-controlled analgesia, and once diet is advanced, oral narcotic pain medication. Ambulation is prescribed after 24 to 48 hours, and hospital discharge is the norm after 72 hours of hospital observation. Nearly 50% of patients are off narcotic-type pain medication by the time of hospital discharge. The labial drains are removed on the day of discharge.

The Foley catheter and vaginal packing are removed on the 6th or 7th postoperative day. Patients are then instructed on dilation. They are expected to dilate three times daily for the first 3 months, then twice daily for 6 to 9 months, then daily thereafter for 15 minutes each session. After 18 months, experimentation with lesser dilation frequencies is possible. The size of the dilator initially is 1 inch but increases to 1½ inches within the first 4 weeks after surgery (Fig. 10.17).

Management of Complications

Intraoperative complications of vaginoplasty include bleeding and injury to surrounding organs, including the rectum, bladder, and urethra. In the immediate postoperative period,

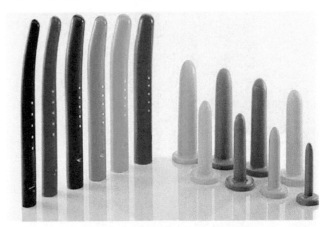

Fig. 10.17 Dilators used for postoperative dilation.

bleeding, hematoma or seroma, wound infection or abscess, wound dehiscence, flap necrosis, or VTE may be observed.

In the immediate postoperative period, bleeding is rare but is usually a result of oozing from the spongiosum edges of the neourethra. This type of bleeding can be addressed with bedside ligature placement or application of a topical coagulant. It is rare to have to take a patient back to the operating room for this type of bleeding. Bleeding could also occur as a result of the neovaginal dissection, which involves disruption of the branches of the inferior gluteal, inferior vesical, and pudendal vascular supply to the levator ani muscles.[21] Tight vaginal packing is important. Interventional radiology embolization of bleeding vessels is generally not recommended, as this may compromise the flaps and result in flap necrosis. Surgical management with direct visualization and ligation of bleeding vessels is preferred in cases of persistent bleeding and hemodynamic compromise.

Most postoperative complications occur within 4 months of the surgery[13] and include neovaginal or introital stenosis, genitourinary or rectovaginal fistula formation, abnormal urinary stream, urethral meatal stenosis, and sexual dysfunction. Outcomes and complications were reported in 1461 patients who underwent penile inversion vaginoplasty in a systematic review of surgical techniques.[6] Stricture of the neovaginal introitus was reported in 12% of patients, vaginal stricture other than the introitus in 7%, vaginal shrinkage in 2% to 10%, partial necrosis of the neovagina in 3% to 4%, clitoral necrosis in 1% to 3%, rectal injury in 2% to 4%, rectovaginal fistula in 1%, neovaginal prolapse in 1% to 2%, urethral meatal stenosis in 5%, wound dehiscence in up to 33%, abscess in 5%, hematoma in 4% to 6%, and surgical bleeding in 3% to 10%. Changes in voiding may occur in 32% of patients, with 19% reporting worse voiding and 19% reporting some degree of incontinence.[22] Vaginal intercourse is reported by 75% of transgender women (range 33% to 87%), and the ability to orgasm in 70% to 84%. Dyspareunia is present in 2% to 6%.

In a review of intestinal vaginoplasty for transgender and gynecologic indications, overall complication rates were 6.4% for sigmoid vaginoplasty, and 8.3% for ileal vaginoplasty.[11] Severe complications occurred in 0.6% of sigmoid vaginoplasties and included necrosis of the sigmoid conduit, necrotizing fasciitis, bilateral lower extremity compartment syndrome, and intraluminal abscess at the neovaginal apex. In addition, a 0.9% incidence of small bowel obstruction was reported. No severe complications were reported following ileal segment vaginoplasty; however, two cases of anastomotic stenosis occurred. Introital stenosis was reported in 8.6% and 1.2% of sigmoid and ileal segment vaginoplasties, respectively, with diffuse stenosis occurring in 3.5% of cases. Review of the literature reveals that intestinal neovaginal stenosis rates may be as high as 43% in the transgender population.[6] Other rare but possible complications may include necrosis, rectovaginal fistula, prolapse of the sigmoid vaginal segment, and excessive discharge or malodor.

A retrospective comparison of laparoscopic intestinal vaginoplasty versus perineal full-thickness skin graft vaginoplasty performed in 50 transgender women and three cisgender women revealed two rectal perforations (10%) and one bladder neck injury in the intestinal group and six rectal perforations (19%; $P = .46$) in the full-thickness perineal skin graft group.[15] Operative time was significantly shorter for the perineal skin graft group (130 ± 35 minutes) than for the laparoscopic intestinal vaginoplasty group (191 ± 45 minutes; $P < .01$). Intraoperative intestinal neovaginal length was significantly greater after intestinal vaginoplasty, but adequate intraoperative depth was able to be achieved in 31 of 32 skin graft vaginoplasties. Both groups were hospitalized for a mean of 8 days. Complications in the laparoscopic intestinal vaginoplasty group leading to prolonged hospitalization included fecal peritonitis in a patient with intraoperative rectal perforation, stenosis of the anastomosis, and intestinal torsion. In the perineal skin graft group, prolonged hospitalization occurred secondary to rectal perforation in three patients, and superficial wound infection in one patient. In long-term follow-up (median 3.8, range 1.1 to 19.7 years), nearly all sigmoid neovaginas (90%) and perineal skin graft neovaginas (80%; $P = .45$) were of adequate depth for intercourse. Two sigmoid neovaginas required removal, one due to compromised vasculature and necrosis, the other due to excessive fibrosis. Five cases of complete stenosis were observed in the perineal skin graft group. Other complications in the intestinal group included one of neovaginal prolapse, and two cases of introital stenosis. In the skin graft group, three patients underwent revision of the labia, and two were treated for granulation tissue at the neovaginal apex.

Complications should be referred to the original surgeon or to a surgeon with experience and expertise in vaginoplasty techniques for assessment and management. In cases of vaginal stenosis, revision surgery may be indicated for severe stenosis (complete neovaginal revision) or an obvious skin bridge or scar obstructing the introits (introitoplasty). Other cases of neovaginal or introital stenosis may be managed conservatively with neovaginal dilation. Urethral meatal stenosis often presents as abnormal urinary stream spraying, and as previously mentioned, may be addressed by release of the stenosis or revision of an obstructing skin bridge.

In cases of intraoperative rectal injury, primary layered closure may be undertaken, and a protective colostomy may be considered to allow for wound healing and the prevention of rectovaginal fistula formation. Postoperative rectovaginal or

pararectal abscess or feculent vaginal discharge should alert the surgeon to the possibility of an undetected rectal injury, and further investigation including imaging and/or examination under anesthesia is recommended. In a retrospective review of 1082 patients who had undergone vaginoplasty surgery, the incidence of rectoneovaginal fistula was 1.2%, with a much higher incidence occurring in patients who had undergone revision vaginoplasty (6.3%) versus primary surgery (0.8%).[23] In this cohort of patients, 23 (2.1%) had a recognized intraoperative rectal injury. Of these patients, 17.3% ($n = 4$) developed a postoperative rectoneovaginal fistula.

Neovaginal prolapse may require local excision in the setting of a sigmoid neovagina if the prolapse is limited to the mucosa only, or neovaginopexy may be performed for complete prolapse. In general, prolapse appears to be a rare complication, and few case reports or series exist reporting on management of this type of outcome.

Minor postoperative complications that can be managed in the office may include vaginal spotting, vaginitis, and hair growth in the neovagina. Vaginal spotting often occurs secondary to granulation tissue formation in the neovagina and can be managed locally with silver nitrate or excision. A trial of vaginal estrogen may be acceptable, although there is no evidence for this intervention. Yeast vaginitis may occur as a result of the warm, moist neovaginal environment, and postoperative skin sloughing may also contribute to symptoms of excessive discharge and malodor. Douching with a vinegar or povidone/iodine solution, or with a mixture of baby soap and warm water, may be recommended for routine hygiene.[24] If preoperative hair removal procedures are not performed or are inadequate, excessive hair growth within the neovagina may lead to tangling and knotting, which requires trimming and removal in the office setting.

Outcomes of Surgery

The recovery period after surgery can be lengthy, but studies looking at patient satisfaction after vaginoplasty surgery show that patients are generally very satisfied after surgery. In a retrospective analysis of postoperative patients, Papdopulos et al. reported that 91% of patients expressed significant improvement in their quality of life, and all patients would undergo surgery again if given the choice.[25]

Regret after GCS is rare, occurring in 0% to 3.8% of patients.[26–28] Cases of regret are usually due to the difficulty of the transition process itself and resultant ongoing discrimination. Transphobia manifests itself as anti-trans violence, discrimination, and subtle hostilities which can make life after transition difficult for some individuals. Factors that have been found to be associated with regret include poor social and family support, late-onset gender transition, suboptimal cosmetic outcome, poor sexual function, concomitant mental health issues, and noncompliance with WPATH SOC guidelines.[27–29]

REFERENCES

1. The World Professional Association for Transgender Health. Standards of Care for the Health of Transsexual, Transgender, and Gender Nonconforming People; 2011. http://www.wpath.org/site_page.cfm?pk_association_webpage_menu=1351&pk_association_webpage=3926. Accessed January 30, 2018.

2. Wanitphakdeedecha R, Alster TS. Physical means of treating unwanted hair. *Dermatol Ther.* 2008;21(5):392–401.
3. Elamin MB, Garcia MZ, Murad MH, et al. Effect of sex steroid use on cardiovascular risk in transsexual individuals: a systematic review and

meta-analyses. *Clin Endocrinol (Oxf).* 2010;72 (1):1–10.
4. Bratzler DW, Dellinger EP, Olsen KM, et al. Clinical practice guidelines for antimicrobial prophylaxis in surgery. *Am J Health Syst Pharm.* 2013;70(3):195–283.

5. Scarborough JE, Mantyh CR, Sun Z, Migaly J. Combined mechanical and oral antibiotic bowel preparation reduces incisional surgical site infection and anastomotic leak rates after elective colorectal resection: an analysis of colectomy-targeted ACS NSQIP. *Ann Surg.* 2015;262(2):331–337.

6. Horbach SE, Bouman MB, Smit JM, et al. Outcome of vaginoplasty in male-to-female transgenders: a systematic review of surgical techniques. *J Sex Med.* 2015;12(6):1499–1512.

7. Wangjiraniran B, Selvaggi G, Chokrungvaranont P, et al. Male-to-female vaginoplasty: Preecha's surgical technique. *J Plast Surg Hand Surg.* 2015;49(3):153–159.

8. Selvaggi G, Ceulemans P, De Cuypere G, et al. Gender identity disorder: general overview and surgical treatment for vaginoplasty in male-to-female transsexuals. *Plast Reconstr Surg.* 2005;116(6):135e–145e.

9. Perovic SV, Stanojevic DS, Djordjevic ML. Vaginoplasty in male transsexuals using penile skin and a urethral flap. *BJU Int.* 2000;86(7):843–850.

10. Bouman MB, van der Sluis WB, Buncamper ME, et al. Primary total laparoscopic sigmoid vaginoplasty in transgender women with penoscrotal hypoplasia: a prospective Cohort study of surgical outcomes and follow-up of 42 patients. *Plast Reconstr Surg.* 2016;138(4):614e–623e.

11. Bouman M, van Zeijl MCT, Buncamper ME, et al. Intestinal vaginoplasty revisited: a review of surgical techniques, complications, and sexual function. *J Sex Med.* 2014;11(7):1835–1847.

12. Bouman MB, Buncamper ME, van der Sluis WB, Meijerink WJ. Total laparoscopic sigmoid vaginoplasty. *Fertil Steril.* 2016;106(7):e22–e23.

13. Gaither TW, Awad MA, Osterberg EC, et al. Postoperative complications following primary penile inversion vaginoplasty among 330 male-to-female transgender patients. *J Urol.* 2018;199(3):760–765.

14. Buncamper ME, van der Sluis WB, van der Pas RS, et al. Surgical outcome after penile inversion vaginoplasty: a retrospective study of 475 transgender women. *Plast Reconstr Surg.* 2016;138(5):999–1007.

15. Van der Sluis WB, Bouman M, Buncamper ME, et al. Revision vaginoplasty: a comparison of surgical outcomes of laparoscopic intestinal versus perineal full-thickness skin graft vaginoplasty. *Plast Reconstr Surg.* 2016;138(4):793–800.

16. Hage JJ, Karim RB. Abdominoplastic secondary full-thickness skin graft vaginoplasty for male-to-female transsexuals. *Plast Reconstr Surg.* 1998;101(6):1512–1515.

17. Huang TT. Twenty years of experience in managing gender dysphoric patients: I. Surgical management of male transsexuals. *Plast Reconstr Surg.* 1995;96(4):921–930. discussion 931–934.

18. Buncamper ME, van der Sluis WB, de Vries M, et al. Penile inversion vaginoplasty with or without additional full-thickness skin graft: to graft or not to graft? *Plast Reconstr Surg.* 2017;139(3):649e–656e.

19. Hembree WC, Cohen-Kettenis P, Delemarre-van de Waal HA, et al. Endocrine treatment of transsexual persons: an Endocrine Society clinical practice guideline. *J Clin Endocrinol Metab.* 2009;94(9):3132–3154.

20. Unger CA. Gynecologic care for transgender youth. *Curr Opin Obstet Gynecol.* 2014;26(5):347–354.

21. Standring S. True pelvis, pelvic floor and perineum. In: Standring S, ed. *Gray's Anatomy: The Anatomical Basis of Clinical Practice.* 41st ed. Churchill Livingstone: Elsevier Limited; 2016:1221–1236. e1.

22. Hoebeke P, Selvaggi G, Ceulemans P, et al. Impact of sex reassignment surgery on lower urinary tract function. *Eur Urol.* 2005;47(3):398–402.

23. Van der Sluis WB, Bouman MB, Buncamper ME, et al. Clinical characteristics and management of neovaginal fistulas after vaginoplasty in transgender women. *Obstet Gynecol.* 2016;127(6):1118–1126.

24. Deutsch MB. *Guidelines for the Primary and Gender-Affirming Care of Transgender and Gender Nonbinary People.* http://transhealth.ucsf.edu/pdf/Transgender-PGACG-6-17-16.pdf; 2016. Accessed 8 February 2017.

25. Papdopulos NA, Lelle JD, Herschblach P, et al. Quality of life and patient satisfaction following male-to-female sex reassignment surgery. *J Sex Med.* 2017;14(5):721–730.

26. Ruppin U, Pfäfflin F. Long-term follow-up of adults with gender identity disorder. *Arch Sex Behav.* 2015;44:1321–1329.

27. Lawrence AA. Factors associated with satisfaction or regret following male-to-female sex reassignment surgery. *Arch Sex Behav.* 2003;32:299–315.

28. Landén M, Wålinder J, Hambert G, et al. Factors predictive of regret in sex reassignment. *Acta Psychiatr Scand.* 1998;97:284–289.

29. Djordjevic ML, Bizic MR, Duisin D, et al. Reversal surgery in regretful male-to-female transsexuals after sex reassignment surgery. *J Sex Med.* 2016;13:1000–1007.

11

Genital Gender Confirmation Surgery for Patients Assigned Female at Birth

MARTA R. BIZIC | MIROSLAV L. DJORDJEVIC

Introduction

Patients suffering from gender dysphoria feel that their gender assigned at birth is in some way "wrong" and therefore seek to take the opposite gender role. Gender dysphoria is a state that requires a multidisciplinary approach to treatment, and the only real management consists of "adjusting the body to the mind."[1] A multidisciplinary approach includes psychiatric evaluation and ongoing care, hormonal therapy, and physical transition with gender affirmation surgery (also known as genital confirmation or sex reassignment surgery [SRS]), as the last possible step in treatment. In terms of readiness and eligibility for the surgery, it is generally recommended that surgeons and patients follow the criteria set forth by the World Professional Association for Transgender Health (WPATH). The Standards of Care advise that patients undergoing genital surgery should provide two letters of recommendation from qualified mental health professionals, provide confirmation that they have been on hormonal therapy for a period of 1 year minimum, and that the patient should be living full-time as their self-affirmed gender for that year as well. Gender reassignment surgery (GRS) refers to all surgical procedures that a patient wishes to undergo in an effort to become similar to the opposite gender. SRS is a part of GRS and refers only to the genital reconstruction.[2]

When choosing to undergo genital confirmation surgery, the patient must bear in mind the desired postoperative result that they wish to achieve and be knowledgeable about the surgical options that are available to them. This is the point where the patient must undergo a thorough preoperative consultation and examination by the surgeon performing the surgery, as well as a detailed discussion with their referring mental health specialist to help them set realistic expectations and prepare for the postoperative recovery after surgery. Along these lines, it is important to preface that there is no single ideal surgical package that will suit every patient. We need to consider the patient's anatomy as well as their personal concerns. This is why the decision to choose a particular surgical package rests not only with the surgeon, but with the patient as well.

The most commonly performed surgeries in female-to-male (FTM) patients are bilateral mastectomy with male chest contouring and genital reconstructive surgery which includes total hysterectomy with bilateral oophorectomy, vaginectomy, reconstruction of the neophallus, urethral reconstruction, and scrotoplasty with implantation of testicular prostheses. Phalloplasty and metoidioplasty are the two options for neophallic reconstruction and we will discuss these procedures in depth in this chapter.

History and Evolution of the Procedure

The goal of penile reconstruction has always been to create a neophallus of satisfactory appearance. The term "phalloplasty" was first mentioned back in the 19th century by Sprengler and referred to the reconstruction of the superficial penile tissue layers.[3] Bogoras first reported the usage of a single abdominal tube for phalloplasty, naming his technique "penis plastic totalis."[1,4] Hoopes was one of the first surgeons to describe his phalloplasty technique using a simple abdominal tube pedicle flap to create the phallus with no urethral extension. He operated on the premise that most patients were strongly motivated by the "anxiety of discovery" and that functionality was not the primary goal of the surgery.[5,6]

Conversely, Gilbert et al. believed in the functionality of the neophallus, and together with other authors defined the goals that should be met in penile reconstruction[3,7–9]:

1. One stage procedure
2. Aesthetically appealing phallus with a normal appearance and adequate length and girth for sexual intercourse (after penile prosthesis implantation)
3. Voiding while standing up with the urethral meatus opening at the tip of the phallus
4. The phallus possessing adequate tactile and erogenous sensation
5. Minimal scaring of the donor area or disfigurement
6. The phallus reconstruction should preferably be reproducible.

From the experience of severely injured patients during the Second World War, new ideas and possibilities for phalloplasty arose. The first FTM GRS was performed in 1946 by Sir Harrold Gillies.[10,11] This operation involved a pedicled groin flap with creation of a neourethra and subsequent implantation of rib cartilage into the penile shaft and became known as the Gillies' technique and remained in common practice for years to come. The technique was later modified by Biber[12] and later by Laub et al.[13] from Stanford University to incorporate a neourethral reconstruction using an outside-in tubularized infraumbilical abdominal flap. Around this time, Bouman, who performed genital reconstruction in intersex patients, described the use of biaxial superficial inferior epigastric midline infraumbilical flaps for neophallic reconstruction in his FTM patients.[14]

In the early 1970s, McGregor and Jackson introduced the use of the groin flap based off of the superficial circumflex iliac artery and vein as a single pedicled flap.[15] In 1978, Puckett similarly described a tubed groin flap for penile reconstruction, which had successful outcomes reported by many surgeons at that time.[16] In Serbia, the groin flap technique was modified by extending the flap and lengthening the pedicle which led to very successful phallic reconstruction outcomes in adolescents and children.[17]

The gracilis flap was also described as a possible option for phallic reconstruction, and Orticochea was the first to report success with its use in a five-stage neophallic reconstruction which resulted in a neophallus of normal size, color, micturition, with normal tactile, thermal, pain and erogenous sensitivity, and the ability for normal erections.[18] Horton et al. also reported their experience with unilateral gracilis flaps in phallic reconstruction.[19]

The radial forearm free flap (RFFF) was initially developed in 1978 by Chinese postgraduate doctors at Shenyang Military Hospital. They used the radial forearm flap as a free flap vascularized by the radial artery for the correction of severe neck burn scar contractures. Later in 1982, their teacher, Song et al., reported this flap in the English literature, naming it the "forearm flap."[20,21] Chang and Hwang first described the use of the radial forearm flap in single-stage phalloplasty surgery incorporating an autogenous cartilage stiffener in seven cases with satisfactory results and only one case of fistula.[22] After their publication, it became known as the "Chinese flap." Biemer later described a modification in which the neourethra was centered over the radial artery to provide it with the best possible perfusion.[23] Semple placed the neourethra centrally over the vascular pedicle, reducing the width of the forearm flap, but resulting in a considerable reduction in neophallic length and a suboptimal donor site scar.[24] Gilbert et al. described a modification to Biemer's modification of the RFFF by centering the urethra on the ulnar forearm and allowing for creation of the glans by widening the "cricket bat" design.[25] Gottlieb proposed a design incorporating a centrally placed neourethra in continuity with the neoglans, eliminating the need for a circumferential meatal suture line, thus avoiding meatal stenosis without sacrificing phallic length.[26] Another modification of the RFFF was the introduction of the radial bone into the phallus as a stiffener.[27] Unfortunately, this modification resulted in a high complication rate including urethral fistula formation (40% to 50%) and need for postoperative urethral reconstruction as well as fractures of the donor forearm in about 9% of the patients.[28] While placement of this type of stiffener seems to be associated with a high complication rate, patients who do not experience complications seem to be satisfied. In recent studies looking at neophallus reconstruction with the use of an osteocutaneous RFFF, 70% of the patients report good to excellent stiffener function during intercourse.[29] Currently, forearm flaps are one of the most popular methods for total penile reconstruction. The majority of centers performing the phallic reconstruction with RFFF are using penile implants to create phallus rigidity to allow for penetrative sexual intercourse.

In 1987, Upton reported the use of a lateral arm flap based on the posterior radial collateral artery for phallic reconstruction, which allowed for an inconspicuous donor site without compromise of the size of the neophallus.[30] The technique includes a prefabricated neourethra which is positioned within the lateral arm to permit the coexistence of an erectile prosthesis alongside a fully vascularized urethra. Khouri et al. later reported 5-year outcomes after phalloplasty using the prefabricated lateral arm flap technique, and all patients were found to have erogenous and tactile sensibility of the neophallus.[31]

The lateral thigh flap was first described by Baek in 1983. This is a fascial flap based on the smaller vessels that extend from the profunda femoris system to the skin.[32] The anterolateral thigh (ALT) flap, first described in 1984 by Song et al., is a fasciocutaneous flap usually based on the musculocutaneous and septocutaneous perforators of the descending branch of the lateral circumflex femoral artery and its venae comitans.[33] As a free flap, ALT was first mentioned by Felici and Felici in 2006, who reported their results in six FTM patients with the possibility of insertion of a penile prosthesis for penetrative sexual intercourse.[34]

Outcomes from the pedicled latissimus dorsi flap were reported in the late 19th century in breast reconstruction following mastectomy.[35] It was first described as a free flap in 1976 by Baudet et al.[36] In 2006, our center in Belgrade reported on its use for neophallic reconstruction in eight boys with a diagnosis of micropenis as a result of exstrophy-epispadias complex.[37] The latissimus dorsi flap has been widely used in reconstructive surgery because of its versatility and reliability. The free flap is used with great success in both adult and pediatric populations because it allows for the creation of a neophallus of adequate length and circumference.

Above we describe the most commonly used flaps. Many other free flaps have been described for phallus reconstruction, including the free deltoid flap, scapular free flap, sensate osteocutaneous free fibula flap, tensor fasciae latae, deep epigastric artery perforator (DIEAP) flap, and the dorsalis pedis flap.[7,38–45]

As the above neophalloplastic techniques were being developed, an alternative to phallic reconstruction using the hormonally enlarged clitoris was also under study. This procedure was first reported by Durfee and Rowland.[46] The term metoidioplasty, as the technique is known today, was introduced by Lebovic and Laub and is derived from Greek words "meta"— "toward" and "oidion"— "male genitalia."[47] Eicher later introduced the term "clitoral penoid" which actually refers to the same surgical procedure.[48] Metoidioplasty involves the creation of a small penis, inadequate for penetration during intercourse, but otherwise involving all the phenotypic characteristics of male genitalia. The first big series of patients (70 FTM patients) undergoing this procedure was published by Hage and Turnhout and revealed that more than two surgical procedures were needed to obtain successful outcomes after surgery.[49]

There are clearly many techniques for penile reconstruction and no true gold standard exists. This emphasizes the point that all techniques are fraught with disadvantages. In this chapter, we will emphasize the most commonly used surgical techniques for genital confirmation in FTM patients and we will elaborate on patient eligibility and readiness criteria for each procedure.

Phalloplasty Surgery: Current Operative Techniques

Phalloplasty involves creating a neophallus from extragenital tissue and is considered one of the most challenging and complex procedures in reconstructive surgery. Phallic reconstruction should ideally create an aesthetically pleasing phallus with sufficient length for vaginal penetration, with tactile and erogenous sensibility, with the ability to void in standing position, and with acceptable donor site morbidity.

Since total penile reconstruction was first described, there have been ongoing endeavors to develop the ideal technique for phalloplasty. Advancements in phalloplastic techniques have mirrored the improvements in reconstructive flap surgery. First experiences involved the use of local flaps, most commonly based off of the inferior epigastric vessels. In the 1980s microsurgical free flaps became very popular in reconstructive surgery, and these techniques are also applied to SRS phalloplasty surgeries.[22–25,41–50] Today, there are many options for phalloplasty, including pedicled flaps (abdominal flap, groin flap, ALT flap) and free transfer flaps (RFFF and the latissimus dorsi flap). The most commonly used flaps in FTM patients are the RFFF and the free musculocutaneous latissimus dorsi (MLD) flap.

ABDOMINAL FLAP PHALLOPLASTY

In this procedure, the donor site is located on the abdomen or waist. A "bird wing" incision is marked with its base in the suprapubic/mons pubic position with lateral extensions up to the lower abdominal skin crease, extending to both flanks. The base-to-limb ratio of the flaps is kept at 4 or 5:1, so that adequate blood supply is ensured to the most distal end. The depth of the incision reaches up to the anterior rectus sheath and the external oblique aponeurosis, from medial to lateral, with blood supply provided by superficial epigastric and circumflex iliac vessels. In abdominal "flap-apposition" and phalloplasty, the two lateral "wings" are approximated in the midline using subcuticular sutures. The clitoris is usually left in its native position to allow for sexual sensation. Urethral reconstruction cannot be performed in the first stage, but it is performed in one of the later stages. In cases where erectile function is desired, a penile prosthesis can be implanted.

Recently Bettocchi et al. published their technique of the pedicled pubic phalloplasty with the neourethra reconstructed from the hairless strip of skin from the clitoris and labia in 85 FTM patients. The authors reported complications in 75% of the patients related to urethral reconstruction, out of which 64% had urethral stricture and 55% had urethral fistula. They also reported that in cases where a two-staged urethroplasty was performed, there was a decrease in the overall complication rate.[51]

The main advantage of the abdominal flap phalloplasty is that it is a relatively easy procedure to perform, with acceptable scaring of the donor area and of the neophallus. The main disadvantage of the procedure is the creation of a relatively small neophallus with poor erotic sensation and undesirable hair growth.

GROIN FLAP PHALLOPLASTY

The base of this flap lies over the femoral artery approximately 2 cm below the inguinal ligament. The flap is then designed to be approximately 22 × 12 cm. The surface of the flap is outlined in three parts: (1) the lateral thin hairless part (approximately 2 cm) for the neourethra; (2) the thick, partially hairy medial part for the neophallus shaft; and (3) the base of the flap (approximately 4 to 5 cm) which is to be de-epithelialized. The flap is elevated beneath the deep fascia, leaving out the rectus or the external oblique fascia, starting from its distal part and proceeding to its base. Dissection is performed medially and the sartorius fascia is lifted together with the deep branch of the superficial iliac circumflex artery. The base of the flap is then mobilized from the lower and medial margin by blunt dissection of the subcutaneous tissue.

De-epithelization is performed at about 4 to 5 cm from the base of the flap, excluding approximately 2 cm of the lateral part, which is to be used for the neourethra. About 2 cm of the lateral part of the flap is separated from the medial part by de-epithelializing a 1 cm margin of skin which is then tubularized over a stent, then sutured with running and interrupted absorbable sutures. The medial part is tubularized over the newly formed urethra in a tube-within-a-tube fashion. After the flap is elevated with a long pedicle, a subcutaneous tunnel measuring 3 fingerbreadths in width is created between the donor and recipient site and the arch of the pedicle is rotated between 90 and 180 degrees without compromising the blood supply of the flap. The neophallus is sutured to the skin of the recipient region and the neourethra is anastomosed to the native urethra after it has been lengthened using the labia minora, while the clitoris is incorporated into the base of the neophallus. Urethral anastomosis may be performed simultaneously, or in a second procedure, following a complete formation of the neourethra. The donor site skin defect can be easily closed by undermining and direct approximation.[17]

Advantages of the groin flap phalloplasty are that it is a relatively short procedure to perform, with a satisfying postoperative result for the patient and acceptable morbidity and scarring of the donor area. Disadvantages are similar to those of the abdominal phalloplasty: poor erogenous sensation, smaller and usually hairy neophallus. In our experience, complications occurred in 5 out of the 24 patients who underwent this procedure. All of these complications were resolved with a minor surgical repair (two urethral fistulas, one stenosis of the urethral anastomosis, and two patients with partial flap necrosis).[17]

ANTEROLATERAL THIGH FLAP PHALLOPLASTY

The mobilization of this flap is performed medial to lateral, with careful mobilization anteriorly between the rectus femoris and vastus lateralis muscles to preserve the perforators through the vastus lateralis muscle. The ALT flap has a rectangular shape with one side shorter and wider and the other longer and narrower, for the neophallus and neourethra, respectively. After the major perforator vessel is identified, pedicle dissection goes through the septum to the descending branch of the lateral circumflex femoral artery. The flap is then marked eccentrically to obtain the maximal pedicle length possible. The lateral cutaneous nerve of the thigh is identified, mobilized, and dissected at about 5 cm proximal to the superior edge of the flap, to preserve an adequate length for the neurorrhaphy part of the procedure.[38,52,53]

The main advantage of the ALT phalloplasty is the avoidance of a microvascular anastomosis, good sensation of the neophallus due to the anastomosis of the lateral cutaneous nerve with the clitoral nerve, as well as low morbidity and "invisible" scar at the donor site, adequate size of the neophallus, as well as better skin tone matching with the genital color compared to the RFFF phalloplasty. Disadvantages include presence of hair on the donor area, which in some cases requires prior laser hair removal, and a large donor defect that requires a split thickness graft for closure. Another limitation of the technique is that the ALT flap phalloplasty can only be done in patients with no excessive fatty tissue. Several authors have published their results of ALT flap phallic reconstruction with the neourethra constructed using the tube-within-a-tube technique with different success rates.[54–56]

RADIAL FOREARM FREE FLAP PHALLOPLASTY

Starting in the late 1980s, the RFFF phalloplasty was considered the gold standard for neophallic reconstruction. This procedure involves the construction of a neophallus from forearm tissue. The neophallus is usually formed from tissue taken from the inner forearm skin (on the patient's nondominant side) as well as vaginal tissue to form the neourethra. The forearm tissue includes nerves and vasculature that are grafted after the neophallus is constructed into a tube around a catheter. The neourethra is anastomosed to the native urethra and allows for urination while standing. The clitoris is left intact beneath the neophallus or within the constructed neoscrotum so that it can be stimulated independently of the neophallus. The use of the RFFF is well described by many surgeons in the genital reconstructive surgery literature.[22–27,57–63]

The RFFF is perfused by the radial artery and venous drainage is provided by the paired venae comitantes which accompany the artery as well as the subcutaneous veins of the forearm including the cephalic vein. The radial artery arises from the brachial artery just distal to the antecubital fossa and travels between the brachioradialis and flexor carpi radialis as it runs distally into the forearm. It runs in the lateral intermuscular septum, which separates the flexor and extensor compartments of the forearm. It supplies the skin over the volar aspect of the forearm from the elbow to the wrist as well as portions of the radius. Generally, the skin is thin, pliable, and usually hairless while the vascular pedicle may be up to 18 cm in length and the vessel diameters are usually large (2 to 4 mm). Medial or lateral antebrachial cutaneous nerves can also be included in this flap and are commonly used when a sensate flap is created.[1,22]

At the preoperative evaluation of the patient, it is necessary to examine the forearm to see where a hairless skin paddle can be taken. An Allen test should be performed with compression of the radial artery to ensure collateral circulation via the ulnar artery.[22]

The flap is raised in the usual fashion. A tube-within-a-tube is created from a single, folded, 13-cm-long radial forearm flap. A 4.5-cm-wide area along the ulnar border of the forearm, without the presence of hair, is tubed inward around a Foley catheter, creating the neourethra. The adjacent radial strip of skin is de-epithelialized to allow the flap to be rolled up. The remaining 12-cm width of the radial part of skin is then used to provide an external cover as it is wrapped around the inner tubed portion. The radial artery, venae comitantes, lateral cutaneous nerve of forearm, and cephalic vein are dissected. The pedicle of the flap is left attached while a second surgical team prepares the recipient groin vessels.

To achieve a normally positioned phallus, inferior to the pubic symphysis, the urethral meatus must be advanced. This lengthening is achieved by raising a labia minora flap in continuity with the external urethral meatus which is tubularized around a Foley catheter. The new urethral opening is brought out onto the mons pubis, and this can be done either as part of a one-stage procedure or as an initial procedure some months prior to the phalloplasty. The clitoris remains undisturbed at the base of the new phallus, retaining its sensation. Once the recipient site is ready, the radial artery flap is transferred to the groin. The neourethra is anastomosed to the advanced female urethra. Vascular anastomosis of the radial artery end to side with the common femoral and of the cephalic vein end to end with

the long saphenous vein is performed. The lateral cutaneous nerve of the forearm is joined to the ilioinguinal nerve (Fig. 11.1).[22]

The Ghent group published their results using the RFFF for phallus reconstruction in 316 FTM patients. Their most common complications were related to urethral reconstruction (40%), with urethral fistula appearing in 17% of the patients requiring revision surgery, 16.7% developing fistulas that healed spontaneously, and 6% resulting in urethral strictures that were treated conservatively. Authors reported erectile prosthesis implantation in 143 patients with a high complication rate of 41% with need for revision surgery. In their study, the authors concluded that a complete penile reconstruction with an erection device can never be performed in a single operation, and that the penile prosthesis can only be placed after healing of the reconstructed neophallus is complete.[64]

The London group has also published their results with RFFF phalloplasty with urethral reconstruction in 115 patients. Of these patients, 112 were satisfied with their postoperative results and 86% reported sensation in the neophallus. Urethral fistula and stricture occurred in 9 and 20 of the patients, respectively, which were resolved with revision surgery. Success of voiding in standing position occurred in 99% of their patients.[65]

The advantages of the RFFF procedure include the creation of a sensate neophallus with the creation of the neourethra at the same stage. The main advantage of this flap is consistent arterial anatomy and a long vascular pedicle with vessels of a large diameter, which facilitates microsurgical anastomoses. However, disadvantages of this flap are related to issues that can occur at the donor site, such as delayed healing, need for skin grafting for closure, unsightly scars, and limited wrist motion. Additional limitations include the size and width of the neophallus, especially in thin patients, which can sometimes hinder the implantation of a penile prosthesis or lead to complications after implantation.

LATISSIMUS DORSI FLAP PHALLOPLASTY

Our group uses the MLD flap because of its reliable and suitable anatomy (good size, volume, and length of neurovascular pedicle) to meet the aesthetic and functional requirements of phallic reconstruction. We report excellent results with MLD flap use in penile reconstruction in children and adolescents with congenital aphallia and penile trauma.[41]

In preoperative preparation, patients are advised to have a special massaging treatment of the donor area (the nondominant side is usually chosen to be the donor site) for at least 3 months preoperatively, to make the donor site skin elastic and soft for the direct closure after flap harvesting. Patients are also advised not to work out to build muscle, as extra muscle bulk can cause problems with vascularization during the tubularization of the flap.[66]

This procedure consists of two or three separate surgical procedures: designing and harvesting a latissimus dorsi musculocutaneous flap from the nondominant side with thoracodorsal artery, vein, and nerve; and, insertion of a penile prosthesis and staged neophallic urethroplasty. The steps of the surgery are described below.

First Stage

Removal of Female Reproductive Organs. The procedure is usually performed by three teams: gynecologists, plastic

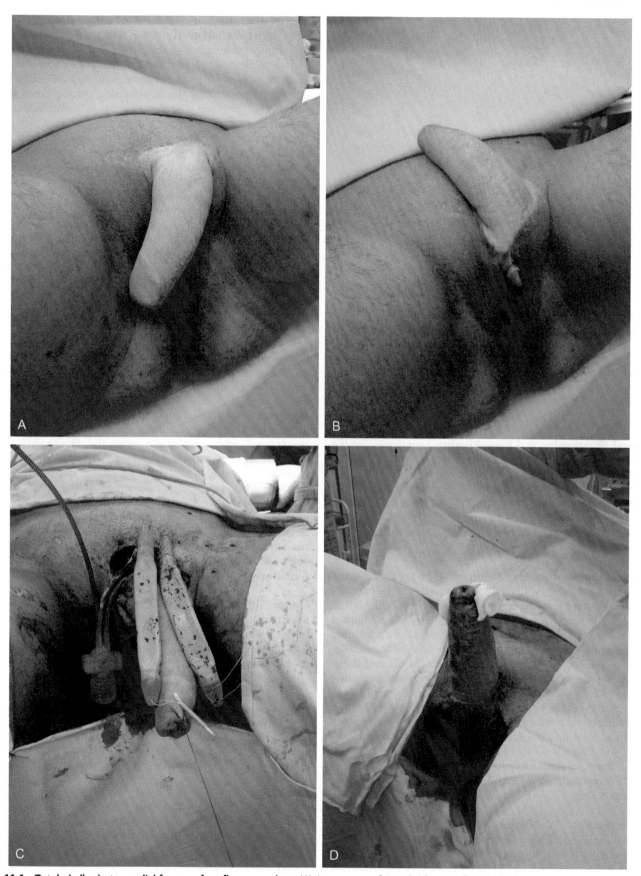

Fig. 11.1   Total phalloplasty—radial forearm free-flap procedure. (A) Appearance after radial forearm flap phalloplasty. (B) Prominent clitoris lies under the neophalic base. Scrotums are empty. (C) Inflatable prostheses are prepared for insertion into then neophallus. (D) Scrotoplasty with testicular implants is done. Clitoris is covered and positioned at the base of the neophallus.

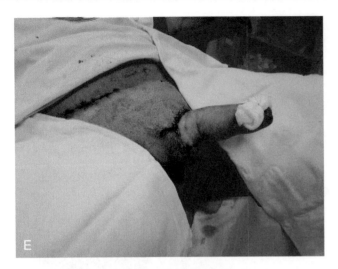

Fig. 11.1, cont'd   (E) Appearance in erect state.

surgeons, and urologists. Hysterectomy and bilateral salpingo-oophorectomy can be performed either before or at the same time as the first stage of phalloplasty. In the majority of cases, the transvaginal approach is used for the removal of female reproductive organs. Complete vaginal mucosa removal is performed by colpocleisis except for the distal anterior vaginal wall close to the native urethral meatus, which is later used for the proximal part of neourethral reconstruction.[66]

Clitoral Lengthening and Repositioning. Lengthening of the clitoris starts with a circular incision between the inner and outer layer of the clitoral prepuce and continues around the urethral plate and native urethral orifice. After complete degloving, the fundiform and suspensory clitoral ligaments are dissected from the pubic bone to advance the clitoris, mobilizing it to enable its fixation in a new position at the base of the neophallus.[66]

Urethral Lengthening. Reconstruction of the proximal part of the neourethra begins with the reconstruction of its bulbar part. A vaginal flap is harvested from the anterior vaginal wall with its base close to the female urethral meatus.[67] This flap is joined with the remaining part of the divided urethral plate, forming the bulbar part of the neourethra. Further urethral reconstruction includes the use of all available hairless vascularized tissue to lengthen the neourethra to the maximum extent, preventing postoperative complications. In this way, the new urethral opening is placed at the base or in the first third of the neophallus, depending on the availability of the hairless tissue. Both varieties of flaps, clitoral, and labial, have fine supportive tissue that prevents fistula formation and yields satisfactory aesthetic results. A suprapubic cystostomy tube is introduced into the bladder and a silicone catheter is placed into the neourethra for a period of 10 days (Fig. 11.2A–E).

Reconstruction of the Perineum and Scrotum. Following colpocleisis, the vaginal space is closed and the perineum is reconstructed to have a male appearance. The two labia majora are joined in the midline over the neourethra creating a one-sac scrotum. Silicone testicular prostheses are inserted into the previously created pockets in the two labia majora, completing the scrotoplasty part of the procedure.[66]

Flap Design. The patient is placed in the lateral position (upper torso placed in a full lateral position at 90° and the pelvis at a 30° angle) to provide access to the groin. The flap consists of two parts: a rectangular part for the neophallic shaft and a semicircular component for glans reconstruction. Flap dissection starts with an incision along the anterior skin margin down to the deep fascia. The plane is developed between the latissimus dorsi and serratus anterior muscles, using sharp and blunt dissection. The flap is divided inferiorly and medially, cauterizing the large posterior perforators of the intercostal vessels, and then lifted to expose the neurovascular pedicle. The pedicle, surrounded by fatty tissue, is identified and dissected proximally up to the axillary vessels. The thoracodorsal nerve is identified and isolated proximally for 3 to 4 cm, preserving its vascularization. The flap is elevated completely, except for the neurovascular bundle, which is not transected until the recipient vessels and nerve have been prepared for microanastomosis. The latissimus muscle is fixed to the edges of the skin at several points to prevent layer separation during further dissection. The flap is tubularized creating the neophallus, while still perfusing on its vascular pedicle. The circularized terminal part is rotated back over the distal body and sutured to create a neoglans. The completely constructed neophallus is detached from the axillar region after the subscapular artery, vein, and thoracodorsal nerve are clamped and divided at their origins, to achieve maximal pedicle length (Fig. 11.3A and B).[66]

Recipient Site—Dissection of the Blood Vessels. Dissection of the recipient area is performed together with the dissection of the femoral artery, saphenous vein, and ilioinguinal nerve. A "Y" incision is made on the mons pubis and a wide tunnel is created between the incisions to receive the pedicle. After identifying all neurovascular structures at the recipient site, the thoracodorsal vessels and nerve are divided, the neophallus is transferred to the pelvic region, and a microsurgical vascular anastomosis is performed immediately. The neophallic base is fixed to the skin at the recipient site with interrupted nonresorbable sutures. The stabilizing recipient skin site is approximated further and closed (see Fig. 11.3C and D).[66]

Donor Site Closure. Whenever possible, the donor site is approximated and closed directly, after adjacent undermining of the wound edges. In cases where there is significant tension that may compromise healing and lead to donor site necrosis, a split thickness skin graft is used to close the defect.[66]

Next Stages

Staged Neophallic Urethral Reconstruction. The next stage of the urethral reconstruction is performed after there is complete healing of the neophallus (usually not earlier than 6 months from the initial surgery). We believe that staging this part of the reconstruction is the best way to successfully reconstruct the neophallic urethra. This principle, introduced by Johanson in the 1950s, is practiced today by many surgeons performing this procedure.[68] The first part includes the creation of a "new urethral plate" using buccal mucosa grafts. The use of buccal mucosa grafts, first described 70 years ago, has become the gold standard for urethral reconstruction. These grafts are very tough, elastic, simple to harvest, easy to handle, and leave no noticeable scar at the donor site. Use of these grafts is also advantageous in cases where the available genital skin is insufficient, such as after multiple failed urethral reconstructions.

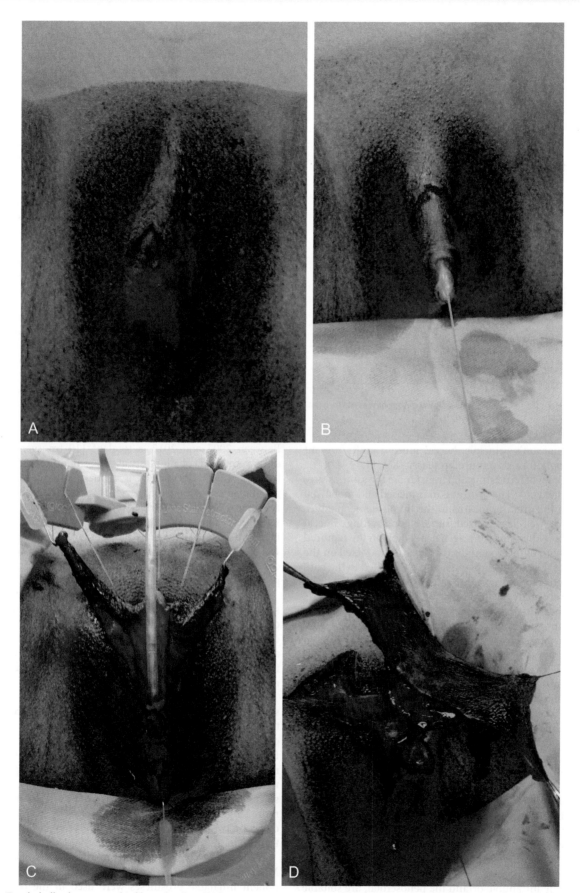

Fig. 11.2   Total phalloplasty—urethral lengthening. (A) Preoperative appearance of female external genitalia. (B) Hairless clitoral skin is marked for urethral lengthening. (C) Harvesting of both labia minora is performed. (D) Vascularized genital flap, created from both labia minora and clitoral skin, is prepared for urethral lengthening.

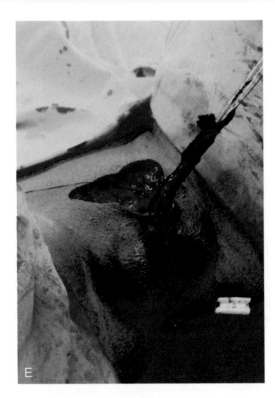

Fig. 11.2, cont'd   (E) Flap is tubularized to create a new urethra. Scrotum with testicular implants is created.

Following Johanson's principle, buccal mucosa grafts present the optimal option in staged urethroplasty (Fig. 11.4A–D).[69]

The principles of harvesting and transfer are the same as previously described.[70,71] The ventral skin is incised and mobilized starting from the urethral meatus to the tip of the neophallus. This creates a well-vascularized surface for grafting. Buccal mucosa grafts (either pairs or single, depending on the required width and length of the neourethra) are placed and fixed on the ventral side of the phallus. All grafts must be quilted to the base for better survival and prevention of graft shrinkage. When the healed grafts are ready for final stage tubularization and closure, it is important to incise the underlying tissue that will support the neourethra and avoid ischemia at the neourethral suture line. It is recommended that a second layer be created from the surrounding tissue, to cover and support the newly created urethra. The key to a successful repair is waiting until the skin is supple enough. The urethral tubularization should be performed when the "new urethral plate" has become soft and thus more easily mobilized for tubularization. Patients are advised to apply moisturizing and antiscar creams to the urethral plate until the next stage of urethral reconstruction. If necessary, additional buccal mucosa grafts can be used for urethral plate augmentation and easier tubularization.

Penile Prosthesis Insertion. Since erectile function cannot be achieved after total phalloplasty, implantation of a penile prosthesis is the only viable option. Its usage has frequently been associated with complications, sometimes in as many as 50% of cases.[72] We currently have two types of penile prostheses available, semi-rigid and inflatable. Only two surgical approaches, the infrapubic or/and the penoscrotal, are suitable for penile prosthesis implantation into the neophallus.

In the case of the infrapubic approach, a longitudinal or a transverse incision is made below the pubis, just above the base of the neophallus. Hegar dilators are used to create the space for insertion of the prosthesis. The prosthesis is fixed to the periosteum of the inferior pubic rami and covered with vascular grafts imitating tunica albuginea to prevent protrusion through the glans (Fig. 11.5A–D). Disadvantages of the infrapubic approach include possible damage of the neurovascular bundle of the neophallus and limited exposure for prosthesis insertion. The pump of the inflatable prosthesis is inserted into the scrotum using a small incision above the scrotum (Fig. 11.6A–D).[66]

With the penoscrotal approach, a vertical or a transverse incision is made ventrally at the penoscrotal junction. Initially, there was concern that this approach might be associated with a higher infection rate than the infrapubic approach; however, there are no data to support this. Advantages of the penoscrotal approach include avoidance of injury to the vascular supply, better exposure for prosthesis insertion, insertion of the pump without additional incisions, and easier anchoring of the prosthesis to the pubic bones. Fixation of the cylinder bases to the periosteum of the inferior pubic rami stabilizes the prosthesis and discourages cylinder protrusion through the neoglans. With the vertical penoscrotal approach, all layers are opened longitudinally allowing for good visualization of all structures, especially the urethra. The scar resulting from this incision is barely visible and is hidden between the two hemiscrotums.

Outcomes of the Musculocutaneous Latissimus Dorsi Phalloplasty

Between 2007 and 2015, a total of 119 transgender patients underwent MLD phalloplasty at our center. In 85 patients, phalloplasty was performed as a primary procedure, and in 27 patients, it was done after previously performed metoidioplasty. Another seven patients underwent MLD phalloplasty as a reversal surgery. The average size of the neophallus was 15 cm (ranging from 12 to 21 cm) and 13 cm in girth (ranging from 12 to 15 cm). In six cases, split-thickness skin grafts were used to cover the ventral side of the neophallus preventing high suture pressure and possible compartment syndrome.

In our series, less than 20% of patients reported tactile sensation of the neophallus, confirming one of the main drawbacks of this procedure. The majority of sensation was limited to the clitoris, which was incorporated at the base of the neophallus, and the proximal part of the urethra, which was created from the hairless flaps of genital skin (clitoral skin and labia minora skin).

Total length of the reconstructed urethra, during the first stage, was measured during the surgery and ranged from 12.1 to 19.7 cm (median 13.8 cm). In 80% of patients, the urethral opening was located in the proximal third of the neophallus. In eight patients, the neourethral opening was placed in the mid part of the neophallus. In the remaining 16 patients, the newly created urethra was opened at the base of the neophallus, since there was not enough vascularized genital hairless skin for more lengthening. Neophallic urethral reconstruction by either one- or a two-stage buccal mucosa graft tubularization was performed in 82 patients.

We used two types of penile prostheses in 48 of our patients. Malleable prostheses were implanted in 29 patients and tricomponent inflatable prostheses were used in the remaining 19. There was more interest in penile prostheses implantation,

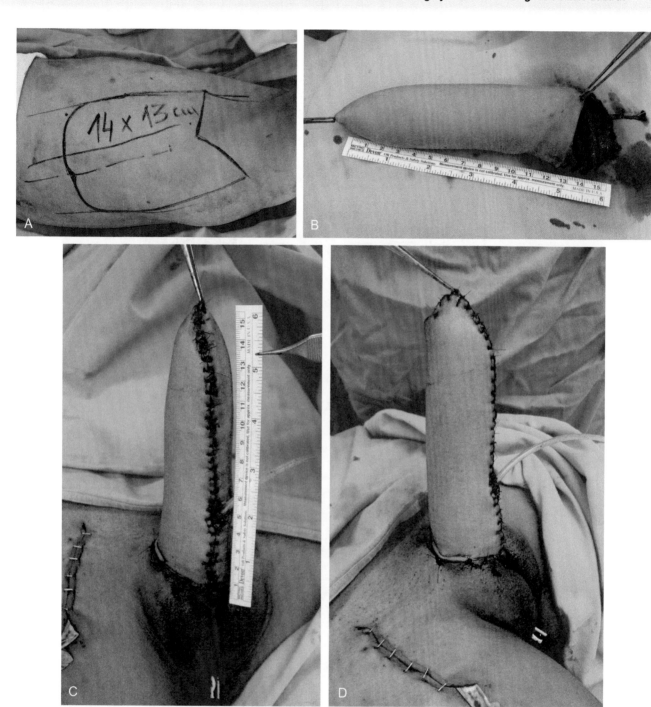

Fig. 11.3   Total phalloplasty—latissimus dorsi flap. (A) Design of the flap. (B) Flap tubularization. (C) Appearance at the end of surgery. A well-sized neophallus is created. (D) Lateral view: normal relationship of the neophallus and scrotum.

but high cost of the prostheses presented a limiting factor for the patients in our series.

A psychologist or a psychiatrist evaluated patients postoperatively. According to patients' self-reports, the majority were pleased with the aesthetic appearance of their male genitalia (101 "completely satisfied," 18 "somewhat satisfied"). Erogenous sensation based on clitoral stimulation was reported by all 119 patients. None of the patients reported problems or difficulties in sexual arousal, masturbation, or orgasms. In all patients who had received penile implants, sexual intercourse with complete penetration was adequate.

Perioperative Considerations and Postoperative Care

Broad-spectrum antibiotics are recommended to prevent infection after any stage. In the first stage of phalloplasty, a special dressing and fixation of the neophallus in an elevated position are used to prevent pedicle kinking. After each stage of urethral reconstruction, a suprapubic catheter is placed for a period of 3 weeks to allow for a satisfactory healing of the neourethra. When the urethral plate is being reconstructed using the buccal mucosa graft, the buccal mucosa graft should undergo a special

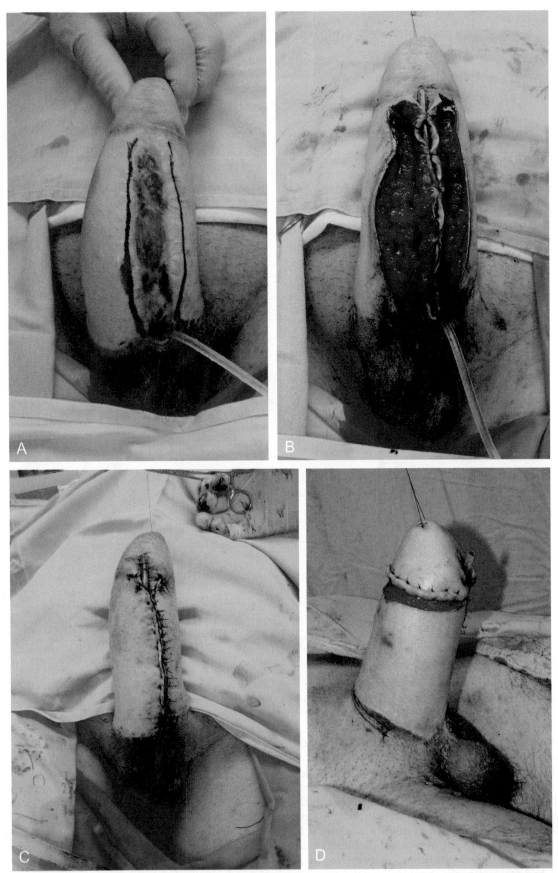

Fig. 11.4 Total phalloplasty—staged urethroplasty. (A) Appearance after phalloplasty and new urethral plate, created by buccal mucosa ventral grafting. (B) Buccal mucosa grafts are dissected and tubularized. (C) Neourethra is created. Ventral part of the neophallus is closed. (D) Outcome after urethroplasty and glansplasty.

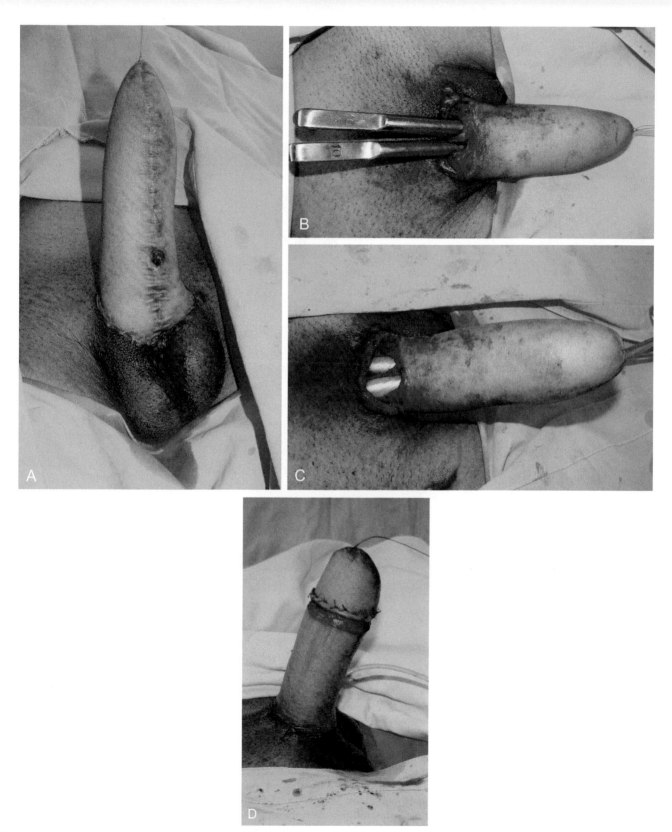

Fig. 11.5 Total phalloplasty—malleable penile prosthesis. (A) Appearance after the first stage. (B) Hegar dilators are used to create the space for implants by dorsal approach. (C) Two malleable implants are inserted into the neophallus. (D) Appearance after surgery. Glans is created using the Norfolk technique.

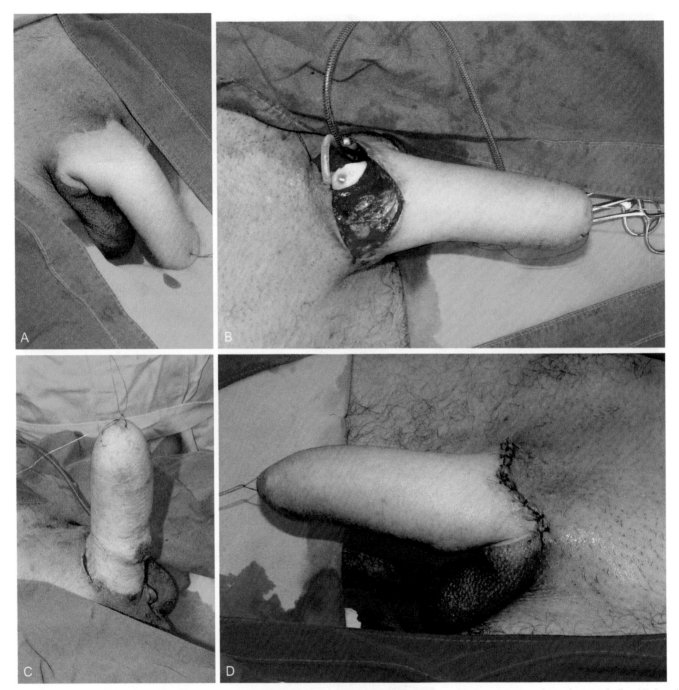

Fig. 11.6 Total phalloplasty—inflatable penile prosthesis. (A) Preoperative appearance. (B) Two cylinders are inserted into the neophallus. (C) Good rigidity is achieved by prosthesis activation. (D) Appearance in the flaccid state.

treatment that includes wetting of the graft every 3 hours during the first 72 hours, and then treatment with antibiotic ointment and moisturizing cream with gentle massage for a period of at least 6 months to prepare the urethral plate for tubularization. After penile prosthesis implantation, special care should be taken to prevent infection and rejection, together with antibiotic prophylaxis.[66] Patients are advised to refrain from physical activity for a period of 2 months after phalloplasty, and sexual intercourse should be avoided after penile prosthesis implantation for a period of 8 weeks postoperatively.

Management of Complications

Complications that might occur after this type of SRS may be classified as minor, that is, those that can be managed nonoperatively; and major, that is, those requiring additional surgery.

Minor postoperative complications include postoperative hematomas, wound infection, partial skin necrosis, urinary retention, urinary tract infections, and complications related to urethral reconstruction (dribbling, spraying, fistulas, and strictures). Hematoma can be avoided by meticulous hemostasis during surgery and afterwards by the application of a self-adherent dressing. In the majority of cases, postoperative hematoma resolves spontaneously and surgical exploration is hardly ever necessary. Partial skin necrosis, which might occur even after careful handling, usually heals spontaneously merely with treatment with fibrinolytic ointment. Prolonged suprapubic drainage precludes urinary retention.

Postoperative complications related to urethroplasty include dribbling and spraying during voiding, which usually disappear during the first 3 months postoperatively. Urethral fistulas and strictures are the main complications that may occur after total phalloplasty with urethral reconstruction. Reasons for fistulization may be insufficient vascular supply of the local flaps and inappropriate width of the neourethra causing increased pressure on the proximal part of the urethra and anastomotic sites, infection, or external pressure to the neourethra by testicular prostheses. The development of fistulas can be prevented by covering the anastomosis with an additional layer of subcutaneous tissue. In some patients with a urethral fistula, leaking resolves spontaneously with no need for surgical repair. The majority of temporary urethral strictures can be managed by periodic dilation for a short period of time postoperatively.

Revision Surgeries

Major postoperative complications include all complications that require secondary revision (hematomas, wound dehiscence, flap necrosis, urethral fistulas, urethral strictures, loss and dislocation of testicle implants, or penile prosthesis). One of the most severe complications is arterial or vein thrombosis, which requires immediate revision surgery to prevent complete or partial flap loss. Urethral fistulas that require surgical intervention are repaired by fistula excision and fistula repair with available local vascularized flaps. Urethral strictures should be confirmed by voiding cystourethrogram (VCUG), thin urine stream, and urine retention. Most of the strictures are located at the site of anastomosis between the native urethra and neourethra. Repair of the stricture can include anastomotic or buccal mucosa graft urethroplasty. Strictures located in the neophallic urethra can be repaired by buccal mucosa graft urethroplasty as well. Complications related to the buccal mucosa harvesting site are extremely rare. Loss of a testicular implant might be related to wound dehiscence, wound infection, or infection of the testicular capsule due to urine leakage. The testicular implants can be dislocated upwards or downwards. The surgical repair always consists of repositioning of the implant and fixation so it may create a new capsule.

In cases where the neophallus is positioned in a higher suprapubic position than is anatomically normal, the revision surgery consists of repositioning the phallus such that further urethral reconstruction is possible, and adequate distance from the reconstructed scrotum must be considered (Fig. 11.7A–D).

Protrusion of the penile prosthesis can occur as a result of wound dehiscence, infection, or prosthesis rejection. The surgical repair consists of repositioning the prosthesis, sometimes removing it, and then performing a reimplantation at a later stage. If a penile prosthesis revision surgery is necessary, it should be performed by the same approach that was used for the initial implant.

Metoidioplasty: Current Operative Techniques

In FTM patients who wish to avoid excessive and stigmatizing scaring of their bodies, but who still want to have male genitalia, the best option is the metoidioplasty operation. Metoidioplasty involves the creation of a small neophallus which resembles a real penis, using only tissue from the patient's own genitals. The reconstructed phallus can achieve an erection when aroused and allows for the possibility of voiding in the standing position if the urethra is reconstructed as well. Penetration during sexual intercourse is usually not possible in patients who opt for metoidioplasty, due to the smaller neophallic size.[73] Metoidioplasty provides a realistic erectile and sensate neophallus, but with a less rigid erection than is found in cisgender males due to the absence of tunica albuginea and smaller cavernosal bodies. Nevertheless, patients self-report that penetration is possible for some individuals.[74]

In preoperative preparation for metoidioplasty, patients are advised to use a vacuum pump in combination with local application of dihydrotestosterone cream to the clitoris for a period of 3 months before the surgery.[74] Metoidioplasty can be performed together with the removal of internal female organs (hysterectomy and bilateral salpingo-oophorectomy) and vaginectomy, but it is not necessary for individuals who want to preserve their reproductive potential and experience parenthood or for those patients who desire vaginal penetration, vaginectomy does not need to be performed.

CLITORAL ANATOMY

When considering metoidioplasty, it is important to identify the homologies in female and male anatomy. The clitoris is composed of two paired erectile bodies, a clitoral corona, and a dorsal neurovascular bundle, similar to the penis, and the deep artery and dorsal artery of the clitoris, branches of the internal pudendal artery, provide its blood supply. Unlike in males, the ventral part of the clitoris is comprised of a short, wide urethral plate. The main difference between female external genitalia and male genitalia is that in females, the genitalia are separate from the urethra. Additionally, the clitoral ligaments are better developed, hiding it further beneath the pubic bone, and giving it its curved shape. The external part of the clitoris attaches the mons pubis to the body and glans and extends into the medial aspect of the labia majora. It is a thick, fibro-fatty structure measuring 7 to 8 cm wide. The deep part connects the clitoral body to the pubic bones. The suspensory ligament significantly differs between the sexes in shape, orientation, and composition. The clitoris can achieve a preoperative length of 2 to 6 cm (measured from the pubic symphysis to the coronal tip) under the influence of testosterone use. The clitoral glans, despite the fact that it is cleaved and inferiorly appended to the labia minora, can engorge to about 2 cm in width.[75,76] The clitoral nerves are positioned at 11 o'clock and 1 o'clock along the shaft of the clitoris and the glans as observed by Ginger et al., Oakley et al., and Baskin et al. in their anatomic studies.[77–79] There is an absence of innervation at the 12 o'clock position and the lowest nerve density is located on the ventral aspect of the glans. The most abundant innervation is located at the top and dorsal portion of the glans clitoris, as reported by Shih et al.[80] The clitoral shaft is curved because of its connection to the labia minora, the suspensory ligament superiorly, and the ventral chordae located underneath the shaft. The urethral plate, located ventrally, is short and wide. All these connections create the curvature of the clitoris, constraining the length of a potential neophallus.[75]

Metoidioplasty relies upon the straightening and lengthening of the hypertrophied clitoris. During the procedure, the chordae are divided and there is release of the cavernosal bodies from their attachments to the labia minora. If urethral lengthening is performed, there is elongation of the short urethral plate. A simple metoidioplasty can be chosen, which only involves creation of a neophallus without urethral reconstruction which does allow for voiding while standing. In the case of the simple metoidioplasty, the urethral plate is simply divided above the

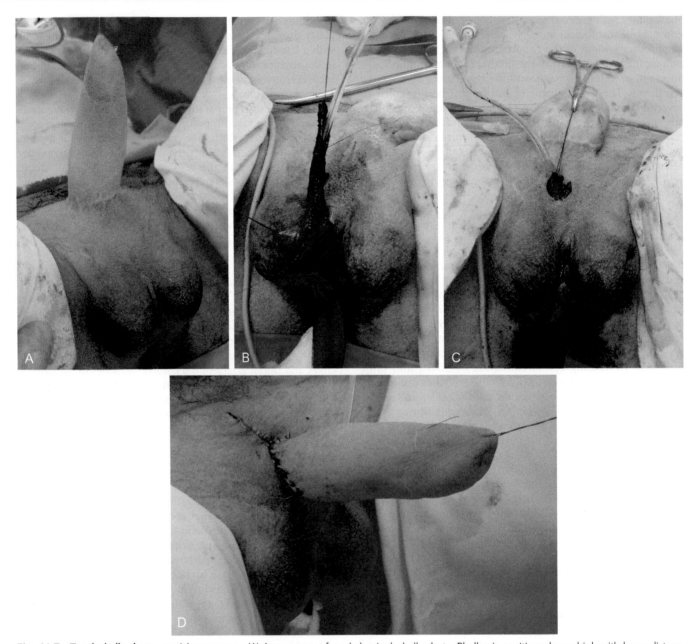

Fig. 11.7 Total phalloplasty—revision surgery. (A) Appearance after abdominal phalloplasty. Phallus is positioned very high with huge distance from the scrotum. (B) Urethral lengthening with vascularized genital flaps. (C) Urethral movement and fixation in new position. (D) Repositioning of the neophallus in a new, better relationship with the scrotum.

native urethral meatus. Metoidioplasty with urethral lengthening includes various surgical techniques to lengthen the urethral plate and to reconstruct the proximal part of the neourethra. These techniques include the use of the buccal mucosa graft, a labial mucosa graft, or a ring flap. The distal urethra is most commonly created from a labial mucosa island flap. The ventral portions of the urethra are derived proximally from a vaginal pedicle flap and distally from the labial mucosa or clitoral skin.

SIMPLE METOIDIOPLASTY

The simple metoidioplasty is performed on the hormonally hypertrophied clitoris. The skin around the clitoral corona is circumferentially incised, followed by degloving of the clitoral body and transection of the suspensory ligaments. The urethral plate is dissected by oblique incisions to move the clitoris more anteriorly. The chordae are divided transversely with electrocautery and the base of the shaft is bulked and closed vertically with interrupted absorbable suture. The subcutaneous labial skin is further attached to the shaft along the corpora until the corona is reached. The degloved corona is reattached to the labia minora skin. In the end, the external surface of the labia minora skin is closed in the midline to reconstruct the ventral skin of the neophallus. Since the native urethral opening stays intact, care must be taken to gauge how low the midline closure is, in order to allow for adequate urine outflow. A Foley catheter is placed to avoid urine contact with the suture lines.[13]

Complications associated with simple metoidioplasty are rare and usually are related to the incisional closure. The procedure is an almost complication-free genital confirmation surgery option for patients that can be done as an outpatient procedure with minimal recovery.

RING METOIDIOPLASTY

The ring metoidioplasty is similar to the simple metoidioplasty in that the chordae are released and the suspensory ligaments transected to straighten the neophallus. Where this procedure differs is in the extension of the urethral plate. In a ring metoidioplasty, a labial ring flap is harvested from the inner surfaces of the bilateral labia minora and the urethral plate. The posterior labial frenulum is included at the distal end of the flap. The flap is then raised, posteriorly to anteriorly, using blunt dissection. The corpora cavernosa clitoridis are straightened and lengthened by excising the chordae. The window of the inner ring flap is closed, and the flap is tubularized around a catheter, and the ventral defect of the neourethra is completed using a mobilized anterior vaginal flap in an oblique fashion to prevent strictures. The neophallic skin is reconstructed using available skin from the outer surface of the labia minora using a Z-plasty technique to avoid ventral scar contracture.[81]

Postoperative complications are mainly related to the urethral reconstruction and include urethral fistula (10% to 28%) and stricture (3% to 7%). Scrotoplasty can be performed together with the ring metoidioplasty or as a second-stage procedure. Postoperative tactile and erogenous sensation is preserved with the natural small neophallus that enables voiding while standing in some, but not in all individuals.[81]

METOIDIOPLASTY WITH URETHRAL EXTENSION

When voiding in standing position is imperative, the creation of a competent neourethra with urethral advancement becomes the main goal of the procedure. The metoidioplasty with urethral reconstruction as a one-stage procedure is based on the repair of the most severe forms of hypospadias in intersex children and combines the use of genital skin flaps with a buccal mucosa graft. Male-like appearance of the external genitalia is achieved with scrotoplasty and insertion of two testicular implants. We published our first results of our one-stage metoidioplasty in 2003 and reported a high success rate in aesthetic but also in functional outcomes in 17 out of 22 patients who were part of the study.[82]

The procedure is performed with the patient in lithotomy position. Vaginectomy is performed by total removal of the vaginal mucosa (colpocleisis), except for the distal anterior vaginal wall near the native urethral opening. This part of the vagina is preserved so that it may be used for proximal urethral reconstruction. Maximal straightening and lengthening of the clitoris can be achieved by complete dissection of the fundiform and suspensory ligaments of the clitoris. On the ventral side of the clitoris, the wide and short urethral plate is carefully divided from the clitoral bodies and separated at the level of glandular corona, additionally lengthening the clitoris, but creating a urethral plate defect (Fig. 11.8A–D).

Reconstruction of the neourethra starts with the reconstruction of the bulbar part. One of the main advantages of this technique is the simultaneous removal of the vaginal mucosa and use of the remaining anterior vaginal wall in creation of the bulbar urethra. The bulbar urethra suffers the highest urinary stream pressure and therefore presents a high-risk point for postoperative fistula development. The joining of the clitoral

bulbs over the neourethra and the additional covering with vascularized surrounding tissue is considered the key for successful fistula prevention. Additional urethral reconstruction is performed using a buccal mucosa graft and vascularized genital skin flaps.[67,83] As previously mentioned, buccal mucosa grafts are a good option for this type of reconstruction and harvesting of these grafts is a safe procedure with low morbidity and complication rate.[70,84] The graft is sutured to cover the urethral defect, and quilted to the clitoral bodies for better graft survival. Urethral reconstruction is completed either by using a longitudinal dorsal clitoral skin flap button-holed ventrally, or a flap harvested from the inner surface of the labia minora. Recently, we have developed a preference for the labial flap due to improved surgical outcomes (Fig. 11.9A–D).[83]

The labial flap is joined with the buccal mucosa graft over a 12 Fr urethral tube to create the neourethra. The penile shaft is reconstructed using the remaining clitoral and labial skin, taking care to create an anatomic penoscrotal angle. The labia majora are joined in the midline to create the scrotal sac, and two silicone testicular prostheses are inserted through bilateral incisions at the top of labia majora. A suprapubic catheter is placed in all cases and left in place for a period of 3 weeks.

METOIDIOPLASTY FOLLOWED BY PHALLOPLASTY

After undergoing metoidioplasty some patients desire to further confirm their masculinity by undergoing phalloplasty, with an adult-size phallus reconstruction. In our center, about 13% of the patients who undergo one-stage metoidioplasty decide to have phalloplasty at a later date and the most commonly reported reason for their decision is their desire to perform penetrative sexual intercourse.

We perform MLD phalloplasty procedures as well for these cases. The design and harvesting of the flap are performed as previously described with the incorporation of the small phallus into the neophallus. The urethral reconstruction is performed as a staged procedure with a buccal mucosa graft to create the urethral plate for the future tubularization and anastomosis with the lengthened urethra of the small phallus. Glans reconstruction is performed by the previously published Norfolk technique.[6] In those patients who desire penetrative sexual intercourse, penile implants are inserted using the previously described approaches (Fig. 11.10A–D).

Outcomes of Metoidioplasty

Between September 2002 and January 2016 we surgically treated 502 patients (mean age 33, 18 to 62 years) with the one-stage metoidioplasty. The first results were published in 2013 (Fig. 11.11A and B).[83]

Hysterectomy and bilateral salpingo-oophorectomy were performed simultaneously in 56 patients. In all of these cases, vaginectomy was performed with preservation of the anterior vaginal wall. For urethral reconstruction, we used two different surgical techniques using genital flaps in combination with buccal mucosa grafts for the penile urethra. In 49 patients we used a buccal mucosa graft and a flap harvested from the dorsal hairless clitoral skin buttonholed ventrally, and in the second group of 453 patients we used buccal mucosa grafts in combination with hairless skin harvested from labia minora. The median postoperative follow-up period in our study was 41 months.

Neophallic length ranged from 4 to 10 cm in maximal extension (median 5.6 cm), with 5.9 cm mean size in the second

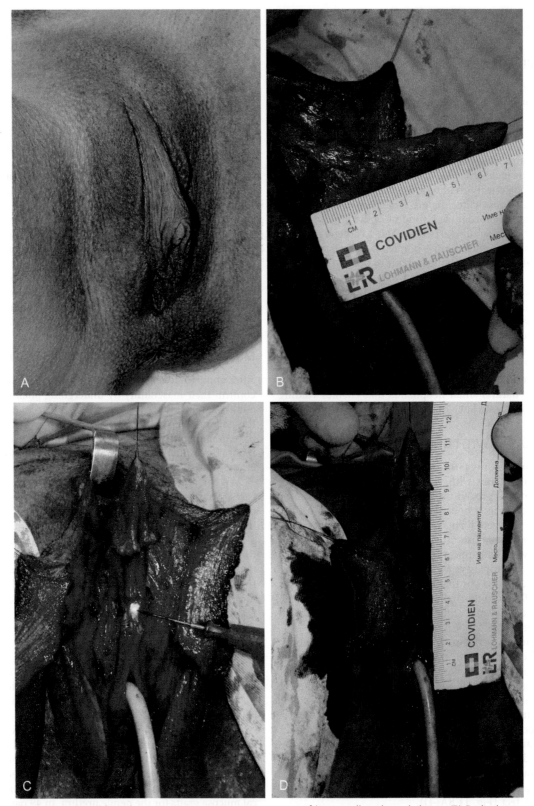

Fig. 11.8 Metoidioplasty—clitoral lengthening. (A) Preoperative appearance of hormonally enlarged clitoris. (B) Radical removal of suspensory ligaments. (C) Division of short urethral plate. (D) Outcome after complete clitoral lengthening.

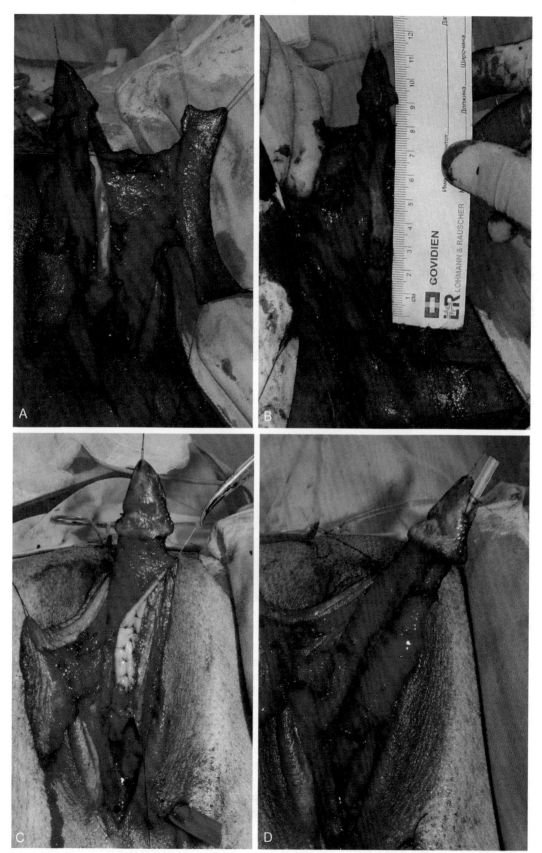

Fig. 11.9 **Metoidioplasty—urethral lengthening.** (A) Harvesting of the left labial skin flap. (B) Insertion of the buccal mucosa graft ventrally as a distal part of the neourethra. (C) Joining of the labial flap with the buccal mucosa graft. (D) Outcome after urethral lengthening. Long neourethra is completely covered by surrounding vascularized subcutaneous tissue.

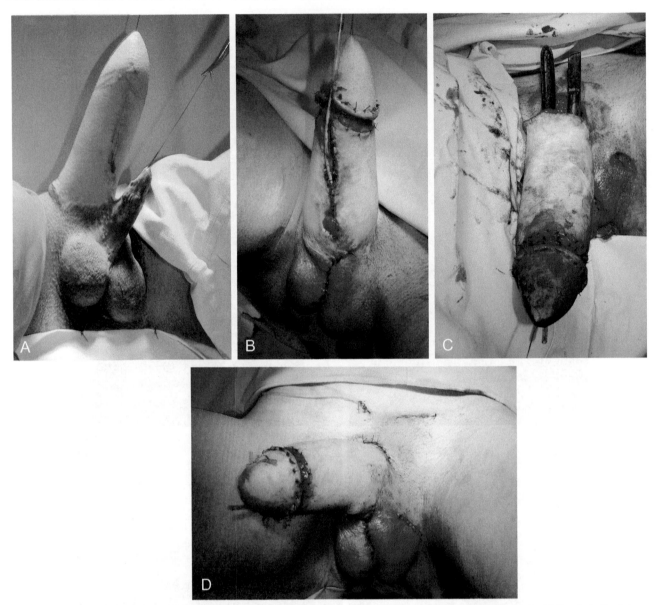

Fig. 11.10 Metoidioplasty followed by phalloplasty. (A) Appearance after metoidioplasty and first-stage phalloplasty. (B) Small phallus is incorporated in new phallus with urethral lengthening. (C) Insertion of inflatable penile prosthesis by dorsal approach. (D) Outcome after surgery.

group, compared to 5.2 cm in the first group.[83] Minor complications, such as dribbling and spraying during voiding, occurred in 34.7% and 29.8% of patients in the first and second groups, respectively. These complications did not require surgical intervention, and resolved spontaneously 3 months after the surgery. Complications that required surgical repair were mainly related to urethral reconstruction. Urethral fistula occurred in 28 patients: 7 patients from the first group and 21 patients from the second group. Urethral stricture was reported in 6 patients from the first group and in 8 patients from the second group. Other complications that required additional surgical intervention were testicular implant rejection in 6 patients, as well as testicular implant displacement in 19 patients. About 11% of the patients from both groups required some minor aesthetical corrections of the neophallic skin, mons pubis, and scrotum.[83]

Adequate urethral diameter was checked in all patients by urethrography and uroflowmetry. Voiding while standing was significantly better in the second group compared to the first.

All patients were evaluated by a psychologist, and according to their self-reports, the majority of them were pleased with the appealing appearance of their new male genitalia (460 "completely satisfied," 42 "somewhat satisfied").[83] Erection of the neophallus was present in all 502 patients and none of the patients reported difficulties or other problems related to sexual arousal, masturbation, or orgasm. One patient reported full penetration during sexual intercourse with his partner.

PERIOPERATIVE CONSIDERATIONS AND POSTOPERATIVE CARE

Broad spectrum antibiotics and anticholinergic drugs are prescribed while a catheter is in place. The urethral stent is removed 10 days after the surgery. Postoperative use of a vacuum pump is advised to prevent retraction of the neophallus, starting 3 weeks after surgery, for a period of at least 6 months, combined with treatment with phosphodiesterase type-5 inhibitors. Patients are

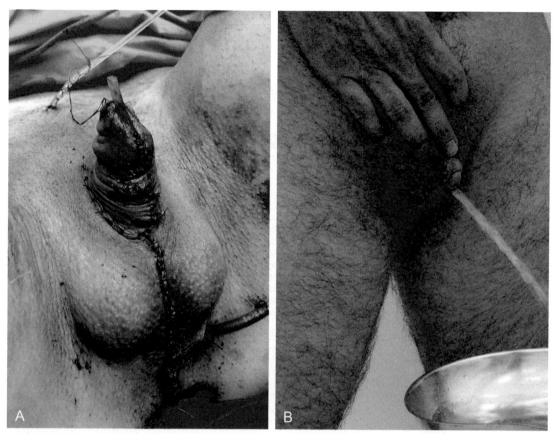

Fig. 11.11   Metoidioplasty—outcomes. (A) Appearance after one-stage metoidioplasty with urethral lengthening and scrotoplasty. (B) Outcome 3 months later with good voiding while standing.

advised to refrain from physical activity after the surgery for a period of 1 month and from bicycle riding and running for a period of 3 months postoperatively.

PERIOPERATIVE COMPLICATIONS

Minor postoperative complications after metoidioplasty include hematoma, wound infections, skin necrosis, urinary tract infections, and complications related to urethral reconstruction (dribbling, spraying, urethral fistula). The reported complication rate ranges from 17.5% to 35%, with spontaneous resolution in the majority of patients.

REVISION SURGERIES

The complications that require secondary revision (flap necrosis, urethral fistulas, urethral strictures, testicular implant displacement) are considered major complications. Urethral fistulas are the most common major complication requiring revision surgery, occurring in 7% to 15% of all cases, and are repaired by excision of the fistula and closure with an available local vascularized flap. When a urethral stricture develops, anastomotic or buccal mucosa graft urethroplasty is performed. In cases of a dislocated testicular implant, repositioning and fixation of the implant into its proper place, along with the creation of a new capsule, is indicated.[33,67,76,83,85]

Conclusion

As a multistage surgical procedure in FTM patients, phalloplasty poses considerable challenges. The goal of phalloplasty is to create adult male genitalia that allows for voiding in the standing position, has a satisfactory aesthetic appearance, and provides good sexual function. In this chapter we describe many reconstructive flap options for phalloplasty. The radial forearm flap phalloplasty is currently accepted as the gold standard phalloplasty procedure.[63] In our center, we more commonly perform the MLD flap phalloplasty as we believe that it is an acceptable choice for FTM patients and yields an excellent penile size, allowing for urethral reconstruction and penile prosthesis implantation. New refinements and improvements of all the techniques described are needed as the patient population requesting these surgeries continues to grow.

Metoidioplasty has been recognized as the method of choice in FTM patients who wish for a male-like appearance of their genitals, without undergoing a complex and multistaged surgery. It is considered a good option in patients with good clitoral growth with testosterone use. The main disadvantage of metoidioplasty is that the created neophallus is usually inadequate in length to allow for penetrative intercourse, and all patients should be informed of this fact prior to surgery.

ACKNOWLEDGMENTS
This chapter is supported by Ministry of Science and Technical Development, Republic of Serbia, Project No. 175048.

REFERENCES

1. Monstrey S, Houtmeyers P, Lumen N, Hoebeke P. Radial forearm flap phalloplasty. In: Djordjevic M, Santucci R, eds. *Penile Reconstructive Surgery.* Saarbrucken: LAP Lambert Academic Publishing; 2012:254–278.
2. The World Professional Association for Transgender Health. *Standards of Care for the Health of Transsexual, Transgender, and Gender Nonconforming People.* 7th Version. <http://www.wpath.org>; 2011. Accessed 24 July 2016.
3. Hage JJ, De Graaf FH. Addressing to ideal requirements by free flap phalloplasty: some reflections on refinements of technique. *Microsurgery.* 1993;14:592–598.
4. Bogoras N. Plastic construction of penis capable of accomplishing coitus. *Zentral Chir.* 1936;63: 1271–1276.
5. Hoopes JE. Operative treatment of the female transsexual. In: Green R, Money J, eds. *Transsexualism and Sex Reassignment.* Baltimore: John Hopkins Press; 1969:335–354.
6. Hoopes JE. Surgical construction of the male external genitalia. *Clin Plast Surg.* 1974; 1(2):325–334.
7. Gilbert DA, Horton CE, Terzis JK, Devine CJ, Jr Winslow BH, Devine PC. New concepts in phallic reconstruction. *Ann Plast Surg.* 1987;18 (2):128–136.
8. Monstrey S, Ceulemans P, Hoebeke P. History of female to male surgery. In: Ettner R, Monstrey S, Eyler EA, eds. *Principles of Transgender Medicine and Surgery.* New York: The Haworth Press; 2007:135–168.
9. Monstrey S, Ceulemans P, Roche N, Houtmeyers P, Lumen N, Hoebeke P. Reconstruction of male genital defects. In: Song DH, Neligan PC, eds. *Plastic Surgery: Lower Extremity, Trunk and Burns.* China: Elsevier Saunders; 2012:297–326. 3rd ed 4.
10. Gillies HD, Harrison RJ. Congenital absence of the penis. *Br J Plast Surg.* 1948;1:8.
11. Gillies H. In: Millard Jr DR, ed. London: Butterworth; 1957:368–388. The Principles and Art of Plastic Surgery; Vol 2.
12. Biber SH. A method for constructing the penis and scrotum. In: *Presented at the VIth International Symposium on Gender Dysphoria, San Diego;* 1979.
13. Laub DR, Eicher W, Laub II DR, Hentz VR. Penis construction in female-to-male transsexuals. In: Eicher W, ed. *Plastic Surgery in the Sexually Handicapped.* Berlin: Springer; 1989: 113–128.
14. Bouman FG. The first step in phalloplasty in female transsexuals. *Plast Reconstr Surg.* 1987;70:662–664.
15. McGregor IA, Jackson IT. The groin flap. *Br J Plast Surg.* 1972;25:3–16.
16. Puckett CL, Montie JE. Construction of male genitalia in the transsexual, using a tubed groin flap for the penis and a hydraulic inflation device. *Plast Reconstr Surg.* 1978;61: 523–530.
17. Perovic S. Phalloplasty in children and adolescent using the extended pedicle island groin flap. *J Urol.* 1995;154:848–853.
18. Orticochea MA. New method of total reconstruction of the penis. *Br J Plast Surg.* 1972;25: 347–366.
19. Horton CE, McCraw JB, Devine CJ, Jr Devine PC. Secondary reconstruction of the genital area. *Urol Clin N Am.* 1977;4:133–141.
20. Kruavit A, Visuthikosol V, Punyahotra N, Srimuninnimit V. Radial forearm free flap. *Thai J Surg.* 2004;25:7–22.
21. Song R, Gao Y, Song Y, Yu Y, Song Y. The forearm flap. *Clin Plast Surg.* 1982;9:21–26.
22. Chang TS, Hwang WY. Forearm flap in one-stage reconstruction of the penis. *Plast Reconstr Surg.* 1984;74:251–258.
23. Biemer E. Penile construction by the radial arm flap. *Clin Past Surg.* 1988;15:425–430.
24. Semple JL, Boyd JB, Farrow GA, Robinette MA. The "cricket bat" flap: a one-stage free forearm flap phalloplasty. *Plast Reconstr Surg.* 1991;88: 514–519.
25. Gilbert DA, Jordan GH, Devine CJ, Jr Winslow BH. Microsurgical forearm "cricket bat-transformer" phalloplasty. *Plast Reconstr Surg.* 1992;90(4):711–716.
26. Gottlieb LJ, Levine LA. A new design for the radial forearm free-flap phallic construction. *Plast Reconstr Surg.* 1993;92(2):276–283.
27. Koshima I, Tai T, Yamasaki M. One-stage reconstruction of the penis using an innervated radial forearm osteocutaneous flap. *J Reconstr Microsurg.* 1986;3(1):19–26.
28. Fang RH, Kao YS, Ma S, Lin JT. Phalloplasty in female-to-male transsexuals using free radial osteocutaneous flap: a series of 22 cases. *Br J Plast Surg.* 1999;52(3):217–222.
29. Kim SK, Lee KC, Kwon YS, Cha BH. Phalloplasty using radial forearm osteocutaneous free flaps in female-to-male transsexuals. *J Plast Reconstr Aesthet Surg.* 2009;62(3): 309–317.
30. Upton J, Mutimer KL, Loughlin K, Ritchie J. Penile reconstruction using the lateral arm flap. *J R Coll Surg Edinb.* 1987;32(2):97–101.
31. Khouri RK, Young VL, Casoli VM. Long-term results of total penile reconstruction with a prefabricated lateral arm free flap. *J Urol.* 1998; 160(2):383–388.
32. Baek SM. Two new cutaneous free flaps: the medial and lateral thigh flaps. *Plast Reconstr Surg.* 1983;71(3):354–365.
33. Song YG, Chen GZ, Song YL. The free thigh flap: a new free flap based on the septocutaneous artery. *Br J Plast Surg.* 1984;37:149–159.
34. Felici N, Felici A. A new phalloplasty technique: the free anterolateral thigh flap phalloplasty. *J Plast Reconstr Aesth Surg.* 2006;59: 153–157.
35. Tansini I. Nuovo processo per l'amputazzione della mammaela per cancre. *Reforma Medica.* 1896;12:3.
36. Baudet J, Guimberteau J, Nascimento E. Successful clinical transfer of two free thoraco dorsal axillary flaps. *Plast Reconstr Surg.* 1976;58: 680–688.
37. Djordjevic ML, Bumbasirevic MZ, Vukovic PM, Sansalone S, Perovic SV. Musculocutaneous latissimus dorsi free transfer flap for total phalloplasty in children. *J Pediatr Urol.* 2006;2: 333–339.
38. Harashina T. Reconstruction of the penis with a free deltoid flap. *Br J Plast Surg.* 1992;45 (3):254–255.
39. Yang MY, Li SK, Li YQ, et al. Penile reconstruction by using a scapular free flap. *Zhonghua Zheng Xing Wai Ke Za Zhi.* 2003;19(2):88–90.
40. Rashid M, Tamimy MS. Phalloplasty: the dream and the reality. *Indian J Plast Surg.* 2013;46 (2):283–293.
41. Sadove RC, Sengezer M, McRoberts JW, Wells MD. One-stage total penile reconstruction with a free sensate osteocutaneous fibula flap. *Plast Reconstr Surg.* 1993;92:1314–1323.
42. Sengezer M, Oztürk S, Deveci M, Odabaşi Z. Long-term follow-up of total penile reconstruction with sensate osteocutaneous free fibula flap in 18 biological male patients. *Plast Reconstr Surg.* 2004;114:439–450.
43. Santanelli F, Scuderi N. Neophalloplasty in female-to-male transsexuals with the island tensor fasciae latae flap. *Plast Reconstr Surg.* 2000;105:1990–1996.
44. Cheng KX, Hwang WY, Eid AE, Wang SL, Chang TS, Fu KD. Analysis of 136 cases of reconstructed penis using various methods. *Plast Reconstr Surg.* 1995;95(6):1070–1080.
45. Seyhan T, Borman H. Pedicled deep inferior epigastric perforator flap for lower abdominal defects and genital reconstructive surgery. *J Reconstr Microsurg.* 2008;24(6):405–412.
46. Durfee R, Rowland W. Penile substitution with clitoral enlargement and urethral transfer. In: Laub DR, Gandy P, eds. Proceedings of the Second Interdisciplinary Symposium on Gender Dysphoria Syndrome Palo Alto: Stanford University Press; 1973:181–183.
47. Lebovic GS, Laub DR. Metoidioplasty. In: Ehrlich RM, Alter GJ, eds. *Reconstructive and Plastic Surgery of the External Genitalia.* Philadelphia: WB Saunders; 1999:355–360.
48. Eicher W. Surgical treatment of female-to-male transsexuals. In: Eicher W, Kubli F, Herms V, eds. *Plastic Surgery in the Sexually Handicapped.* Berlin: Springer; 1989:106–112.
49. Hage JJ, Turnhout WM. Long-term outcome of metoidioplasty in 70 female to male transsexuals. *Ann Plast Surg.* 2006;57:312–316.
50. Ranno R, Veselý J, Hýza P, et al. Neophalloplasty with re-innervated latissimus dorsi free flap: a functional study of a novel technique. *Acta Chir Plast.* 2007;49(1):3–7.
51. Bettocchi C, Ralph DJ, Pryor JP. Pedicled pubic phalloplasty in females with gender dysphoria. *BJU Int.* 2005;95(1):120–124.
52. Descamps MJ, Hayes PM, Hudson DA. Phalloplasty in complete aphallia: pedicled anterolateral thigh flap. *J Plast Reconstr Aesthet Surg.* 2009;62:e51–e54.
53. Rubino C, Figus A, Dessy LA, et al. Innervated island pedicled anterolateral thigh flap for neophallic reconstruction in female-to-male transsexuals. *J Plast Reconstr Aesthet Surg.* 2009;62: e45–e49.
54. Morrison SD, Son J, Song J, et al. Modification of the tube-in-tube pedicled anterolateral thigh flap for total phalloplasty: the mushroom flap. *Ann Plast Surg.* 2014;72(suppl 1): S22–S26.
55. Hasegawa K, Namba Y, Kimata Y. Phalloplasty with an innervated island pedicled anterolateral thigh flap in a female-to-male transsexual. *Acta Med Okayama.* 2013;67(5):325–331.
56. Lumen N, Monstrey S, Ceulemans P, van Laecke E, Hoebeke P. Reconstructive surgery for severe penile inadequacy: phalloplasty with a free radial forearm flap or a pedicled anterolateral thigh flap. *Adv Urol.* 2008;704343. https://doi.org/10.1155/2008/704343.
57. Matti BA, Matthews RN, Davies DM. Phalloplasty using the free radial forearm flap. *Br J Plast Surg.* 1988;41(2):160–164.

58. Hage JJ, Bouman FG, de Graaf FH, Bloem JJ. Construction of the neophallus in female-to-male transsexuals: the Amsterdam experience. *J Urol*. 1993;149(6):1463–1468.

59. Baumeister S, Sohn M, Domke C, Exner K. Phalloplasty in female-to-male transsexuals: experience from 259 cases. *Handchir Mikrochir Plast Chir*. 2011;43(4):215–221.

60. Garaffa G, Ralph DJ, Christopher N. Total urethral construction with the radial artery-based forearm free flap in the transsexual. *BJU Int*. 2010;106(8):1206–1210.

61. Monstrey S, Hoebeke P, Selvaggi G, et al. Penile reconstruction: is the radial forearm flap really the standard technique? *Plast Reconstr Surg*. 2009;124(2):510–518.

62. Schaff J, Papadopulos NA. A new protocol for complete phalloplasty with free sensate and prelaminated osteofasciocutaneous flaps: experience in 37 patients. *Microsurgery*. 2009;29(5):413–419.

63. Leriche A, Timsit MO, Morel-Journel N, Bouillot A, Dembele D, Ruffion A. Long-term outcome of forearm flee-flap phalloplasty in the treatment of transsexualism. *BJU Int*. 2008;101(10):1297–1300.

64. Doornaert M, Hoebeke P, Ceulemans P, T'sjoen G, Heylens G, Monstrey S. Penile reconstruction with the radial forearm flap: an update. *Handchir Mikrochir Plast Chir*. 2011;43:208–214.

65. Garaffa G, Christopher NA, Ralph DJ. Total phallic reconstruction in female-to-male transsexuals. *Eur Urol*. 2010;57(4):715–722.

66. Djordjevic ML, Bizic MR, Stanojevic D. Phalloplasty in female-to-male transsexuals. In: Djordjevic M, Santucci R, eds. *Penile Reconstructive Surgery*. Saarbrucken: LAP Lambert Academic Publishing; 2012:279–304.

67. Djordjevic ML, Bizic M, Stanojevic D, et al. Urethral lengthening in metoidioplasty (female-to-male sex reassignment surgery) by combined buccal mucosa graft and labia minora flap. *Urology*. 2009;74:349–353.

68. Johanson B. Reconstruction of the male urethra in strictures. Application of the buried intact epithelium tube. *Acta Chir Scand*. 1953;176:1.

69. Barbagli G, Palminteri E, De Stefani S, Lazzeri M. Penile urethroplasty. Techniques and outcomes using buccal mucosa grafts. *Contemp Urol*. 2006;18:25–33.

70. Markiewicz MR, Margarone III JE, Barbagli G, Scannapieco FA. Oral mucosa harvest: and overview of anatomic and biologic considerations. *EAU-EBU Update Series*. 2007;5:179–187.

71. Djordjevic ML, Majstorovic M, Stanojevic D, et al. Combined buccal mucosa graft and dorsal penile skin flap for repair of severe hypospadias. *Urology*. 2008;71:821–825.

72. Jordan GH, Alter GJ, Gilbert DA, et al. Penile prosthesis implantation in total phalloplasty. *J Urol*. 1994;152:410–414.

73. Selvaggi G, Bellringer J. Gender reassignment surgery: an overview. *Nat Rev Urol*. 2011;8:274–282.

74. Djordjevic ML, Stanojevic D, Bizic M, et al. Metoidioplasty as a single stage sex reassignment surgery in female transsexuals: Belgrade experience. *J Sex Med*. 2009;6:1306–1313.

75. Stojanovic B, Djordjevic ML. Anatomy of the clitoris and its impact on neophalloplasty (metoidioplasty) in female transgenders. *Clin Anat*. 2015;28:368–375.

76. Vukadinovic V, Stojanovic B, Majstorovic M, Milosevic A. The role of clitoral anatomy in female to male sex reassignment surgery. *ScientificWorldJournal*. 2014;2014:437378.

77. Ginger VA, Cold CJ, Yang CC. Structure and innervation of the labia minora: more than minor skin folds. *Female Pelvic Med Reconstr Surg*. 2011;17:180–183.

78. Oakley SH, Mutema GK, Crisp CC, et al. Innervation and histology of the clitoral-urethal complex: a cross-sectional cadaver study. *J Sex Med*. 2013;10:2211–2218.

79. Baskin LS, Erol A, Li YW, et al. Anatomical studies of the human clitoris. *J Urol*. 1999;162:1015–1020.

80. Shih C, Cold CJ, Yang CC. Cutaneous corpuscular receptors of the human glans clitoris: descriptive characteristics and comparison with the glans penis. *J Sex Med*. 2013;10:1783–1789.

81. Takamatsu A, Harashina T. Labial ring flap: a new flap for metaidoioplasty in female-to-male transsexuals. *J Plast Reconstr Aesthet Surg*. 2009;62:318–325.

82. Perovic SV, Djordjevic M. Metoidioplasty: a variant of phalloplasty in female transsexuals. *BJU Int*. 2003;92:981–985.

83. Djordjevic ML, Bizic MR. Comparison of two different methods for urethral lengthening in female to male (metoidioplasty) surgery. *J Sex Med*. 2013;10:1431–1438.

84. Barbagli G, Vallasciani S, Romano G, Fabbri F, Guazzoni G, Lazzeri M. Morbidity of oral mucosa graft harvesting from a single cheek. *Eur Urol*. 2010;58:33–41.

85. Rohrmann D, Jakse G. Urethroplasty in female to male transsexuals. *Eur Urol*. 2003;44:611–614.

Primary and Preventative Care for Transgender Patients

CHRISTOPHER WOLF-GOULD | CAROLYN WOLF-GOULD

Introduction

Primary care clinicians can learn the skills to provide high-quality, affirming medical care to transgender patients the same way they learn to care for other patients with specific health needs. Clinicians may choose to provide the full spectrum of transition-related medical care, including hormonal therapy and pubertal blockers, or offer only primary care services. Regardless of scope, competency in care for transgender people is essential in our changing world. This skill set requires knowledge about barriers to care, steps for creating a trans-affirming office environment, cultural competency, medical treatment options for transition-related care, and an understanding for how medical transitions impact routine primary care. Most primary care providers are trained within a biopsychosocial framework—meaning that one's health is considered in the context of mind, body, family, work, and culture. This holistic approach is particularly well suited for transgender patients, who may have complex medical and social concerns. In this chapter, we will review basic competencies and strategies for incorporating transgender health into primary care practice.

Barriers to Care

Transgender and gender nonconforming people face relentless discrimination in employment, family life, education, housing, and public accommodation, but some of the most appalling discrimination occurs when these individuals reach out for help—in health-care settings. Transgender people have well-defined health needs but, for many reasons, are often unable to access appropriate medical care. A recent survey of 27,715 transgender people across the United States shows minimal gains in access to health care for transgender people compared with data from 2010.[1,2] Twenty-five percent of those surveyed experienced a problem in the last year regarding their insurance, 33% who saw a health-care provider reported at least one negative experience related to being transgender, 55% of those who sought coverage for transition-related surgery were denied, and 23% of respondents did not see a doctor when they needed to because of fear of maltreatment.[2] Provider-based barriers to care include lack of training or experience with transgender health issues, paucity of evidence-based data to guide therapy, personal discomfort, religious or cultural prohibitions, ethical concerns, fear of complications, fear of litigation, and reluctance to prescribe medications for off-label indications. Patient-based barriers include stigma, lack of adequate insurance coverage, coming-out issues (e.g. fear of violence, rejection, ambivalence), financial problems, mistrust of the medical establishment, absence of knowledgeable providers, and inability to present for sustained monitoring and follow up due to lifestyle issues.

The lack of quality epidemiologic studies creates a significant barrier to care.[3] Uncounted, the size of the transgender population remains unknown, and we are unable to inform public policy or allocate resources. Lesbian, gay, bisexual and transgender (LGBT) people are referred to as a hidden minority, as sexual orientation and gender identity are not readily apparent and patients may be reluctant to reveal themselves to clinicians.[4] Thirty-one percent of transgender people are not out to any of their health-care providers.[2] Most existing epidemiologic studies are flawed by conflicting definitions of what it means to be transgender and only those who seek treatment at gender clinics are accounted for in these studies.[5] One population-based survey reported a 0.5% rate of individuals who self-identified as transgender, indicating a relatively high prevalence.[6] Conway estimates that 0.5% to 2% of the general population have feelings of being transgender and 0.1% to 0.5% have taken steps to transition.[7] As societal norms have changed, gender clinics across the country are reporting increased numbers of patients requesting services, but the ability to find primary care services remains low. Transgender people will remain underserved unless proper epidemiologic studies define the scope of the population.

Intrapersonal and interpersonal stigma presents another barrier to care for transgender people.[8] The concept of minority stress is used to describe the health effects of stigmatization. Makadon outlines the causes of minority stress as "(a) an external, objective traumatic event, such as being assaulted or fired from a job; (b) the expectation of rejection and development of vigilance in interactions with others; (c) the internalization of negative societal attitudes; and (d) the concealment of gender identity or sexual orientation out of shame or guilt or to protect oneself from harm."[9] The concept of intersectionality demonstrates how individuals hold multiple identities, defined in terms of relative sociocultural power and privilege, which shape their experience with stigma.[10] Differences in power and privilege associated with these identities ensure that an unemployed transgender woman of color will have a different experience attempting to access health care than a wealthy, white, transgender man.

Stigma has a direct effect on health. In one study, sexual minorities who lived in communities with high levels of anti-gay prejudice had a higher hazard of morbidity, an 18-year difference in the average age of completed suicide, and a 12-year shorter life expectancy.[8] Transgender patients have increased rates of substance abuse, psychiatric illness, unemployment, HIV infection, and homelessness, which adds stigma to this population and increases the difficulty of accessing or sustaining medical care. Training in cultural competency, while essential, fails to address the larger health-care disparities created by institutionalized sources of stigma which result from cultural, economic, and political conditions.[11]

Traditionally, LGBT health issues receive scant attention in medical training programs.[12] In a survey of 176 medical schools, students received an average of 5 hours of LGBT health training over 4 years.[13] Most medical students receive minimal training on taking a sexual history, leaving them uneasy and unprepared to handle the diversity of human sexual experience.[14] When trainings on LGBT health topics are offered, medical students agree they are relevant to their future work as physicians.[15] Unless the next generation of clinicians receives focused training on the specific health needs, transgender patients will continue to have difficulty accessing clinically and culturally competent care. The resulting "informational and institutional erasure" will lead to ongoing alienation and distrust of medical systems, with a devastating effect on health.[16]

The paucity of evidence-based treatment guidelines, studies on the long-term safety of gender-affirming hormone therapy (GAHT), and guidance for complex medical cases also leads to barriers to care. Few studies exist to define the long-term risks of treatment with GAHT.[17,18] LGBT people have been explicitly excluded from some clinical trials, particularly those related to sexual function.[19] Pathologists and laboratory professionals lack guidelines on how to interpret surgical and cytologic specimens from transgender people, and norms for lab data are based on binary gender definitions.[20] Use of GAHT or pubertal blocking medications for the treatment of gender dysphoria is not FDA approved, which may make clinicians reluctant to prescribe, or fearful of litigation. Over the last decade, a number of professional organizations have released comprehensive treatment guidelines, but recommendations are based on expert opinion, as evidence-based data are lacking.[5,21,22] Clinicians who encounter complex biomedical cases may struggle without evidence-based guidance.[23] Further clinical based research is needed to support informed medical decision-making in the office setting.

Problems with insurance coverage present significant barriers to care. Fourteen percent of transgender people are uninsured, and one in four reported problems related to insurance due to being transgender.[2] These problems included refusal by insurance companies to change name and gender when requested (17%), denial of coverage for gender-specific services such as Papanicolaou (Pap) smears or mammograms (13%), and denial of coverage for routine care (7%), transition-related surgery (55%), and hormone therapy (25%). Many policies deny coverage for transition-related care, which has a disproportionate impact on the social, economic, legal, political, medical, and mental health of low income transgender communities and people of color.[24]

Over the last few years, attention to transgender people in the media has reached a tipping point, with an increase in the coverage of their personal stories, societal issues, and governmental interventions.[25,26] As a result, public debate around the rights of transgender people has swelled, with opponents pitted against proponents from the corridors of public schools all the way to the supreme court. The news is full of stories about bathroom bills and gender-based bullying. Hate groups masquerading as professional organizations publish their own recommendations for care, which are read by vulnerable parents and providers.[27] Religious groups also contribute to the national debate, speaking out in favor or against affirming one's gender identity. Although trained to evaluate the medical literature, providers, medical ethics committee members, and hospital administrators are all products of the same culture and bring implicit bias to exam and board rooms.

These many barriers to care arise as transgender people attempt to negotiate the medical system. *Will the office staff treat me badly? Will my insurance cover my care? Will the doctor understand who I am, what I need? Is it worth the effort to try to get care?*

Removing Barriers to Care: Creating Trans-Affirming Medical Environments

Hospitals and outpatient clinics can intentionally address barriers to care and create welcoming and inclusive patient-centered medical systems.[28] Steps involve choosing a model for care, constructing appropriate visual cues, providing cultural competency training, capturing appropriate demographic information, updating policies and procedures, and learning to provide clinically appropriate services.

Intentional provision of care for LGBT patients usually employs one of two models: LGBT-specific care delivery (a clinic designed to serve this population), or LGBT-embedded care delivery (inclusive services offered within a general ambulatory care practice). In large cities, LGBT-specific clinics are often Federally Qualified Health Centers in neighborhoods with a high proportion of LGBT individuals. They usually advertise well, offer a sense of community and expertise regarding LGBT health concerns, and hire staff who are committed to serving this population.[29,30] In the LGBT-embedded care delivery model, services are provided within the context of a general ambulatory practice.[31] These types of practices vary from site to site in the scope of services offered and expertise of providers. They offer anonymity to patients who prefer not to self-identify, can be established in communities with smaller LGBT patient populations, and may be able to offer more general medical services.

The creation of welcoming environments includes attention to on-site physical structures and visual cues. Welcoming signs and trans-inclusive literature in the waiting room will signal that patients can be open with staff and providers. Gender neutral bathrooms should be installed and properly labeled. Anti-discrimination policies should be prominently displayed. Health centers can identify themselves as LGBT-affirming in hospital directories and marketing campaigns.

Staff should be trained to recognize and address the common problems transgender patients face around insurance coverage. Staff must learn how to bill for gender specific services, such as Pap smears for transgender men and prostate screening for transgender women. Clinicians can request appeals when insurance companies insist that patients conform to outdated standards of care. Patient navigators can direct patients toward policies with inclusive coverage, and advocate for patients who are denied services. Providers should familiarize themselves with local legal or insurance advocacy organizations to assist, when necessary.[32]

Electronic medical records have traditionally offered a binary system for capture of demographic information, missing the opportunity to describe and measure data on sexual and gender minorities (SGM). The Institute of Medicine, under the auspices of the National Institutes of Health (NIH), now recommends routine capture of sexual orientation and gender identity data in all medical records.[33] The Department of Health and Human Services (HHS) has included sexual orientation and gender identity data collection in its requirements for Electronic Health

Records certified by Meaningful Use.[34] Health centers that capture this data will be able to identify and target regional health inequities.

Cultural competency training for staff is essential to creating welcoming and inclusive environments. Training should cover explicit and implicit bias, trans-affirming language, behaviors, and interviewing techniques. Staff and providers are usually unaware of the implicit bias they have absorbed from their cultures. Most healthcare personnel pride themselves on being "accepting of everyone," but true understanding of the lives of those different from ourselves includes acknowledgement of the institutionalized racism, sexism, genderism, ableism, and classism that is an integral part of our culture. These concepts are challenging to address in short cultural competency trainings, and require a willingness on the part of trainees for honest self-assessment. Explicit bias, in the form of racist, transphobic, or homophobic remarks or actions, are easier to identify, but may be equally challenging to address, particularly in clinics with embedded care delivery models, where staff were not necessarily recruited for their commitment to LGBT patients. Culturally competent care includes the recognition that each patient has a unique journey, with differing goals, timelines, and ability/willingness to disclose. Clinicians must learn how to involve family members in the transition process, when appropriate, or support patients who are rejected by family. They must also be aware of the challenges many transgender people face around housing, education, employment, and societal stigma.

Attention to trans-affirming language is an essential part of cultural competency training. Individuals present with an increasing number of terms for self-identification. All office staff must be comfortable asking patients their preferred name and pronouns, and familiar with the common names for identities that fall under the transgender umbrella. They must be comfortable with the concepts of sex assigned at birth, gender expression, and sexual orientation, and understand that patient experience may be fluid. Training manuals are available with teaching tools and lists of definitions, as well as pictorial representations, such as the widely used "genderbread person."[35,36] Clinicians should learn the terms transgender people use to describe common practices, such as "packing" (wearing genital prosthesis), "tucking" (hiding the penis and testicles), and "binding" (wearing compressive chest garments).

Clinical competency is essential to creating a welcoming environment, and a holistic, biopsychosocial approach to care works best. Clinicians should learn to recognize the health-care disparities faced by transgender people of different ethnicities, race, ability, literacy, and socioeconomic status. They should familiarize themselves with common health problems, hormone treatment protocols, and primary care protocols for transgender people. They must learn to take accurate sexual histories, and assess for high risk behaviors and substance abuse. They must develop skills in assessing psychosocial stressors, which includes knowing to ask about common legal, spiritual, social, and emotional problems. Clinicians can partner with mental health providers, creating a therapeutic team to assist struggling patients. Professional medical education programs are available for providers who wish to develop these skills.[37–39]

Clinicians and staff should be aware of transgender-specific community resources and post this information in waiting rooms or on websites, or distribute it via handouts. Patients benefit from access to support groups, pride centers, legal advocacy centers, affirming places of worship, and other social services.

Clinicians can also refer patients to legal groups who assist with changing gender markers on documents. We recommend developing close connections to legal organizations that represent transgender people who face discrimination, such as the America Civil Liberties Union, Lambda Legal, the Transgender Legal Defense and Education Fund, and the National Center for Lesbian Rights.[40–43]

Patient feedback is important to assess the effectiveness of efforts to create welcoming and inclusive spaces. Patients can be asked to participate in focus groups or community advisory boards to comment on their healthcare experience and make recommendations for improvement. Patient satisfaction surveys should include specific questions regarding the experience of transgender patients within the healthcare system.

The US Department of Health and Human Services (HHS) has taken significant steps to advance the health of LGBT communities by implementing article 1557 of the Affordable Care Act, which prohibits discrimination in health care on the basis of sexual orientation and gender identity.[44] The NIH has officially designated SGM as a health disparity population for research, and a new position for a Senior Advisor for LGBT Health has been created within the Office of the Assistant Secretary for Health (OASH).[44] As a result, new services are being evaluated and developed at the federal and state level. The Healthcare Equality Index/Human Rights Campaign offers an online benchmarking tool to assist institutions as they update these policies and then advertise best practices in LGBT health to their community.[45] The first step to reducing barriers to care is to ensure that LGBTQ health care is valued as part of an organization's commitment to quality.[28]

Principles of Primary Care for Gender Nonconforming and Transgender Patients

PATIENT CARE OVER THE LIFE CYCLE

Primary care providers are uniquely positioned to attend to the medical needs of transgender and gender nonconforming patients throughout all stages of life. Patient needs are age-specific, and individuals may initiate care for primary care and/or gender related services at any stage. Clinicians who routinely ask questions about gender identity for all patients will facilitate the coming-out process by signaling the importance of gender health as part of primary care.

Parents often present asking for guidance with young children exhibiting gender nonconforming behaviors. Some parents present with curiosity and interest, while others struggle with denial, fear, grief, shame, guilt, or partners who have different parenting styles. Clinicians who learn to support parents kindly and without judgment are best able to help families negotiate through normal stages of resistance and acceptance.

Clinicians can counsel that gender exploration is normal and that gender diversity in childhood may or may not persist into adulthood. In studies of prepubertal children referred to gender clinics for assessment, only 6% to 27% of children demonstrated dysphoria that persisted into adulthood.[46–49] In other studies, gender nonconforming boys were more likely to identify as gay than trans as adults. However, many transgender adults report consistent, insistent, and persistent cross-gender identification from a young age. Clinicians can encourage parents to adopt a supportive, gender-affirming approach for all children, refer to mental health providers when appropriate, and encourage schools to accommodate gender diverse students.

Adolescence is a particularly challenging time for transgender individuals. The development of secondary sex characteristics in the assigned, rather than experienced, gender may trigger gender dysphoria, and pubertal youth often seek medical care for anxiety, depression, substance abuse, eating disorders, behavioral concerns, or suicidal ideation. Teens may be struggling with self-esteem, bullying, body image, coming out, dating, sexuality, peer interactions, homelessness, and family rejection. Clinicians should ask all teens about gender and sexuality as part of routine anticipatory guidance and assessment for distress. Recognizing gender dysphoria is an important intervention, if done with the intention of creating a safe space for addressing related issues. Informed clinicians may facilitate prompt mental health referrals, discuss indications for pubertal blocking medications or hormone therapy, and normalize the youths' experience.

Transgender adults face a different set of challenges, depending on when they come out and how/if they choose to transition. We recommend asking all adults about their sexual orientation/gender identity as part of routine care, remembering that it may take years to come out to a provider. Many adults struggle with internal distress related to gender dysphoria, and suffer from high rates of suicidal ideation, substance abuse, depression, and anxiety. They may face external challenges, including problems with employment, education, housing, family rejection, parenting, and harassment. Some adults need guidance and referrals for preservation of fertility. Others need assistance accessing mental health services, support groups, voice therapy, hormones, or surgical procedures. Transgender men may need help accessing obstetrical care. Adults with concurrent medical problems will often need support in finding trans-affirming specialists.

The care of older transgender patients requires sensitivity to the fact that these patients may face more barriers to care. As the rate of health problems increases, access to a trans-affirming support network often decreases. Transgender elders came of age in a time when there were fewer options and resources, and may have lived years without affirmation. They may experience grief and regret about lost opportunities or compromises they were forced to make. It may be more difficult, medically and socially, to transition later in life. Transgender elders struggle with ageism as well as transphobia. Many face shock and rejection from family members. Informed clinicians can address and normalize the experience of transgender elders, assist with transitions, and help with access to affirming specialty services.

End-of-life care presents a new set of challenges. LGBT-affirming elder care facilities are often unavailable or difficult to access. Home healthcare personnel and medical specialists may lack training in cultural competency. Nontraditional partners are often excluded from end-of-life decisions and care. Clinicians can insist that elder transgender patients have access to appropriate inpatient and outpatient resources, and that their partners and families are respected. Clinicians can also play an important role by educating community support services.

THE PATIENT ENCOUNTER

Staff and providers can intentionally behave in ways to create safe and affirming medical encounters for transgender patients. Staff should greet patients in a friendly manner, ask about preferred name and pronouns, and document this information in the medical record. Staff must understand that patients have differing degrees of disclosure/"outness," and some may prefer that the clinician use different names/pronouns than the staff. All should follow strict guidelines for confidentiality, and obtain consent to speak about care plans with identified family and friends. Office forms should be designed to capture information about gender diverse patients and nontraditional families.

Medical History

Medical assessments to initiate primary care or transition-related health services follow the same general outline used for all medical encounters, but must also include attention to the common health issues of transgender people. Acute visits for illness unrelated to gender should follow the usual brief format used for all patients. One should avoid questions related to gender transition, unless relevant to the presenting problem.

For comprehensive primary care, including the initiation or management of GAHT, we recommend that providers first obtain a general history, to include the primary concerns of the patient—which may or may not be related to gender. We follow this with the open-ended question, "Tell me your gender history," to learn about the patient's journey in an unstructured manner, with the patient offering the information that is most important/pertinent to them. This can be followed by more direct questions about steps they have taken to transition, with an inventory of body parts present/absent which will be used for routine health maintenance screening recommendations. We ask about how gender dysphoria has impacted aspects of the patient's life, such as family, personal relationships, education, and employment. We query about barriers to transition and hopes for moving forward. We ask about past medical history, including psychiatric care and mental health issues. We carefully assess for suicidality, when appropriate, with the knowledge that 41% of transgender people have attempted suicide at some point in their life.[1] Surgical history should include transition-related procedures, and satisfaction with results. We ask about medications, both prescribed by clinicians and self-prescribed, with the expectation that some patients have self-treated with hormones obtained without medical supervision. In our social histories, we ask about substance abuse, understanding that risks of tobacco, alcohol, and drug abuse are higher in this population. We solicit information about education, jobs, housing, safety, abuse, and social supports. We create genograms to document family histories, a process useful for capturing medical information as well as an understanding of family systems and supports.[50] When appropriate, we ask about plans for childbearing, and whether the patient wants referrals for the preservation of fertility.

Careful and complete sexual histories are essential, with attention to sexual orientation, contraceptive needs, and high-risk behaviors. The stress of gender dysphoria and medical transition may have a profound impact on sexuality and intimacy. A sensitive intake signals that a provider is comfortable discussing sexual health. Testosterone therapy often increases libido. Estradiol may decrease libido and lead to erectile dysfunction, which pleases some patients and frustrates others. Surgical procedures may impact sexuality in positive or negative ways. Some are more comfortable with sex in a body that aligns with gender identity, while others struggle with surgical sequelae. Clinicians can coordinate with surgeons and qualified sex therapists to assist patients with sexual concerns.

For transition related care, we suggest that clinicians first ask about treatment goals, and use this discussion to tailor recommendations for care. Options for care include (1) changes in gender expression or role, (2) hormone therapy to masculinize or feminize the body, (3) surgery to change primary or secondary sex characteristics, and (4) psychotherapy.[5] Some wish to transition from one gender binary to the other as quickly as possible. Others may endorse a nonbinary gender identity, with the goal of an androgynous gender expression. Some patients want gender-affirming surgery; others do not. Some patients will want full social and medical transition; others may wish to take hormones but still present in their assigned gender.

The Physical Exam

Many transgender patients are anxious about physical exams, and mindful clinicians can intentionally behave in ways to help alleviate discomfort and fear. Patient anxiety may be related to anatomical dysphoria regarding primary and secondary sex characteristics, previous experiences with unsupportive clinicians, or a history of trauma. The first step for clinicians is to acknowledge one's own level of comfort. Clinicians who lack self-awareness may avoid or provide inadequate exams, or project awkwardness. We recommend asking each patient, "How do you feel about having an exam?" and "Is there anything I can do to make you more comfortable?" Pay attention to the use of gowns and drapes, and offer clothed exams for those who cannot tolerate disrobing. Some patients will prefer a nurse chaperone in attendance, and others will not. Clinicians can ask how patients refer to their body parts, and use affirming language such as "chest" rather than "breasts" or "genitals" instead of "penis/vagina."

Primary care providers may be asked to provide routine postoperative care for patients who travel long distances for surgery. Establishing a collaborative relationship with the surgeon is essential, and many of the surgeons are adept at advising local providers on postop care from afar.

Physical findings vary depending on the status of hormonal and surgical treatment.[51] We will describe common physical findings for the nonoperative and postoperative patient. Extensive postoperative care is beyond the scope of this chapter.

Physical Exam for Transgender Women

Transgender women may present at any stage of transition. Some will have only typically male physical findings; others will have feminizing changes.

Some women will present with decreased facial/body hair from shaving, depilation, laser, or electrolysis treatments. Clinicians should ask about or note the presence of male pattern baldness, and address this, if problematic. Some women present with local skin irritation, due to adhesives for wigs or breast forms. Feminizing hormones produce varying degrees of breast development, according to genetic predisposition and body habitus. Testes usually diminish in size and get softer with hormonal therapy. Some women practice "tucking" of their testes into the inguinal canals to reduce the genital bulge, and testes may need to be gently pressed back into the scrotum for exams. Although routine testicular exams are not recommended as a screening test for cisgender men, we consider these for transgender women, who may not be comfortable with genital self-exams.[23]

Some transgender women inject with free-form silicone ("pumping"), to enhance their breasts and hips—a practice with many dangerous short-term and long-term complications, including silicone migration, infection, immune reactions, pulmonary embolism, or end-organ damage. Consider and ask about a history of silicone injection for patients presenting with skin conditions, unexplained inflammation, or acute illness.

Postop care for transgender women includes attention to scars from breast implants or facial feminization surgery. Patients are routinely sent home from "bottom" surgeries (orchiectomy, penectomy, and vaginoplasty) before complete healing occurs and may require local follow up. In the immediate postop period, swelling, mild vaginal bleeding, and/or discharge may occur and can be treated supportively. After vaginoplasty, patients are advised to dilate the neovagina on a fixed schedule. Some require assistance/reassurance around the dilation process. The neovagina should be inspected for granulation tissue, which can be removed with silver nitrate, after appropriate surgical consultation. Postop fever, hemorrhage, wound infection, dehiscence, or increasing pain should lead to immediate surgical consultation. Wound separation can occur 6% of time and is usually treated conservatively.[52] Infections, strictures, and fistulas are rare but known complications of vaginoplasty, and clinicians should remain alert to these possibilities.[52]

Transgender women who have had a vaginoplasty should have regular pelvic exams to assess for vaginal health, strictures, STDs, or sexual difficulties. Pap smears are not necessary. We find breast exams useful for transgender women, who have unknown risks of breast cancer and often have questions about breast development.

Physical Exam for Transgender Men

Transgender men may also present at any stage of transition, some with only typically female physical findings and others with full masculinization.

After hormone therapy, transgender men usually have an increase in facial/body hair, masculinization of the bony facial structure, deepening of the voice, increased muscle mass, and clitoromegaly.

We perform chest examination based on the presence or absence of breast tissue. Some surgeons leave residual breast tissue during chest reconstruction, and some transgender men choose not to pursue top surgery. Pelvic exams and Pap smears should be performed for transgender men with a cervix. Some transgender men have anxiety, pain, or anatomical dysphoria around pelvic exams. Clinicians should ask about comfort level and discuss ways to mitigate distress.

An increase in acne is common, especially for younger men in early stages of treatment.

Some transgender men suffer from rashes, or acne/excoriations of the trunk from chest binding. Some may have irritation to the symphysis pubis or genitals from "soft" or "hard" packers (penile prosthesis).[51] Transgender men are at increased risk of male pattern baldness.

Postoperative care from chest reconstruction includes attention to scars and nipple grafting. Look for infection, keloid formation, and nipple graft failure. Seromas, collections of fluid, are common after chest reconstruction and sometimes require drainage or compression. Some patients require top surgery revisions to correct inadequate removal of breast tissue, "dog ears," or other aesthetic problems.

Postoperative care from hysterectomy is routine and can be carried out with assistance from trans-affirming gynecologists. Attention to the presence or absence of ovaries (some surgeons remove and some do not) is essential when evaluating abdominal processes, or assessing bone health.

Postoperative care after phalloplasty/metoidioplasty may be complex and is best performed in close collaboration with the surgeon. The risk of complications depends on surgical technique. Urethral lengthening procedures have a high incidence of stricture and fistula formation. Primary care clinicians should assess for graft viability, strictures, infections, scarring, fistulas, and mental health concerns, which may emerge around protracted postoperative complications.

DIAGNOSIS OF GENDER DYSPHORIA

The criteria for medical treatment with hormones or surgery include "persistent, well-documented gender dysphoria."[5] Clinicians with limited experience may question their ability to accurately diagnose or evaluate a patient for the appropriateness of medical transition. Evolving definitions for gender variance further complicate diagnosis.

Historically, the medical community has viewed transgender people as mentally ill, and vestiges of this pathologizing approach remain deeply embedded in our culture. The evolution of diagnoses used in consecutive editions of the *Diagnostic and Statistical Manual of Mental Disorders* (DSM) offers a window into both professional and popular conceptions about SGM.[53,54] When first published in 1968, the DSM listed homosexuality as a mental disorder. In 1973, the American Psychiatric Association (APA) declassified homosexuality as a mental illness, by a vote of its members. As per Richard Green, "on that fateful day in 1973, in America alone, several million mentally ill persons were cured." It took until 1980 before the diagnosis of ego-dystonic homosexuality (e.g. unhappiness with homosexual feelings) was recognized as biased and removed.[55]

Similarly, diagnoses have evolved in the DSM to reflect a healthier and more nuanced view of gender diversity. In 2015, the DSM 5 replaced the diagnosis *Gender Identity Disorder* with *Gender Dysphoria*, indicating the shift to viewing gender diversity as normal, and *Gender Dysphoria* as a treatable condition. Many clinicians object that the term *Gender Dysphoria* is also limited and pathologizing. Some patients have no dysphoria and still wish to transition. To address this, the World Health Organization has recommended that the term *Gender Incongruence* be used in the International Classification of Diseases (ICD-11). Others argue that because gender variation in children is normal, a distinct diagnosis has no medical utility.[56] The quest for appropriate diagnostic terms is complicated by insurance companies who demand a medical or psychiatric diagnostic code to cover treatment.

The World Professional Association for Transgender Health (WPATH) Standards of Care 7 recommends a gender assessment from a qualified clinician prior to the initiation of gender affirming hormone therapy, to ensure that patients meet criteria for gender dysphoria and have informed treatment expectations.[5] A gender assessment, usually a shorter, more focused process than psychotherapy, may be completed by a mental health or medical provider, and provides an important opportunity to address any relevant social or mental health issues prior to medical transition.[57] Historically, this was performed by mental health providers, who would refer patients to medical providers with a referral letter and recommendations for care. We welcome these referrals in our medical practice, as they offer an opportunity for close coordination of care for patients who need extra support. However, not all patients want, need, or are able to access mental health services, and gender assessments may also be performed by a qualified medical provider under the informed consent model. For patients who are self-treating with hormones obtained from the Internet, we recommend expediting entry to medically supervised care, without gender assessment, a process known as the Harm Reduction Model of Care. We refer those who need mental health services after ensuring that they are medically stable and their hormone regimen is safe.

For new providers who are uncertain of their diagnostic skills, we recommend formal training and close collaboration with mentors and/or experienced providers.

COORDINATION OF CARE

The primary care clinician can play an essential role in the coordination of care for transgender patients. This may include collaboration with mental health providers, surgeons, advocates, voice therapists, electrologists and laser therapy technicians, and medical specialists.

Our practice is to ask patients about their care teams and routinely request releases so that we may coordinate care, when appropriate. We forward office notes to significant providers on the care team. We establish email connections with consulting clinicians when there is a need to communicate regularly for patients with special needs. We review cases with our collaborating mental health providers on a regular basis, either in staff meetings or online. We collaborate both pre- and postoperatively with surgeons.

We strive to keep communication efficient and focused, as collaboration is time consuming. But the benefits to our patients are enormous, and we as clinicians also benefit from the opportunity to partner with our colleagues across disciplines.

Assistance With Document Changes

Transition often involves legal name changes and changes in gender markers on documents. These documents include, but are not limited to, passports, social security cards, driver's licenses, birth certificates, and insurance cards.

Patients require a letter from a licensed physician to change their gender marker on a US Passport. The letter must state that the person has had "appropriate clinical treatment for gender transition." Templates for the required letter are available on the State Department Website.[58] The definition of "appropriate clinical treatment" is intentionally broad, as some patients do not elect medical transitions. Hormone therapy and surgery are not required for most gender marker changes, including those on passports, and the details of treatment should not be included in this letter. A birth certificate, or driver's license with appropriate gender markers, can be substituted for this passport letter.

Physicians can also supply letters for changes in gender markers on Social Security records.[59] There is no gender marker on the Social Security card, but the record in the government file includes a marker, which may be transmitted to employers.

Individual state law determines the process for changes in the gender marker on birth certificates. While some states accept broad definitions for "appropriate clinical treatment," others mandate precise and limited definitions of gender transition, including GAHT or gender-affirming surgery. This practice is discriminatory against people who are unable or do not wish to have medical or surgical interventions.

Gender-Affirming Hormone Therapy: Basics for the Primary Care Clinician

Hormonal therapy is highly effective in enhancing psychological well-being for transgender people.[60] Quality of life is enhanced, and symptoms of depression, anxiety, body discomfort, and psychopathology are reduced.[61–64] All primary care clinicians should have a basic understanding of hormonal therapy. Gender-affirming hormone therapy is considered medically necessary, and is the standard of care for the treatment of gender dysphoria.[5] We will provide a brief overview of masculinizing and feminizing hormones, and discuss the metabolic effects of these medications (Table 12.1). The Endocrine Society recommends initiation of hormone therapy at age 16 or older.[21] Parental consent is required until age 18. Most experts advocate for flexibility around the age for prescribing hormones, and may start hormones before age 16, for youth who meet criteria for gender dysphoria.

MASCULINIZING THERAPY

Testosterone is used by transgender men to develop masculine secondary sex characteristics. Testosterone was first used

TABLE 12.1	Effects of Testosterone and Estradiol on Metabolic and Other Parameters	
Parameter	**Effect**	**Comment**
TESTOSTERONE		
Cholesterol (total)	No significant change	
High-density lipoprotein (HDL)	Decrease by 12 mg/dL	
Low-density lipoprotein (LDL)	No significant change	
Triglycerides	Increase by 35 mg/dL	
Blood pressure	Possible 3–5 mm Hg increase	Antihypertensives as needed
Erythrocytosis	4% increase in hematocrit	Adjust dose. Keep below 50%
Bone density	No increase in osteoporosis risk	
Liver function tests	2%–8% increase in enzymes	
Male pattern alopecia	May or may not be desirable	Consider low dose finasteride
Acne	Reported severe in 16%	Treat or refer if severe
ESTRADIOL		
Cardiovascular mortality	Possible increase in risk	Intensive treatment of cardiovascular risk factors
Venous thromboembolism	Increase	Consider stopping estradiol prior to surgery, use patch in older patients and high risk patients
Lipids	Increase in triglycerides	Patch causes less elevation
Blood pressure	No significant effect	
Bone density	No change	

clinically in the 1930s to relieve vasomotor symptoms and urinary disorders in women.[65] The earliest documented use of testosterone for female-to-male gender transition occurred in 1939 in England, for Michael Dillon.[66]

Testosterone acts directly on androgen receptors, or can be converted to two active metabolites. Aromatization by aromatase produces 17beta-estradiol, while reduction by 5alpha-reductase produces dihydrotestosterone (DHT).[67] Estradiol plays a dominant role in bone health in cisgender man, and contributes to sexual functioning.[68,69] DHT may cause acne and androgenetic alopecia.[68,70]

Testosterone causes an increase in muscle mass, libido, facial and body hair, and acne.[68] The face undergoes masculinizing skeletal changes and body fat redistributes to a masculine shape. The clitoris enlarges, the voice drops, and menses are suppressed.[71,72] Many studies confirm that testosterone administration improves psychological functioning and reduces gender dysphoria, anxiety, and depression in transgender men.[64,73,74]

Testosterone is usually administered subcutaneously (SQ) and intramuscularly (IM). Patients can be trained to self-inject by nursing staff so that medications can be administered safely at home.

For patients averse to injection, other delivery methods include testosterone implants (Testopel) and topical patches or gels. Topical preparations tend to be pricey and may not be covered by insurance. Patients should be advised to use caution to avoid inadvertent administration of topical testosterone to others via skin-to-skin contact. This is especially true for contact with women and children, who may virilize from accidental exposure. Patients should be counseled to apply the gel to the upper arm or shoulder, to wash before skin contact with another person, and to avoid sharing clothing that may be compromised. Dosing for gel preparation depends on which of the four available preparations are used (Androgel, Axiron, Fortesta, and Testim in the United States).[75] Testosterone undecanoate, an oral preparation that circumvents the first pass through the liver, is available in other countries, but is not FDA approved in the United States.[76] Clinicians may encounter patients who are self-treating with this preparation by purchasing medications on the Internet.

Total serum testosterone levels can be monitored periodically during treatment. The lab draw is obtained midway between injections. If the patch or gel is used, levels should be checked between 2 and 12 hours after application. Doses may be titrated up or down based on serum levels and/or clinical results. The Endocrine Society recommends keeping testosterone in the physiologic range for natal adult males. Lab reference ranges for serum testosterone are approximately 320 to 1,000 ng/dL.[22] Clinicians who are constrained by a lack of insurance coverage may choose to adjust dosing based only on clinical results and forgo the measurement of testosterone levels. However, periodic monitoring of the hematocrit remains essential.

METABOLIC EFFECTS OF MASCULINIZING HORMONES

In the short and medium term, hormonal transition for transgender men appears to be safe and effective.[77] Data on the long-term risks of testosterone therapy are limited, and more research is needed for conclusive evidence regarding the long-term safety of this intervention.[71] We will review existing studies on testosterone's known metabolic effects on overall mortality, cardiovascular (CV) health, hematologic risk, bone health, libido, reproductive organs, fertility, skin, hair, and mood.

Overall Mortality and Cardiovascular Risk

The few existing studies that examine all-cause mortality rates for transgender men show conflicting results, and are limited by the failure to separate the effects of testosterone from those of surgical treatment. One study from the Netherlands showed no increase in mortality compared with the general population.[78] A second study showed a late increase in mortality 10 years after gender affirmation surgery,[79] an effect that was attributed to an unexplained higher rate of suicide in the transgender population.[71,79]

Existing studies show no increase in CV events from testosterone therapy for transgender men, although surrogate markers for CV risk may be increased.[80–82] Studies of lipid profiles show decreases in high-density lipoprotein (HDL) of 4 to 13 mg/dL, increases in triglycerides of 6 to 32 mg/dL, and possible elevation of low-density lipoprotein (LDL) and total cholesterol with testosterone treatment. The clinical significance of these changes is unknown.[71,81–86] Testosterone therapy has not been shown to cause significant increases in blood pressure or diabetes, although the quality of these studies is low due to the use of retrospective cohorts.[81,87] Testosterone treatment increases lean body mass while estrogen deficiency causes increased intra-abdominal and subcutaneous body fat.[68] Weight gain is common, and may predispose to medical conditions associated with obesity.

Erythrocytosis

Erythrocytosis, an increase in absolute red blood cell mass, is a known effect of androgen treatment and increases the risk of stroke.[88–90] Strokes caused by erythrocytosis can be thrombotic or embolic.[91] Measurement of actual red cell mass involves isotopic methods, which are beyond the usual scope of practice. Hematocrit and hemoglobin are easily measured and used as surrogate markers for an absolute increase in red blood cell mass.[92] Increased hematocrit (polycythemia) may also be caused by disease processes, such as polycythemia vera, chronic hypoxia, or a decrease in plasma volume due to dehydration, diuretic use, or burns (relative polycythemia).[93] All causes must be considered before assuming polycythemia is due to testosterone use.

The Center of Excellence for Transgender Medicine protocol recommends measuring hematocrit prior to initiating GAHT, at 3, 6, and 12 months, and then every 6 to 12 months.[22] Testosterone dosing can be reduced in the setting of polycythemia. Some protocols suggest changing to topical testosterone, which may be less erythrogenic. Therapeutic phlebotomy can be used to treat hematocrit levels greater than 53%, with a goal of less than 50% to 52%. For patients with significant risk factors for stroke, such as smoking and advanced age, a lower goal for the hematocrit may be more appropriate.[94]

Bone Health

Most studies show either a neutral effect or increased bone mineral density (BMD) with testosterone therapy.[95,96] Data show decreased BMD after oophorectomy, so adequate testosterone dosing must be prescribed after gender affirming oophorectomy.[97]

Libido

Most patients on testosterone therapy develop varying degrees of clitoral enlargement. Some patients are bothered by hypersensitivity of the enlarging clitoris, or are troubled by erections. Some transgender men apply small amounts of topical testosterone to the clitoris to enhance growth, though this practice is not evidence-based. Most patients report an increase in libido, and a change in the quality of orgasm.

Menses, Vagina, and Uterus

Testosterone therapy suppresses ovulation and causes endometrial atrophy.[98] Amenorrhea is expected within 6 to 9 months of initiation of treatment. Many transgender men on testosterone report crampy pelvic pain for reasons that are not well defined.

Fertility and Pregnancy

Although testosterone therapy usually eliminates ovulation and menses, pregnancy has been known to occur. Transgender who engage in vaginal intercourse with partners who have a penis should be counseled about the use of birth control. Birth control options include barrier methods, progesterone oral contraceptives, intrauterine devices (IUD) or implantable hormone devices. If pregnancy is suspected, testosterone should be stopped immediately.

There is a lack of studies that examine the effects of testosterone on fertility for transgender men.[99] Historically, clinicians have counseled patients to consider embryo or oocyte cryopreservation prior to initiating hormone therapy.[22] More recently, reports indicate that transgender men have achieved successful pregnancies and some are able to chestfeed.[100] Further studies are needed before we can counsel patients on the risks of prior use of testosterone on fetal health.

Although not evidence-based, most providers recommend stopping testosterone 6 months prior to conception. Pregnancy can occur prior to the return of menses. Transgender men remain off testosterone until after delivery, or after cessation of chest-feeding. The length of testosterone treatment may influence the likelihood of becoming pregnant.

Hair/Skin

Testosterone will increase facial and body hair in transgender men with this genetic predisposition. It may take 2 to 5 years for maximal facial hair growth. Testosterone often induces a male pattern hair line, with a central peak in the midbrow, and lateral recession. It may induce male-pattern baldness, which, if severe, can be treated with finasteride or topical minoxidil.

Acne is a common problem for transgender men on testosterone. Acne usually peaks at 6 months, and shows significant improvement by 12 months. Hormone-induced acne usually responds well to conventional acne treatments.[101]

Mood Effects

Testosterone therapy has been shown to consistently lead to reductions in anxiety, depression, and dysphoria in transgender men. However, mood changes may also occur, and some report increased irritability, anger, or agression.[102] Doses should be decreased or therapy stopped for patients who complain of worsening mood.

Drug Interactions

There are relatively few significant drug interactions with testosterone therapy. Testosterone has been shown to increase the hypoglycemic effects of diabetic medications, enhance anticoagulant effects of warfarin, and increase fluid retention in patients on corticosteroids.[103,104] Clinicians should monitor patients on these medication combinations appropriately.

FEMINIZING THERAPY

Feminizing hormones are used to stimulate the development of feminine secondary sex characteristics. Typically estradiol is used for feminization and androgen blockers are used to block receptors for testosterone and its metabolites. Clinicians should be familiar with feminizing regimens, routes of administration, dosing, and the metabolic effects of feminizing hormones on CV and other systems.

The use of estrogen with an antiandrogen is the standard of care for feminizing therapy.[105,106] Estrogens can be delivered orally, topically, or intramuscularly. Recommended preparations include 17beta-estradiol (estradiol) given orally or via topical patch.[105] Ethinyl estradiol is no longer recommended due to high rate of thrombotic events.[107]

While estradiol alone will suppress testosterone, antiandrogen medications are usually added to suppress testosterone levels to the natal female range and block the effects of testosterone. Spironolactone and cyproterone acetate (frequently used in Canada and Europe) are the most commonly used antiandrogens. Medroxyprogesterone acetate and Lupron and may also be used for their antiandrogenic effects. Patients on spironolactone should be monitored for hypotension, renal insufficiency, and hyperkalemia, although these are infrequent complications.[108] Antiandrogen therapy should be stopped after orchiectomy.

At times, clinicians add progesterone to the feminizing regimen, although little data are available about the effectiveness or risks to this intervention. The Women's Health Initiative shows that estrogen plus progestin is associated with increased risks of breast cancer, heart attacks, stroke, and venous thromboembolism (VTE) in postmenopausal cisgender women.[109] It is unknown if these risks can be extrapolated to transgender women. Patients often request progesterone, due to reports that it may enhance breast development. However there is no published data supporting this effect.

The Endocrine Society Guidelines recommend monitoring estradiol and testosterone levels, with a goal of normal physiologic range for natal females.[21] They recommend suppression of testosterone levels to less than 50 ng/dL, and maintenance of estradiol levels in the 100-200 pg/mL range. Once testosterone levels have been adequately suppressed, it is unclear whether increasing the estradiol levels into the high-normal range will bring additional feminization.

METABOLIC EFFECTS OF FEMINIZING HORMONES

Active estrogen-sensitive cancer is an absolute contradiction to estrogen. Relative contraindications for estradiol include prior venous thrombosis, and family history of breast cancer in two or more relatives, coronary artery or cerebrovascular disease, severe liver disease (transaminases greater than three times upper level of normal), and severe migraine headaches.[110] We will review the metabolic effects of feminizing therapy on CV risk, VTE, prolactinemia, bone health, libido, prostate and penis, hair/skin, and mood.

Overall Mortality and Cardiovascular Risk

One long-term study demonstrated an increase in all-cause mortality in transgender women, but the increase was not attributed to hormone use.[78] Another long-term study showed no increase in all-cause mortality in a transgender women.[77]

Data on the effects of feminizing therapy on CV health are mixed. Some retrospective studies show increased risk for myocardial infarctions, cardiac mortality, and strokes in transgender women on estrogen, while others show no increase in risk.[111] Feminizing therapy has been shown to increase serum triglycerides without changes in other lipid parameters.[81] However, the overall quality of relevant studies is low, and further prospective studies are needed to delineate the level of increased risk for CV events.[81,112]

Venous Thromboembolism

When oral ethinyl estradiol was used for feminization, the rate of VTE was up to 45 times the expected rate.[18] Follow-up studies demonstrated that oral 17beta-estradiol and transdermal estradiol had lesser prothrombotic effects.[111,113] Currently, oral 17beta-estradiol, transdermal estradiol, or injectable estradiol are the recommended estrogen preparations for GAHT.[110]

Transdermal estrogen has the lowest rates of VTE in postmenopausal cisgender women on estrogens.[114] We recommend transdermal preparations for all patients at increased risk for VTE. Screening for thrombophilia and prophylactic aspirin for prevention of VTE is not recommended (though aspirin may be recommended for prevention of cardiac events).

Transgender women who develop VTE while on oral estradiol should be changed to transdermal estrogen, if they choose to continue hormonal therapy. VTE risk may also be reduced by lowering estrogen dosage. Some clinicians recommend the indefinite use of anticoagulation for those who choose to continue estrogen after VTE.[115]

Perioperative protocols for patients on estradiol are controversial and not evidence-based. Some experts recommend stopping estrogen 2 weeks before surgery and waiting 3 weeks to resume treatment, due to perioperative risk of VTE.[80,115] Others allow continuation of estrogen perioperatively, with or without anticoagulation.[22]

Prolactinemia and Prolactinomas

Patients on estrogen therapy should be monitored clinically for signs of pituitary prolactinoma, such as galactorrhea, visual changes, and headache. While no clear correlation has been established, there are numerous case reports of pituitary prolactinomas in transgender women.[116–118]

Hyperprolactinemia occurs frequently in patients on feminizing hormones, with rates of 4% to 30%.[116,119] Estrogens cause increased prolactin levels by stimulating the proliferation of lactotroph cells and upgrading transcription of prolactin genes.[118] Typically the prolactin levels increase in the first year and then gradually decrease. The antiandrogen cyproterone acetate may also play a role in the development of hyperprolactinemia.[117] Although hyperprolactinemia occurs frequently, pituitary prolactinomas occur in less than 0.1% of patients.[118]

Routine monitoring of serum prolactin levels is controversial. The Endocrine Society and other experts recommend obtaining a prolactin level at baseline and then every 1 to 2 years.[110,120] However, others recommend monitoring clinically for symptoms of prolactinoma without routine blood testing.[22] One disadvantage of screening is the unnecessary alteration of feminizing treatment. Small, asymptomatic prolactinomas do not always require treatment, and large prolactinomas typically respond well to dopamine blockers, so there may be limited benefit to early diagnosis. It is not necessary to reduce or stop estrogen therapy for hyperprolactinemia. Prolactin levels may return to the normal range after orchiectomy.[119]

Bone and Muscle

Transgender women who have had orchiectomy are at increased risk for osteoporosis. In one long-term study, osteoporosis of the spine was observed after 10 years in 23.4% of postoperative transgender women on GAHT.[121] Another study showed that nonoperative transgender women had a lower bone mineral density compared with cisgender men prior to initiating GAHT, but that skeletal status was well preserved on feminizing hormones.[122]

Feminizing hormone use is associated with significant muscle loss in the first 2 years of treatment.[122] Approximately 4 kg of lean body mass are lost following the initiation of androgen deprivation in transgender women.[123]

Libido

Most transgender women report decreased libido on feminizing therapy, as well as decreased frequency of spontaneous erections and decreased ejaculation. Erectile dysfunction is common, and patients may benefit from treatment with sildenafil or tadalafil. Some women report the ability to achieve orgasm without erection, or a different quality to their orgasm.

Penis, Testes, Prostate, and Fertility

The penis may appear smaller for patients on feminizing hormones. Estradiol leads to testicular atrophy and diminished production of testosterone. Atrophy of the prostate can lead to transient postvoid dribbling in the initial year of therapy.[110] Some clinicians report increased incidence of prostatitis during the first years of hormonal transition.[124] Semen volume is decreased or absent. Cases of prostate cancer have been reported in transgender women on feminizing hormones, though the risk may be decreased.[124]

Feminizing hormones may affect fertility, and most clinicians discuss options for sperm banking prior to treatment. Therapy does not guarantee infertility, however, and transgender women can impregnate a sexual partner if contraception is not used.

Hair and Skin

Feminizing hormones cause softening of the skin and decreased hair growth on the body. Facial hair is less affected, and many transgender women seek electrolysis or laser treatment for the face.

The effect on male pattern baldness is variable, but some women have decreased hair loss or even regrowth of hair on feminizing therapy. Hair follicles convert testosterone to dihydrotestosterone (DHT), which causes hair follicles to shrink in people with a genetic predisposition for alopecia. Finasteride decreases serum and scalp DHT by inhibiting conversion of testosterone to DHT, and may be used to treat alopecia in transgender women.[125] Finasteride alone is not an adequate antiandrogen for feminizing regimes.

Mood

Many transgender women report an increased sense of well-being on feminizing hormones. Subjective reports of increased tearfulness, emotional sensitivity, and an awareness of a broader emotional landscape are common. Some patients describe a decrease in aggression and irritability.

Preventative Care

The approach to preventative care for transgender patients is based on various combinations of the patient's age, their experienced gender, their sex assigned at birth, the use of GAHT, and the presence or absence of specific organs. Due to the paucity of long-term, evidence-based studies, preventative screening recommendations are often based on limited data, extrapolation from the cisgender population, and expert opinion. Clinicians must complete a careful history, as well as an inventory of organs present for each patient, including breasts, cervix, testes, prostate, and ovaries to determine which screening tests are indicated. Primary care providers should offer routine screening tests at appropriate intervals during all stages of transition.[110] See Tables 12.2 and Table 12.3 for a summary of screening recommendations for transgender patients.

USE OF GUIDELINES

Preventative care guidelines are published by many professional medical associations, specialty societies, governmental agencies, national task forces, and professional consensus panels. We base the recommendations in this chapter on the United States Preventative Services Task Force (USPSTF) guidelines.[126]

The USPSTF systematically reviews evidence for the effectiveness of screening tests, and develops recommendations for clinical preventative services. Although their recommendations are sometimes controversial, these guidelines are widely followed. Other countries may follow different national standards. The USPSTF does not make specific recommendations for screening tests for transgender patients.

TABLE 12.2	Preventative Care and Monitoring for Patients on Testosterone (Female-to-Male)
Parameter	**Recommendation**
Erythrocytosis	Complete blood count every 3 months first year, then annually
Cholesterol	Periodic screening ages 40–75
Hypertension	Usual treatment
Testosterone level	Consider yearly screen to avoid levels greater than 1,000 ng/dL (check midway between shots)
Breast cancer screening	No screening mammograms after mastectomy Routine mammography starting age 50 prior to mastectomy
Colon cancer screening	Colonoscopy or fecal occult testing starting age 50
Osteoporosis	Screen if post-oophorectomy, or has had an interruption in testosterone therapy
Liver function	Consider annual screening
Diabetes screening	Per usual guidelines for general population

TABLE 12.3	Preventative Care and Monitoring for Patients on Feminizing Hormones (Male-to-Female)	
Parameter	**Recommendation**	
Cholesterol	Periodic screening ages 40–75	
Hypertension	Treat intensively, to keep blood pressure below 140/90	
Breast cancer	Screening not universally recommended; consider screening age 50–75 in patients with other risk factors, or who request screening after discussion of risks and benefits	
Colon cancer	Colonoscopy or fecal occult testing starting age 50	
Prostate cancer	Screening not recommended	
Osteoporosis	Screen if postorchiectomy	
Prolactin	Obtain baseline level and monitor for clinical signs	
Hormone levels	Monitor testosterone (goal <50 ng/dL) and estradiol (goal 100-200 pg/mL) at 3, 6, and 12 months, then annually	
Creatinine, potassium	Periodically if on spironolactone to monitor for hyperkalemia and renal insufficiency	
Diabetes screening	Per usual guidelines for the general population	

PREVENTION OF CARDIOVASCULAR DISEASE

Routine clinical guidelines for the screening and treatment of obesity, hyperlipidemia, hypertension, diabetes, and tobacco abuse are followed for all transgender patients. If patients have significant CV risk factors, clinicians should recommend therapeutic lifestyle changes, such as increased exercise, dietary changes, and weight loss.

Postmenopausal cisgender woman on hormone replacement therapy have increased rates of stroke, CV events, and VTE, with excess cardiac events occurring in women greater than 10 years post-menopause.[127] Studies of transgender women on estrogen show mixed results. One case-control study showed an increase in cerebrovascular events, but not cardiovascular events.[80] A second long-term study (over 11 years) showed a 12% rate of CV and/or thromboembolic complications.[121] The majority of patients with CV events were smokers. A third study found an increased CV risk in transgender women on estrogen compared with the standardized risk of the general population, but only in those using ethinyl estradiol, an estrogen preparation no longer recommended for GAHT.[78] The overall quality of relevant studies is low as most data come from observational studies rather than randomized controlled trials.

Further prospective studies are needed to delineate levels of increased risk for CV events with feminizing treatment.[81,112] As the benefits of GAHT are well established, efforts should be taken to minimize CV risk to allow for continuation of therapy. We recommend counseling all transgender women with CV risk factors on risk reduction prior to initiating GAHT, and monitoring them closely over time.[110] While not evidence-based some experts recommend the use of prophylactic aspirin (81 mg) for transgender women over 50 who are on estrogen.

HYPERLIPIDEMIA

The USPSTF recommends periodic screening for hyperlipidemia for all patients between the ages of 40 and 75, with one or more CV risk factors.[126] For those at high risk for CV disease, earlier screening is recommended. Statins should be prescribed if the risk of a CV event provided by a risk calculator is greater than 7.5% over 10 years.[128]

Use of a CV risk calculator brings up three questions: (1) Which calculator to use? (2) What is the accuracy of the estimated risk? And (3) which gender should be used in the calculation? Over 25 different risk calculators exist, providing inconsistent absolute risk estimates.[129] The Framingham Risk Calculator and the American College of Cardiology/American Heart Association (ACC/AHA) CV calculator are most often used, but data suggest that calculators overestimate risk for CV events, and no studies have been performed to assess the accuracy of these tools for transgender people.[130] When asked to choose a gender for CV calculations, choices include (1) the sex assigned at birth, (2) the experienced gender, if the patient has had hormonal or surgical interventions, or (3) the calculation of two separate scores (male and female) with determination of an average score of the two.

We recommend using gender assigned at birth in risk calculators. There is a difference in CV risk between cisgender men and cisgender women, with cisgender men having a higher risk than cisgender women. Estrogen used by transgender women does not decrease the risk of CV events, while testosterone also may be neutral in terms of CV risk for transgender men.[78] Thus gender-affirming hormonal treatment does not narrow the difference in risk between natal males and natal females. For this reason, using the gender assigned at birth rather than the experienced gender in risk calculators may give a more accurate assessment of CV risk. Due to a lack of data, this recommendation is not yet evidence-based.

HYPERTENSION

Preliminary research shows no clinically significant effect of GAHT on blood pressure.[81] Clinicians should follow standard monitoring and treatment protocols. Spironolactone use in transgender women may have useful antihypertensive effects.

DIABETES

One published study shows increased insulin resistance or glucose intolerance in transgender women on estrogen, although the actual risk for diabetes is not defined.[87] Some experts recommend annual diabetic screening for transgender women on estrogen.[110] Screening options include fasting glucose, hemoglobinA1C, or 2-hour oral glucose tolerance test.[131]

For transgender men, routine diabetic screening guidelines should be followed. Recommendations include periodic screening for overweight or obese individuals (BMI greater than 25 kg/m^2) between the ages of 40 and 70.[131]

SMOKING

Thirty percent of transgender people use tobacco, compared with 20% of the general population.[1] Seventy percent of the transgender smokers report a desire to quit, similar to the general population.[1] We counsel all patients to stop smoking, and offer appropriate pharmacotherapy and/or referrals for behavioral interventions.

CANCER SCREENING

Although studies are limited, GAHT has not been associated with an increase in overall cancer mortality.[78] Screening recommendations are usually based on the presence or absence of body parts, rather than sex assigned at birth or experienced gender. Few studies have been done to assess the efficacy of cancer screening in transgender people. Despite the fears of patients and clinicians, only a few cases of hormone-related cancers have been reported in transgender people, and the risks of hormone-dependent cancers in this population are unknown.[132]

Breast Cancer Screening for Transgender Women on Estrogen

Data regarding the risk/benefit of screening mammograms for transgender women are inconclusive. Cisgender men have a breast cancer rate of 2/100,000 years, and cisgender women have a rate of 125/100,000 years. The rate of breast cancer in transgender women on estrogens has not been defined. Three studies show little increase in risk of breast cancer in transgender women treated with GAHT.[80,133,134] We advise caution in generalizing from this data, as few of the studies were prospective, and in some, the average age of patients was young, leading to possible underestimation of cancer rates.

Some experts recommend mammograms every 2 years for transgender women over the age of 50, who have been on feminizing hormone for 5 to 10 years.[112] One may consider more aggressive screening for transgender women with additional risk factors, such as a strong family history or carriers of the BRCA mutations. Many providers take a cautious approach, which includes routine screening following the guidelines for cisgender women. However, the risks of mammography, including false positives with associated emotional distress and unnecessary procedures/cost, may outweigh the potential benefits, if breast cancer rates are closer to cisgender men than cisgender women. Ongoing research is required to determine the benefit of mammography in this population.

There is insufficient evidence to recommend clinician breast exams or self-breast examination in cisgender or transgender patients.[135] In our office, we perform breast exams as part of general education or to address other concerns women have regarding their breasts.

Breast Cancer Screening for Transgender Men

The risk of breast cancer for transgender men on testosterone has not been defined. Screening recommendations for transgender men who have not had chest reconstruction surgery are the same as for cisgender women: biennial screening mammograms from age 50 to 74.[126]

Chest surgery for transgender men usually includes subcutaneous mastectomy with masculine chest reconstruction. Residual breast tissue is often left in the nipple-alveolar complex and other parts of the chest.[110] Both patients and providers must be aware that breast cancer can develop in this residual tissue. Some experts recommend periodic examinations for axillary lymphadenopathy and chest masses.[110] Screening mammography after bilateral mastectomy is not recommended.[136]

Gynecologic Cancer Screening for Transgender Men

Pap smears and human papilloma virus (HPV) testing are recommended for transgender men with a cervix, following the same guidelines for cisgender women.[137] Due to patient and provider discomfort, Pap tests are performed less frequently on transgender men than on cisgender women.[138] In addition, there is a higher rate of unsatisfactory Pap smears (10%) in transgender men, due to the physical changes resulting from testosterone, and from discomfort with exams.[139] Insurance companies may deny coverage for Pap smears due to a mismatch between gender markers and this gender-specific testing. Clinicians should counsel all transgender men on the importance of regular cervical cancer screening, and discuss ways to assist patients with anxiety around testing. We offer relaxation techniques or light oral sedation to those patients who are fearful of vaginal inspection and speculum exams.

The USPTF recommends that clinicians defer all Pap screening until age 21. Between ages of 21 and 29, they recommend Pap smears without HPV testing every 3 years.[126] For patients aged 30 to 65 at low risk for cervical cancer, recommendations include cotesting with Pap smear and HPV testing every 3 to 5 years.[126,140] More frequent screening can be offered to people who are at higher risk due to sexual behavior.[139]

For patients at low risk for cervical cancer (e.g. never sexually active) and high levels of anxiety with vaginal exam, we recommend a discussion regarding the risks/benefits of screening. Less frequent or curtailment of screening may be appropriate.[110] Consider hysterectomy for transgender men with a high risk of cervical cancer who have persistent unsatisfactory Pap smears, or are unable to tolerate exams.

The HPV vaccination is recommended for all adolescents and young adults up to age 26.[141] The two-dose schedule can be used when initiated between ages 9 and 14. For ages 15 to 26, the three-dose schedule is recommended.

Screening for endometrial cancer in asymptomatic transgender men is not recommended.[22] Persistent vaginal bleeding despite 6 to 12 months of testosterone therapy, or return of menses after a significant period of amenorrhea without missed doses of testosterone, should initiate a workup for abnormal uterine bleeding. If no pathological etiology is identified, clinicians can treat menstrual bleeding with progesterone or aromatase inhibitors, or consider endometrial ablation or hysterectomy.[22]

Some raise theoretical concerns about the risk of endometrial hyperplasia in transgender men, resulting from unopposed estrogen through aromatization of testosterone. One case report describes endometrial cancer that presented in a 51-year-old transgender man with vaginal spotting after 7 years of testosterone therapy.[142] However, no increased risk for endometrial cancer has been shown, and endometrial atrophy, rather than hyperplasia, is seen in a large proportion (45%) of transgender men on testosterone.[132] Providers should be aware that obesity, advanced age, family history of uterine cancer, and polycystic ovary syndrome increase the risk for endometrial cancer, and carry a higher index of suspicion for patients with these risk factors.[143]

The USPSTF does not recommend screening for ovarian cancer in cisgender women.[126] While there have been case reports of ovarian cancer in transgender men and concerns about testosterone's effect on ovarian architecture, a meta-analysis did not show any association between polycystic ovary syndrome and ovarian cancer.[143–145] There is no evidence to support screening transgender men for ovarian cancer.

Screening for Colon Cancer

Screening recommendations for colon cancer in transgender patients are the same as for the general population. Screening with colonoscopy, sigmoidoscopy, or fecal occult blood testing should be performed between the ages of 50 and 75.[146]

Prostate Cancer Screening for Transgender Women

The USPSTF recommends that clinicians have a discussion with cisgender men ages 55-69 about the benefits and risks of prostate-specific antigen (PSA) screening and not screen those who do not express a preference for screening. For cisgender men older than 69, PSA screening is not recommended. Digital rectal exam is not recommended for screening for prostate cancer.[126]

There is no indication that GAHT or gender-affirming surgeries increase the rate of prostate cancer. Due to a lack of evidence-based recommendations for transgender women, we follow the above USPSTF recommendations. Patients at higher risk due to ethnicity (e.g. African Americans) or family history may benefit from screening. Providers should remember that even after full hormonal and surgical transition, transgender women still have prostates, which can become hypertrophic and/or malignant. Estrogen therapy does not appear to induce hyperplasia in the prostate.[147] There are case reports of benign prostatic hypertrophy and prostate cancer in transgender women. Clinicians should be aware that orchiectomy and some antiandrogen medications reduce PSA levels, making this a less reliable tool for evaluating symptomatic patients or individuals at high risk for prostate cancer.[148]

Screening for Testicular Cancer

Testicular exams are not recommended as a screening tool for testicular cancer in cisgender men.[126] There are a few reports of testicular tumors in transgender women, but the risks of cancer in this population are not well defined.[23] For patients with severe anatomical dysphoria, testicular exams may be appropriate, but there is no evidence to support routine testicular exams for transgender women.

OSTEOPOROSIS SCREENING

Both estrogen and testosterone therapy help maintain bone density. Recommendations for screening for osteoporosis depend on the presence or absence of gonads, and the use of GAHT.

The USPSTF does not recommend screening cisgender men with average risk for osteoporosis. Studies for transgender women show a neutral or positive effect on BMD with GAHT.[149–151] Therefore, we do not recommend screening for osteoporosis in transgender women on feminizing hormones with intact testes.

Consistent testosterone therapy maintains or increases the density of bones in transgender men.[151,152] However, the magnitude of testosterone's effect on bone density is unclear. We consider screening transgender men on testosterone at age 65 with dual-energy X-ray absorptiometry (DEXA) scans if they have had a significant interruption in their testosterone therapy.[110] Transgender men who have not taken testosterone should be screened at age 65, or earlier, if additional risk factors are present.

The risk of osteoporosis increases in patients who have had oophorectomy or orchiectomy, as sex hormones are instrumental in maintaining bone health. All patients with gonadectomies should be screened with DEXA scans starting at age 65, even if on GAHT. Younger patients who have had gonadectomy, and who have been off GAHT for 5 or more years, should be screened starting at age 50.[110]

Screening can also be offered to transgender patients who have increased risk factors for osteoporosis. Risks for osteoporosis include smoking, alcohol use, lack of exercise, Caucasian or Asian ethnicity, and parental fracture history. Adequate dietary calcium and vitamin D intake and weight-bearing exercise should be encouraged in all individuals.

Lifelong therapy with GAHT is recommended for all individuals who have had an orchiectomy or oophorectomy.[110] Low doses of estrogens or testosterone may be adequate for protection of bone density in these patients.[124] Luteinizing hormone (LH) may be used as a measure for adequacy of hormone replacement related to bone health, since low LH levels correlate closely with high bone density (inverse correlation).[97]

Conclusion

As primary care clinicians, we our uniquely situated to assist transgender patients, due to our breadth of training, our ability to bring a biopsychosocial perspective into the office, and our commitment to learn new skills to meet the needs of diverse patients. Clinicians with a basic knowledge about the medical, social, legal, and spiritual challenges of transgender people can reduce barriers to care, create affirming environments, and have a profound impact on the health of these patients.

Management of gender dysphoria requires a different medical paradigm. Typically patients from the general population present to us because they are sick, and we assist in managing their disease. But gender variance is not an illness. These patients may suffer, but they are not sick. The goal of medical interventions is an enhanced sense of well-being, and a decrease in gender dysphoria. Yes, we prescribe therapies and monitor response to treatment, but for our patients, gender transition is a journey of self-discovery and the pursuit of authentic expression. Bearing witness to this process is a profound and moving experience for us, as clinicians and human beings. It challenges us to question and explore our own attitudes and beliefs—another transformative process—and one that enriches our lives.

Some transgender people use the term *gender euphoria* to describe the relief and well-being that comes from medical treatment. A transgender medical student described his experience to us like this:

Gender euphoria is the opposite of gender dysphoria. A transgender person experiences dysphoria when their body or presentation causes them distress—for instance, when they are reminded of the presence of their original, primary, or secondary sex characteristics, or when others incorrectly assume their gender identity. Gender dysphoria is unique and exquisitely painful, and gender euphoria is equally unique and exquisitely soothing. It is a sense of "rightness" in the same way dysphoria is "wrongness," and just as dysphoria may provoke a magnitude of distress that should not be known to any person, euphoria is often accompanied by joy of a kind unexpected by a transgender person before they undergo treatment. The burden of years is gone; before treatment the burden is so omnipresent that it begins to seem inescapable, so the escape is something like a miracle. It might seem mysterious to a cisgender person how the feeling that one's body correlates with one's gender could be so remarkable—cisgender people, after all, feel this all the time—but to a transgender person who starts out at the bottom of a dark pit of dysphoria, even the elevation to level ground seems like an incredible leap. The most innocuous things to a cisgender person—being addressed by the correct pronouns, wearing swimsuits to the beach, signing a document with the correct name—are sources of great pleasure for a trans person, and because these innocuous things are everywhere, there is much to take pleasure in. (R. Richards, personal communication, April 4, 2017)

As clinicians, we apply for and are granted hospital "privileges," implying that the work of caring for other human beings is a source of honor and joy. We are privileged by our window into the lives of our patients—the births, the deaths, the struggles, the joys. We encourage all primary care clinicians to develop the skills that will enable them to care for transgender patients in their practices.

REFERENCES

1. Grant JM, Mottet L, Tanis JE, Harrison J, Herman J, Keisling M. *Injustice at every turn: a report of the National Transgender Discrimination Survey.* National Center for Transgender Equality: Washington; 2011.
2. James SE, Herman JL, Rankin S, Keisling M, Mottet L, Anafi M. *The report of the 2015 US Transgender Survey.* National Center for Transgender Equality: Washington; 2016.
3. Zucker KJ, Lawrence AA. Epidemiology of gender identity disorder: recommendations for the standards of care of the World Professional Association for Transgender Health. *Int J Transgenderism.* 2009;11:8–18.
4. Hart D. Toward better care for lesbian, gay, bisexual and transgender patients. *Minn Med.* 2013;96:42–45.
5. Coleman E, Bockting W, Botzer M, et al. Standards of care for the health of transsexual, transgender, and gender-nonconforming people, version 7. *Int J Transgenderism.* 2012; 13:165–232.
6. Conron KJ, Scott G, Stowell GS, Landers SJ. Transgender health in Massachusetts: results from a household probability sample of adults. *Am J Public Health.* 2012;102:118–122.
7. Olyslager, F, Conway L. (2007) On the Calculation of the Prevalence of Transsexualism, paper presented at the World Professional Association of Transgender Health 20th International Symposium, Chicago, Illinois; September, 2007. http://ai.eecs.umich.edu/people/conway/TS/Prevalence/Reports/Prevalence%20of%20Transsexualism.pdf. Accessed 18.11.18.
8. Hatzenbuehler ML, Bellatorre A, Lee Y, Finch BK, Muennig P, Fiscella K. Structural stigma and all-cause mortality in sexual minority populations. *Soc Sci Med.* 2014;103: 33–41.
9. Makadon HJ, Mayer KH, Potter J, Goldhammer H. *The Fenway Guide to Lesbian, Gay, Bisexual, and Transgender Health.* Philadelphia: ACP Press; 2008.
10. Parent MC, DeBlaere C, Moradi B. Approaches to research on intersectionality: perspectives on gender, LGBT, and racial/ethnic identities. *Sex Roles.* 2013;68:639–645.
11. Metzl JM, Hansen H. Structural competency: theorizing a new medical engagement with stigma and inequality. *Soc Sci Med.* 2014;103: 126–133.
12. Rondahl G. Students inadequate knowledge about lesbian, gay, bisexual and transgender persons. *Int J Nurs Educ Scholarsh.* 2009;6. https://doi.org/10.2202/1548-923X.1718 article11.
13. Obedin-Maliver J, Goldsmith ES, Stewart L, et al. Lesbian, gay, bisexual, and transgender-related content in undergraduate medical education. *JAMA.* 2011;306:971–977.
14. Solursh DS, Ernst JL, Lewis RW, et al. The human sexuality education of physicians in North American medical schools. *Int J Impot Res.* 2003;15:S41.
15. Sequeira GM, Chakraborti C, Panunti BA. Integrating lesbian, gay, bisexual, and transgender (LGBT) content into undergraduate medical school curricula: a qualitative study. *Ochsner J.* 2012;12:379–382.
16. Bauer GR, Hammond R, Travers R, Kaay M, Hohenadel KM, Boyce M. "I don't think this is theoretical; this is our lives": how erasure impacts health care for transgender people. *J Assoc Nurses AIDS Care JANAC.* 2009;20:348–361. https://doi.org/10.1016/j.jana. 2009.07.004.
17. Asscheman H, Giltay EJ, Megens JA, et al. A long-term follow-up study of mortality in transsexuals receiving treatment with cross-sex hormones. *Eur J Endocrinol.* 2011; 164: 635–642.
18. Asscheman H, Gooren LJG, Eklund PLE. Mortality and morbidity in transsexual patients with cross-gender hormone treatment. *Metabolism.* 1989;38:869–873.
19. Egleston BL, Dunbrack Jr L, Hall MJ. Clinical trials that explicitly exclude gay and lesbian patients. *N Engl J Med.* 2010;362: 1054–1055.
20. Gupta S, Imborek KL, Krasowski MD. Challenges in transgender healthcare: the pathology perspective. *Lab Med.* 2016;47(3):180–188.
21. Hembree WC, Cohen-Ketteris P, Gooren L, et al. Endocrine Treatment of Gender-Dysphoric/Gender-Incongruent Persons: An Endocrine Society Clinical Practice Guideline. *J Clin Endocrinol Metab.* 2017;102:3869–3903.
22. Guidelines for the primary and gender-affirming care of transgender and gender non-binary people. http://transhealth.ucsf.edu/trans?page=guidelines-home; n.d. Accessed 22.03.2017.
23. Wolf-Gould CS, Wolf-Gould CH. A transgender woman with testicular cancer: a new twist on an old problem. *LGBT Health.* 2015;3: 90–95. https://doi.org/10.1089/lgbt.2015.0057.
24. Gehi PS, Arkles G. Unraveling injustice: race and class impact of Medicaid exclusions of transition-related health care for transgender people. *Sex Res Soc Policy.* 2007;4:7–35.
25. Garofalo R. Tipping points in caring for the gender-nonconforming child and adolescent. *Pediatr Ann.* 2014;43:227–229. https://doi.org/10.3928/00904481-20140522-06.
26. Steinmetz, K. 2014, 'The Transgender Tipping Point', *Time* 9 June, 2014.
27. Cretella MA, Van Meter Q, McHugh P. Gender ideology harms children. American College of Pediatricians. https://www.acpeds.org/the-college-speaks/position-statements/gender-ideology-harms-children; 2017. Accessed 05.03.17.
28. Bau I. *Building Patient-Centered Medical Homes for Lesbian, Gay, Bisexual, and Transgender Patients and Families.* National LGBT Health Education Center: Boston, MA; 2016.
29. *Fenway Health.* Fenway health: your care your community. http://fenwayhealth.org/; n.d. Accessed 23.03.17.
30. *Mazzoni Center.* <https://www.mazzonicenter.org/>; n.d. Accessed 23.03.17.
31. *Bassett Healthcare Network.* Transgender health services. http://www.bassett.org/medical/services/transgender-health-services/; n.d. Accessed 23.03.17.
32. LGBT Task Force. Examining transgender insurance coverage. *Health Care N Y.* 2015. http://hcfany.org/lgbt-task-force-examining-transgender-insurance-coverage/. Accessed 17.11.18.
33. Institute of Medicine. *The Health of Lesbian, Gay, Bisexual, and Transgender People: Building a Foundation for Better Understanding.* Washington: National Academies Press; 2011.
34. *Human Rights Campaign.* HHS to include sexual orientation & gender identity in meaningful use of electronic health program. http://www.hrc.org/blog/hhs-to-include-sexual-orientation-gender-identity-in-meaningful-use-of-elec/; n.d. Accessed 02.04.17.
35. Green ER, Maurer L. *The Teaching Transgender Toolkit: A Facilitator's Guide to Increasing Knowledge, Decreasing Prejudice & Building Skills.* Planned Parenthood of the Southern Finger Lakes: Ithaca, NY; 2015.
36. The Genderbread Person v3. Its Pronounced Metrosexual. http://itspronouncedmetrosexual.com/2015/03/the-genderbread-person-v3/; n.d. Accessed 02.04.17.
37. Hollenbach A, Eckstrand K, Dreger A. *Implementing Curricular and Institutional Climate Changes to Improve Health Care for Individuals Who Are LGBT, Gender Nonconforming, or Born with DSD.* Association of American Medical Colleges: Washington; 2014.
38. Safer J, Pearce E. A simple curriculum content change increased medical student comfort with transgender medicine. *Endocr Pract.* 2013;19:633–637.
39. Goldberg JM. Training community-based clinicians in transgender care. *Int J Transgenderism.* 2006;9:219–231. https://doi.org/10.1300/J485v09n03_10.
40. TLDEF. About TLDEF. http://tldef.org/page.php?id=2; n.d. Accessed 18.03.17.
41. *American Civil Liberties Union.* https://www.aclu.org/; n.d. Accessed 18.03.17.
42. Kendell K. Homepage. National Center for Lesbian Rights. http://www.nclrights.org/; n.d. Accessed 18.03.17.
43. *Lambda Legal.* http://www.lambdalegal.org/node/24885; n.d. Accessed 18.03.17.
44. HHS.gov. Advancing LGBT health and well-being: 2016 report of the HHS LGBT Policy Coordinating Committee. 2016. https://www.hhs.gov/programs/topic-sites/lgbt/reports/health-objectives-2016.html. Accessed 01.04.17.
45. *Human Rights Campaign.* Healthcare equality index 2017. http://www.hrc.org/hei/; n.d. Accessed 29.03.2017.
46. Cohen-Ketenis PT. Gender identity disorder in DSM? *J Am Acad Child Adolesc Psychiatry.* 2001;40:391.
47. Zucker KJ, Bradley SJ. *Gender Identity Disorder and Psychosexual Problems in Children and Adolescents.* New York: Guilford Press; 1995.
48. Drummond KD, Bradley SJ, Peterson-Badali M, Zucker KJ. A follow-up study of girls with gender identity disorder. *Dev Psychol.* 2008;44:34.
49. Wallien MS, Cohen-Ketenis PT. Psychosexual outcome of gender-dysphoric children. *J Am Acad Child Adolesc Psychiatry.* 2008; 47:1413–1423.
50. McGoldrick M, Gerson R, Petry SS. *Genograms: Assessment and Intervention.* New York: WW Norton & Company; 2008.

51. Williamson C. Providing care to transgender persons: a clinical approach to primary care, hormones, and HIV management. *J Assoc Nurses AIDS Care*. 2010;21:221–229. https://doi.org/10.1016/j.jana.2010.02.004.

52. Bowers M, Post-op care (GRS). Male to female. http://marcibowers.com/mtf/your-surgery/post-op-care/; n.d. Accessed 14.03.17.

53. Herek GM. Facts about homosexuality and mental health 1997. http://psychology.ucdavis.edu/rainbow/html/facts_mental_health.html. Accessed 15.03.17.

54. Group for advancement of psychiatry. LGBT mental health syllabus. http://www.aglp.org/gap/1_history/; n.d. Accessed 15.03.2017.

55. Green R. In Memoriam: Judd Marmor, M.D. *Arch Sex Behav*. 2004;33:327–328. https://doi.org/10.1023/B:ASEB.0000029073.76131.59.

56. Gender incongruence of childhood. ILGA. http://ilga.org/what-we-do/gender-identity-and-gender-expression-program/gender-incongruence-childhood/; n.d. Accessed 22.03.17.

57. Wylie K, Knudson G, Khan SI, Bonierbale M, Watanyusakul S, Baral S. Serving transgender people: clinical care considerations and service delivery models in transgender health. *Lancet*. 2016;388:401–411. https://doi.org/10.1016/S0140-6736(16)00682-6.

58. Change of Sex Marker. https://travel.state.gov/content/passports/en/passports/information/gender.html; n.d. Accessed 24.05.17.

59. How do I change my gender on Social Security's records? https://faq.ssa.gov/en-us/Topic/article/KA-01453; n.d. Accessed 17.11.18.

60. Leavitt F, Berger JC, Hoeppner JA, Northrop G. Presurgical adjustment in male transsexuals with and without hormonal treatment. *J Nerv Ment Dis*. 1980;168:693–697.

61. Gómez-Gil E, Zubiaurre-Elorza L, Esteva I, et al. Hormone-treated transsexuals report less social distress, anxiety and depression. *Psychoneuroendocrinology*. 2012;37:662–670. https://doi.org/10.1016/j.psyneuen.2011.08.010.

62. Gorin-Lazard A, Baumstarck K, Boyer L, et al. Hormonal therapy is associated with better self-esteem, mood, and quality of life in transsexuals. *J Nerv Ment Dis*. 2013;201:996–1000. https://doi.org/10.1097/NMD.0000000000000046.

63. Fisher AD, Castellini G, Bandini E, et al. Cross-sex hormonal treatment and body uneasiness in individuals with gender dysphoria. *J Sex Med*. 2014;11:709–719. https://doi.org/10.1111/jsm.12413.

64. Colizzi M, Costa R, Todarello O. Transsexual patients' psychiatric comorbidity and positive effect of cross-sex hormonal treatment on mental health: results from a longitudinal study. *Psychoneuroendocrinology*. 2014;39:65–73. https://doi.org/10.1016/j.psyneuen.2013.09.029.

65. Mocquot P, Moricard R. Etude préliminaire des effects provoques par l'hormone male sur les troubles fonctionnels urinaires de femme et de l'utilisation males en gynecologie. *Bull Soc Obst Gynéc*. 1936;25:787.

66. Dillon M, Jivaka L, Stryker S. *Out of the Ordinary: A Life of Gender and Spiritual Transitions*. 1st ed. New York: Fordham University Press; 2016.

67. Snyder PJ. Testosterone treatment of male hypogonadism. UpToDate. https://www.uptodate.com/contents/testosterone-treatment-of-male-hypogonadism?source=search_result&search=testosterone&selectedTitle=5~150; n.d. Accessed 26.02.17.

68. Finkelstein JS, Lee H, Burnett-Bowie S-AM, et al. Gonadal steroids and body composition, strength, and sexual function in men. *N Engl J Med*. 2013;369:1011–1022. https://doi.org/10.1056/NEJMoa1206168.

69. Khosla S, Melton LJ, Riggs BL. Estrogens and bone health in men. *Calcif Tissue Int*. 2001;69:189–192.

70. Donovan J, Goldstein BG, Goldstein AO. Androgenetic alopecia in men: pathogenesis, clinical features, and diagnosis. UpToDate. https://www.uptodate.com/contents/androgenetic-alopecia-in-men-pathogenesis-clinical-features-and-diagnosis?source=see_link; n.d. Accessed 26.02.17.

71. Irwig MS. Testosterone therapy for transgender men. *Lancet Diabetes Endocrinol*. 2017;5(4):301–311. https://doi.org/10.1016/S2213-8587(16)00036-X.

72. Unger CA. Hormone therapy for transgender patients. *Transl Androl Urol*. 2016;5:877–884. https://doi.org/10.21037/tau.2016.09.04.

73. Keo-Meier CL, Herman LI, Reisner SL, Pardo ST, Sharp C, Babcock JC. Testosterone treatment and MMPI-2 improvement in transgender men: a prospective controlled study. *J Consult Clin Psychol*. 2015;83:143–156. https://doi.org/10.1037/a0037599.

74. Manieri C, Castellano E, Crespi C, et al. Medical treatment of subjects with gender identity disorder: the experience in an Italian Public Health Center. *Int J Transgenderism*. 2014;15:53–65. https://doi.org/10.1080/15532739.2014.899174.

75. Ullah MI, Riche DM, Koch CA. Transdermal testosterone replacement therapy in men. *Drug Des Devel Ther*. 2014;8:101–112. https://doi.org/10.2147/DDDT.S43475.

76. Surampudi P, Swerdloff RS, Wang C. An update on male hypogonadism therapy. *Expert Opin Pharmacother*. 2014;15:1247–1264.

77. Gooren LJ, Giltay EJ, Bunck MC. Long-term treatment of transsexuals with cross-sex hormones: extensive personal experience. *J Clin Endocrinol Metab*. 2008;93:19–25.

78. Asscheman H, Giltay EJ, Megens JAJ, de Ronde WP, van Trotsenburg MAA, Gooren LJG. A long-term follow-up study of mortality in transsexuals receiving treatment with cross-sex hormones. *Eur J Endocrinol*. 2011;164:635–642. https://doi.org/10.1530/EJE-10-1038.

79. Dhejne C, Lichtenstein P, Boman M, Johansson ALV, Långström N, Landén M. Long-term follow-up of transsexual persons undergoing sex reassignment surgery: cohort study in Sweden. *PLoS One*. 2011;6. e16885. https://doi.org/10.1371/journal.pone.0016885.

80. Wierckx K, Elaut E, Declercq E, et al. Prevalence of cardiovascular disease and cancer during cross-sex hormone therapy in a large cohort of trans persons: a case-control study. *Eur J Endocrinol*. 2013;169:471–478. https://doi.org/10.1530/EJE-13-0493.

81. Elamin MB, Garcia MZ, Murad MH, Erwin PJ, Montori VM. Effect of sex steroid use on cardiovascular risk in transsexual individuals: a systematic review and meta-analyses. *Clin Endocrinol (Oxf)*. 2010;72:1–10. https://doi.org/10.1111/j.1365-2265.2009.03632.x.

82. Mueller A, Haeberle L, Zollver H, et al. Effects of intramuscular testosterone undecanoate on body composition and bone mineral density in female-to-male transsexuals. *J Sex Med*.

2010;7:3190–3198. https://doi.org/10.1111/j.1743-6109.2010.01912.x.

83. Pelusi C, Costantino A, Martelli V, et al. Effects of three different testosterone formulations in female-to-male transsexual persons. *J Sex Med*. 2014;11:3002–3011. https://doi.org/10.1111/jsm.12698.

84. Quirós C, Patrascioiu I, Mora M, et al. Effect of cross-sex hormone treatment on cardiovascular risk factors in transsexual individuals. Experience in a specialized unit in Catalonia. *Endocrinol Nutr*. 2015;62:210–216. https://doi.org/10.1016/j.endonu.2015.02.001.

85. Wierckx K, Van Caenegem E, Schreiner T, et al. Cross-sex hormone therapy in trans persons is safe and effective at short-time follow-up: results from the European network for the investigation of gender incongruence. *J Sex Med*. 2014;11:1999–2011. https://doi.org/10.1111/jsm.12571.

86. Fernández-Balsells MM, Murad MH, Lane M, et al. Adverse effects of testosterone therapy in adult men: a systematic review and meta-analysis. *J Clin Endocrinol Metab*. 2010;95:2560–2575. https://doi.org/10.1210/jc.2009-2575.

87. Elbers JMH, Giltay EJ, Teerlink T, et al. Effects of sex steroids on components of the insulin resistance syndrome in transsexual subjects. *Clin Endocrinol (Oxf)*. 2003;58:562–571.

88. Kennedy BJ, Gilbertsen AS. Increased erythropoiesis induced by androgenic-hormone therapy. *N Engl J Med*. 1957;256:719–726. https://doi.org/10.1056/NEJM195704182561601.

89. Gardner FH, Gorshein D. Regulation of erythropoiesis by androgens. *Trans Am Clin Climatol Assoc*. 1973;84:60–70.

90. Spivak JL. Polycythemia vera: myths, mechanisms, and management. *Blood*. 2002;100:4272–4290. https://doi.org/10.1182/blood-2001-12-0349.

91. Zoraster RM, Rison RA. Acute embolic cerebral ischemia as an initial presentation of polycythemia vera: a case report. *J Med Case Reports*. 2013;7:131. https://doi.org/10.1186/1752-1947-7-131.

92. Alvarez-Larrán A, Ancochea A, Angona A, et al. Red cell mass measurement in patients with clinically suspected diagnosis of polycythemia vera or essential thrombocythemia. *Haematologica*. 2012;97:1704–1707. https://doi.org/10.3324/haematol.2012.067348.

93. Tefferi A. Polycythemia vera: a comprehensive review and clinical recommendations. *Mayo Clin Proc*. 2003;78:174–194. https://doi.org/10.4065/78.2.174.

94. Pearson TC, Wetherley-Mein G. Vascular occlusive episodes and venous haematocrit in primary proliferative polycythaemia. *Lancet Lond Engl*. 1978;2:1219–1222.

95. Turner A, Chen TC, Barber TW, Malabanan AO, Holick MF, Tangpricha V. Testosterone increases bone mineral density in female-to-male transsexuals: a case series of 15 subjects. *Clin Endocrinol (Oxf)*. 2004;61:560–566. https://doi.org/10.1111/j.1365-2265.2004.02125.x.

96. Schlatterer K, Auer DP, Yassouridis A, von Werder K, Stalla GK. Transsexualism and osteoporosis. *Exp Clin Endocrinol Diabetes*. 1998;106:365–368. https://doi.org/10.1055/s-0029-1211999.

97. van Kesteren P, Lips P, Gooren LJ, Asscheman H, Megens J. Long-term follow-

up of bone mineral density and bone metabolism in transsexuals treated with cross-sex hormones. *Clin Endocrinol (Oxf)*. 1998;48: 347–354.

98. Perrone AM, Cerpolini S, Maria Salfi NC, et al. Effect of long-term testosterone administration on the endometrium of female-to-male (FtM) transsexuals. *J Sex Med*. 2009;6: 3193–3200. https://doi.org/10.1111/j.1743-6109.2009.01380.x.

99. Obedin-Maliver J, Makadon HJ. Transgender men and pregnancy. *Obstet Med*. 2016;9:4–8.

100. Light AD, Obedin-Maliver J, Sevelius JM, Kerns JL. Transgender men who experienced pregnancy after female-to-male gender transitioning. *Obstet Gynecol*. 2014;124:1120–1127.

101. Wierckx K, Van de Peer F, Verhaeghe E, et al. Short- and long-term clinical skin effects of testosterone treatment in trans men. *J Sex Med*. 2014;11:222–229. https://doi.org/10.1111/jsm.12366.

102. Futterweit W. Endocrine therapy of transsexualism and potential complications of long-term treatment. *Arch Sex Behav*. 1998;27:209–226.

103. Kapoor D, Goodwin E, Channer KS, Jones TH. Testosterone replacement therapy improves insulin resistance, glycaemic control, visceral adiposity and hypercholesterolaemia in hypogonadal men with type 2 diabetes. *Eur J Endocrinol*. 2006;154:899–906. https://doi.org/10.1530/eje.1.02166.

104. Lorentz SM, Weibert RT. Potentiation of warfarin anticoagulation by topical testosterone ointment. *Clin Pharm*. 1985;4:332–334.

105. Gooren L. Hormone treatment of the adult transsexual patient. *Horm Res*. 2005;64 (suppl 2):31–36. https://doi.org/10.1159/000087751.

106. Levy A, Crown A, Reid R. Endocrine intervention for transsexuals. *Clin Endocrinol (Oxf)*. 2003;59:409–418.

107. Asscheman H, T'Sjoen G, Lemaire A, et al. Venous thrombo-embolism as a complication of cross-sex hormone treatment of male-to-female transsexual subjects: a review. *Andrologia*. 2014;46:791–795. https://doi.org/10.1111/and.12150.

108. Graber EM. K+larity for spironolactone: at last!. *JAMA Dermatol*. 2015;151:926–927. https://doi.org/10.1001/jamadermatol.2015.35.

109. Rossouw JE, Anderson GL, Prentice RL, et al. Writing Group for the Women's Health Initiative Investigators. Risks and benefits of estrogen plus progestin in healthy postmenopausal women: principal results from the Women's Health Initiative randomized controlled trial. *JAMA*. 2002;288:321–333.

110. Ettner R, Monstrey S, Eyler E. eds. *Principles of Transgender Medicine and Surgery. 1st reprint ed*. New York: Routledge; 2007.

111. Van Kesteren PJ, Asscheman H, Megens JA, Gooren LJ. Mortality and morbidity in transsexual subjects treated with cross-sex hormones. *Clin Endocrinol (Oxf)*. 1997;47: 337–343.

112. Gooren LJ, Giltay EJ, Bunck MC. Long-term treatment of transsexuals with cross-sex hormones: extensive personal experience. *J Clin Endocrinol Metab*. 2008;93:19–25. https://doi.org/10.1210/jc.2007-1809.

113. Toorians A, Thomassen M, Zweegman S, et al. Venous thrombosis and changes of hemostatic variables during cross-sex hormone treatment in transsexual people. *J Clin Endocrinol Metab*. 2003;88:5723–5729.

114. Canonico M, Plu-Bureau G, Lowe GD, Scarabin P-Y. Hormone replacement therapy and risk of venous thromboembolism in postmenopausal women: systematic review and meta-analysis. *BMJ*. 2008;336:1227–1231.

115. Shatzel JJ, Connelly KJ, DeLoughery TG. Thrombotic issues in transgender medicine: a review. *Am J Hematol*. 2017;92:204–208. https://doi.org/10.1002/ajh.24593.

116. Asscheman H, Gooren LJ, Assies J, Smits JP, de Slegte R. Prolactin levels and pituitary enlargement in hormone-treated male-to-female transsexuals. *Clin Endocrinol (Oxf)*. 1988;28: 583–588.

117. García-Malpartida K, Martín-Gorgojo A, Rocha M, Gómez-Balaguer M, Hernández-Mijares A. Prolactinoma induced by estrogen and cyproterone acetate in a male-to-female transsexual. *Fertil Steril*. 2010;94:1097. e13–15, https://doi.org/10.1016/j.fertnstert.2010.01.076.

118. Cunha FS, Domenice S, Câmara VL, et al. Diagnosis of prolactinoma in two male-to-female transsexual subjects following high-dose cross-sex hormone therapy. *Andrologia*. 2015;47:680–684. https://doi.org/10.1111/and.12317.

119. Nota NM, Dekker MJHJ, Klaver M, et al. Prolactin levels during short- and long-term cross-sex hormone treatment: an observational study in transgender persons. *Andrologia*. 2017;49(6) https://doi.org/10.1111/and.12666.

120. *National LGBT Health Education Center*. The medical care of transgender persons. https://www.lgbthealtheducation.org/publication/transgender-sod/; n.d. Accessed 02.04.17.

121. Wierckx K, Mueller S, Weyers S, et al. Long-term evaluation of cross-sex hormone treatment in transsexual persons. *J Sex Med*. 2012;9:2641–2651.

122. Van Caenegem E, Wierckx K, Taes Y, et al. Preservation of volumetric bone density and geometry in trans women during cross-sex hormonal therapy: a prospective observational study. *Osteoporos Int*. 2015;26:35–47.

123. Gooren LJ. Hormonal sex reassignment. *Int J Transgenderism*. 1999;3:1–7.

124. Feldman J, Goldberg JM. Transgender primary medical care. *Int J Transgenderism*. 2006;9:3–34. https://doi.org/10.1300/J485v09n03_02.

125. Kaufman KD, Olsen EA, Whiting D, et al. Finasteride in the treatment of men with androgenetic alopecia. *J Am Acad Dermatol*. 1998;39:578–589.

126. *US Preventive Services Task Force*. Published recommendations. https://www.uspreventiveservicestaskforce.org/BrowseRec/Search; n.d. Accessed 25.03.17.

127. Martin KA, Rosenson RS. *Menopausal Hormone Therapy and Cardiovascular Risk*. Waltham, MA: UpToDate; 2017.

128. Stone NJ, Robinson JG, Lichtenstein AH, et al. 2013 ACC/AHA guideline on the treatment of blood cholesterol to reduce atherosclerotic cardiovascular risk in adults: a report of the American College of Cardiology/American Heart Association Task Force on Practice Guidelines. *J Am Coll Cardiol*. 2014;63: 2889–2934. https://doi.org/10.1016/j.jacc.2013.11.002.

129. Allan GM, Nouri F, Korownyk C, Kolber MR, Vandermeer B, McCormack J. Variation among cardiovascular risk calculators in relative risk increases with identical risk factor increases. *BMC Res Notes*. 2015;8:417. https://doi.org/10.1186/s13104-015-1401-8.

130. DeFilippis AP, Young R, Carrubba CJ, et al. An analysis of calibration and discrimination among multiple cardiovascular risk scores in a modern multiethnic cohort. *Ann Intern Med*. 2015;162:266. https://doi.org/10.7326/M14-1281.

131. *US Preventive Services Task Force*. Recommendations for primary care practice. https://www.uspreventiveservicestaskforce.org/Page/Name/recommendations; n.d. Accessed 22.05.17.

132. Mueller A, Gooren L. Hormone-related tumors in transsexuals receiving treatment with cross-sex hormones. *Eur J Endocrinol*. 2008;159: 197–202. https://doi.org/10.1530/EJE-08-0289.

133. Gooren LJ, van Trotsenburg MAA, Giltay EJ, van Diest PJ. Breast cancer development in transsexual subjects receiving cross-sex hormone treatment. *J Sex Med*. 2013;10: 3129–3134. https://doi.org/10.1111/jsm.12319.

134. Brown GR, Jones KT. Incidence of breast cancer in a cohort of 5,135 transgender veterans. *Breast Cancer Res Treat*. 2015;149: 191–198.

135. Tu S-P, Reisch LM, Taplin SH, Kreuter W, Elmore JG. Breast self-examination: self-reported frequency, quality, and associated outcomes. *J Cancer Educ Off J Am Assoc Cancer Educ*. 2006;21:175–181. https://doi.org/10.1207/s15430154jce2103_18.

136. Phillips J, Fein-Zachary VJ, Mehta TS, Littlehale N, Venkataraman S, Slanetz PJ. Breast imaging in the transgender patient. *Am J Roentgenol*. 2014;202:1149–1156.

137. *ACOG*. Health care for transgender individuals. http://www.acog.org/Resources-And-Publications/Committee-Opinions/Committee-on-Health-Care-for-Underserved-Women/Health-Care-for-Transgender-Individuals; n.d. Accessed 29.03.17.

138. Peitzmeier SM, Khullar K, Reisner SL, Potter J. Pap test use is lower among female-to-male patients than non-transgender women. *Am J Prev Med*. 2014;47:808–812. https://doi.org/10.1016/j.amepre.2014.07.031.

139. Peitzmeier SM, Reisner SL, Harigopal P, Potter J. Female-to-male patients have high prevalence of unsatisfactory Paps compared to non-transgender females: implications for cervical cancer screening. *J Gen Intern Med*. 2014;29:778–784. https://doi.org/10.1007/s11606-013-2753-1.

140. Schlichte MJ, Guidry J. Current cervical carcinoma screening guidelines. *J Clin Med*. 2015;4:918–932. https://doi.org/10.3390/jcm4050918.

141. Meites E. Use of a 2-dose schedule for human papillomavirus vaccination—updated recommendations of the Advisory Committee on Immunization Practices. *MMWR Morb Mortal Wkly Rep*. 2016;65(49):1405–1408. https://doi.org/10.15585/mmwr.mm6549a5.

142. Urban RR, Teng NNH, Kapp DS. Gynecologic malignancies in female-to-male transgender patients: the need of original gender surveillance. *Am J Obstet Gynecol*. 2011;204:e9–e12. https://doi.org/10.1016/j.ajog.2010.12.057.

143. Barry JA, Azizia MM, Hardiman PJ. Risk of endometrial, ovarian and breast cancer in women with polycystic ovary syndrome: a systematic review and meta-analysis. *Hum Reprod Update*. 2014;20:748–758. https://doi.org/10.1093/humupd/dmu012.

144. Hage JJ, Dekker JJ, Karim RB, Verheijen RH, Bloemena E. Ovarian cancer in female-to-male transsexuals: report of two cases. *Gynecol Oncol*. 2000;76:413–415. https://doi.org/10.1006/gyno.1999.5720.

145. Grynberg M, Fanchin R, Dubost G, et al. Histology of genital tract and breast tissue after long-term testosterone administration in a female-to-male transsexual population. *Reprod Biomed Online*. 2010;20:553–558. https://doi.org/10.1016/j.rbmo.2009.12.021.

146. *US Preventive Services Task Force*. Final update summary: colorectal cancer: screening. https://www.uspreventiveservicestaskforce.org/Page/Document/UpdateSummaryFinal/colorectal-cancer-screening; n.d. Accessed 10.05.17.

147. van Kesteren P, Meinhardt W, van der Valk P, Geldof A, Megens J, Gooren L. Effects of estrogens only on the prostates of aging men. *J Urol*. 1996;156:1349–1353.

148. Gooren L, Morgentaler A. Prostate cancer incidence in orchidectomised male-to-female transsexual persons treated with oestrogens. *Andrologia*. 2014;46:1156–1160. https://doi.org/10.1111/and.12208.

149. Wierckx K, Mueller S, Weyers S, et al. Long-term evaluation of cross-sex hormone treatment in transsexual persons. *J Sex Med*. 2012;9:2641–2651. https://doi.org/10.1111/j.1743-6109.2012.02876.x.

150. Jones RA, Schultz CG, Chatterton BE. A longitudinal study of bone density in reassigned transsexuals. *Bone*. 2009;44:S126. https://doi.org/10.1016/j.bone.2009.01.278.

151. Haraldsen IR, Haug E, Falch J, Egeland T, Opjordsmoen S. Cross-sex pattern of bone mineral density in early onset gender identity disorder. *Horm Behav*. 2007;52:334–343. https://doi.org/10.1016/j.yhbeh.2007.05.012.

152. Van Caenegem E, Wierckx K, Taes Y, et al. Bone mass, bone geometry, and body composition in female-to-male transsexual persons after long-term cross-sex hormonal therapy. *J Clin Endocrinol Metab*. 2012;97:2503–2511. https://doi.org/10.1210/jc.2012-1187.

13

Gynecologic Care for Transgender Patients

JUNO OBEDIN-MALIVER | GENE DE HAAN

Introduction: Role of the Gynecologist

Obstetricians, gynecologists (OBGYNs), and other women's health providers have a critical role in the care of transgender people. Transgender people, both transgender men and transgender women, have biophysiological and sociocultural needs, which can be addressed by the comprehensive and caring attention of the OBGYN provider.

For transgender men, the need for OBGYN care fits perfectly within an OBGYN's scope of practice; while 80% of transmale patients use hormones as part of medical transition, only 20% undergo surgical transition and so many retain their pelvic organs.[1] Providers should be aware that as transition progresses, attending a "women's health" care–focused space or receiving "gynecological" care may be uncomfortable or may worsen baseline dysphoria in their trans male patients.[2,3] Conversely, for transgender women, regardless of stage of transition, gynecologic care is often very affirming for them, and the experience may be very different.[3]

Organizations that have historically been defined as "Womens' health provider" organizations, including the American Congress of Obstetricians and Gynecologists (ACOG) and American College of Nurse-Midwives (ACNM) and associated educational institutions such as the Council on Resident Education in Obstetrics and Gynecology (CREOG) recognize the importance of providing care for transgender individuals. ACOG's Committee Opinion on the topic states, "obstetrician-gynecologists should be prepared to assist or refer transgender individuals for routine treatment and screening as well as hormonal and surgical therapy. Basic preventative services, like sexually transmitted infection testing and cancer screening, can be provided without specific expertise in transgender care. Hormonal and surgical therapies for transgender patients may be requested, but should be managed in consultation with health care providers with expertise in specialized care and treatment of transgender patients."[4] The ACNM statement similarly recognizes that "the most important thing all midwives can do to improve the health care outcomes of gender variant individuals is to use their skills to create care that is welcoming and accessible." The ACNM's statement also recognizes that "most members of this community require the same primary, mental, and sexual health care that all individuals need. Musculoskeletal, cardiovascular, breast, and pelvic care for individuals who have undergone hormonal and/or surgical therapy is typically straightforward but in some cases requires additional training. Similarly, administration of hormone therapy for gender affirmation is appropriate for primary care providers, including certified nurse-midwives/certified midwives (CNMs/CMs) who have undergone appropriate training."[5] Both of these organizations recognize that transgender health care is within the scope of practice for women's health care providers, but they also recognize that additional training might be necessary.

Education in this area is critically important as about half of transgender patient respondents in a large national survey reported having to educate their health providers about their health needs.[1] The World Professional Association for Transgender Health (WPATH) "strongly encourages the increased training and involvement of primary care providers in the area of feminizing/masculinizing hormone therapy."[6] Similarly, ACOG calls for increased education in its Committee Opinion 512 entitled "Health Care for Transgender Patients."[4] Meeting these calls for education, training objectives have been incorporated into the CREOG curriculum in order to cover core competencies for obstetrics and gynecology residents.[7] These guidelines are included in the "focused areas of gynecological care" under the larger theme of Primary and Preventative Ambulatory Health Care (Unit 2, Section 2.E).[7] Concerns regarding the phrasing of these CREOG objectives exist as it is unclear whether the objectives as they stand actually recognize and guide the care of transgender men (individuals who identify as male but were assigned female at birth)—they are mistakenly referred to as "women" in the guidelines. The guidelines are currently limited, but they are well intentioned as they recognize the importance of OBGYN care for people of all genders.[8] With time, they are likely to evolve and will become more accurate and comprehensive.

Currently, transgender health training for OBGYNs is not sufficient. Grimstad et al. surveyed OBGYN residency program directors and found that among the 39% of program directors that responded, 82% reported transgender health objectives were "very or somewhat important." However, only 70% were aware of CREOG specific objectives, and fewer still used specific educational activities such as lectures (63%) and reading materials (52%) to train residents on these topics.[9] Reassuringly, many more desired educational materials to be made available to their residents including enhanced reading materials, online modules, and patient exposure.[9] Similar findings are presented by Unger who surveyed practicing OBGYNs in nine academic obstetrics and gynecology departments in the United States about provider experience with and knowledge about caring for transgender individuals. Among the 141 respondents, most of whom were generalists and many practicing in an academic environment, approximately 74% of whom had been in practice for more than 5 years, 80% did not receive training on caring for transgender individuals during training.[10] She also reported that 11% of providers were unwilling to perform cervical cancer screening with Pap smear on transgender men, and 20% were unwilling to perform a routine breast examination on a transgender woman.[10] As information became more specific in the survey, fewer individuals were knowledgeable or able to extend their knowledge base to transgender patients—with 66% not knowing the requirements transgender patients must meet for gender affirming surgeries and 62% not knowing routine health maintenance screening recommendations (prostate cancer, diabetes, and hyperlipidemia for transgender women).[10] There is clearly a need to reassess how more current education objectives such as the CREOG guidelines influence the comfort level and preparedness of the practicing clinician. With time, this type of education should improve, and providers will hopefully be better equipped to care for this patient population.

Though education may be lacking, OBGYNs and other women's health providers already have the skills necessary to provide care for transgender individuals. It is simply the context of that care that must change. In the book Trans Bodies Trans Selves, Simon Adriane Ellis, a genderqueer certified nurse midwife, provides important information about acquiring the skillset necessary to practice within this new context and describes, "Five Tips for 'Women's Health' Providers Working with Gender-Variant Clients": (1) Focus on your skills and biases—by recognizing already existent skills necessary to care for gender-variant people and acknowledging potential triggers about patient's gender identity (GI) or expression that challenge comfort and professionalism; (2) Build trust and offer accommodations; (3) Keep your wording inclusive and honor patient preferences—by replacing terms like "women with the term people," considering appropriate pronoun use, and incorporating these changes into forms and ensuring consistent staff usage; (4) Don't let curiosity get the best of you—by maintaining "professional integrity" and "asking only what you need to know to provide excellent care"; (5) Don't pass the buck—by resisting the "urge to refer patients to 'someone who has more experience.'"[3]

Creating a Trans Friendly Practice

OBTAINING SEXUAL ORIENTATION AND GENDER IDENTITY INFORMATION

It is important to incorporate a comprehensive assessment of both sexual orientation (SO) and gender identity (GI) into one's practice. Sexual and gender minority individuals are underserved, understudied, and vulnerable to poor health[1,11,12] and notable disparities exist for these patients, including: housing, employment, poverty, violence, trauma, and discrimination in the use of public accommodations. For example, transgender individuals experience double the rates of unemployment compared to the general population with 26% reporting that they have lost a job due to their transgender status. Additionally, 19% have reported experiencing homelessness in their lives because of being either transgender or gender nonconforming.[1] Social and economic marginalization also results in poor access to quality health care and results in severe health disparities among this patient population. One finding from the National Transgender Health Discrimination Survey draws attention to the association between employment status and suicide attempts and reports that in 51% of unemployed transgender individuals, 56% of those who lost their job due to bias, and 60% who had worked in the underground economy (e.g., using transactional sex for survival) had attempted suicide at least once.[1]

A critical foundational step in caring for these high-risk patients is identifying and assessing who is transgender and

gender nonconforming and inquiring about patients' sense of self and their identities. The importance of obtaining this SO/GI information in the clinical setting as part of basic demographics has been supported by the 2015 incorporation of the collection of SO/GI into the Centers for Medicare and Medicaid and the Office of the National Coordinator for Health Information Technology requirements for Meaningful Use certified electronic health record incentive programs for optional implementation in 2017 and mandatory implementation in 2018.[13,14] Incorporation into Meaningful Use mandates that all eligible providers, eligible hospitals, and critical access hospitals receiving federal monies as part of their electronic health record incentive programs follow guidelines on collection and tracking of certain information. As a result, most large academic institutions, hospitals, and clinics now fall under this purview. For the solo or private practice practitioners, this is also important in that it enhances care.

Recommendations vary on how to ideally collect SO/GI information. In part this will depend on practice model and the point of data collection. The Williams Institute, The University of California San Francisco Center of Excellence for Transgender Health, and The Fenway Institute have created excellent models from which practitioners can work.[15–18] These frameworks recommend utilizing three to five questions to obtain SO/GI data: one question for current GI, sex assigned at birth, SO, and then two additional questions to assess sexual behavior and sexual attraction (Box 13.1). These questions can be modified depending on how they are used in practice (e.g., by in-person interview by a clinician or staff member or through data collection forms).

It is also important to consider in what order and what context these questions are asked. It is recommended that GI be assessed prior to sex assigned at birth to place emphasis on a person's self-identity.[18] It is also recommended that additional answer categories be allowed wherever possible in recognition of the changing and expanding lexicon, allowing for further self-definition. For questions regarding SO, we recommend assessing the three different domains (e.g., identity, behavior, and attraction) of SO separately from one another as well as distinctly from marital status and assessment of partnership or cohabitation.

Different practices use different methods of obtaining SO/GI depending on the methods used in a particular clinical setting for gathering other demographic measures. Information may be gathered prior to a clinical encounter through a web-based portal or paper questionnaire, on a paper form prior to seeing a clinician, or in an interview setting with a medical assistant prior to seeing the primary clinician. Finally, the clinician may ask or review these details in person. Data show that uniform clinical intake or registration forms help ensure quality and ubiquity of all data collected.[19] and we recommend that practices incorporate SO/GI data collection into all patient assessments and intakes.

Despite concerns of stigma, discrimination, privacy, and confidentiality, there is high acceptability of SO/GI questions in clinical practice settings.[20,21] Patients are able to recognize that there are benefits to disclosure in terms of enhanced quality of care and establishment of doctor-patient relationships.[22,23] Clinicians may be concerned about asking patients to disclose their identities to them, but in general, patients desire to be asked about it. This is evidenced by the work of Cahill et al. who found that out of 301 randomly selected patients who were

BOX 13.1   PROPOSED SEXUAL ORIENTATION AND GENDER IDENTITY QUESTIONS FOR INCORPORATION INTO CLINICAL PRACTICE

What is your current gender identity? (Check all that apply):
- ☐ Male
- ☐ Female
- ☐ Trans male/Trans man
- ☐ Trans female/Trans woman
- ☐ Gender queer/Gender nonconforming
- ☐ Additional Category (Please specify): _____
- ☐ Decline to state

What sex were you assigned at birth, on your original birth certificate?
- ☐ Male
- ☐ Female
- ☐ Decline to state

Self-identification: how one identifies one's sexual orientation (gay, lesbian bisexual, or heterosexual)

Do you think of yourself as:
- ☐ Lesbian, gay, or homosexual
- ☐ Straight or heterosexual
- ☐ Bisexual
- ☐ Something else
- ☐ Don't know
- ☐ Another (Please specify):_____
- ☐ Decline to state

Additional questions to refine sexual behavior and sexual attraction:

Sexual behavior: the gender(s) of sex partners (e.g., individuals of the same gender, different gender, or multiple genders). Note: additional information about specific sexual activities and body parts used for sex should also be assessed.

In the past (time period e.g., year) who have you had sex with?
- ☐ Men only (cisgender men and/or transgender men)
- ☐ Women only (cisgender women and/or transgender women)
- ☐ People with various gender identities: please specify
- ☐ I have not had sex

Sexual attraction: the gender(s) of individuals that someone feels attracted to

People are different in their sexual attraction to other people. Which best describes your feelings? Are you:
- ☐ Only attracted to females?
- ☐ Mostly attracted to females?
- ☐ Equally attracted to females and males?
- ☐ Mostly attracted to males?
- ☐ Only attracted to males?
- ☐ Not sure?

See references 15–18.

asked about their SO/GI information in four different clinical practice sites, only 1% declined to answer the GI question, only 2% declined to answer the sex assigned at birth question, and 1% had missing answers for SO questions. In that same cohort, 14% of respondents did not respond to the ethnicity question.[15] Most questionnaires do not contain a question about preferred pronouns, which we believe is also an important part of the patient intake. Some individuals may use pronouns that differ from

their legal gender or which may appear inconsistent with their gender expression. It remains critical to use the pronouns requested by that patient. There are many sets of pronouns available and asking which pronouns an individual uses will help establish rapport and communicate respect. Becoming competent in this area does take practice and there are clinical best practices that exist on assessing SO/GI in practice. Training opportunities are provided in Box 13.2.

BOX 13.2   TRAINING RESOURCES FOR PROVIDERS

Association of American Medical Colleges. Diversity 3.0 Learning Series. Section: LGBT, Gender Nonconforming, and DSD Health. Includes over 20 videos on integrating LGBT health into medical education, interviewing techniques, strategies for teaching learners, development activities, curricular, and health promotion strategies. https://www.aamc.org/initiatives/diversity/learningseries/.

Deutsch MB, ed. *Guidelines for the Primary and Gender-Affirming Care of Transgender and Gender Nonbinary People.* 2nd ed. University of California, San Francisco—Center of Excellence for Transgender Health. http://transhealth.ucsf.edu/trans?page=guidelines-home. Accessed June 17, 2016.

Pronouns Matter. http://callen-lorde.org/transhealth. Callen Lorde. June 2016.

NYC Health and Hospitals (2011). LGBT Healthcare Training Video: To Treat Me, You Have to Know Who I Am. https://www.youtube.com/watch?v=NUhvJgxgAac&feature=kp. Accessed September 5, 2016.

University of California Center of Excellence for Transgender Health (2014). Online Learning: Acknowledging Gender and Sex. Transgender Health Learning Center. http://transhealth.ucsf.edu/video/story.html. Accessed September 7, 2015.

National LGBT Health Education Center (2015). Achieving Health Equity for Lesbian, Gay, Bisexual, and Transgender People. http://www.lgbthealtheducation.org/lgbt-education/continuing-education/?y=130. Accessed September 5, 2016.

National LGBT Health Education Center (2012). Meeting the Health Care Needs of Transgender People. http://www.lgbthealtheducation.org/lgbt-education/online-courses/continuing-education/?y=13. Accessed September 5, 2016.

National LGBT Health Education Center (2013). Providing Care and Support for Transgender Rural Latino/as and Migrant Farmworker. http://www.lgbthealtheducation.org/lgbt-education/continuing-education/?y=53. Accessed September 5, 2016.

National LGBT Health Education Center (2015). Supporting LGBTQ Youth: Providing Affirmative and Inclusive Care Across the Spectrum of Gender and Sexual Identity. http://www.lgbthealtheducation.org/lgbt-education/continuing-education/?y=123. Accessed September 5, 2016.

National Center for Transgender Equality (2016). An Introduction to Transgender People. https://www.facebook.com/TransEqualityNow/videos/vb.40078161989/10153582088701990/?type=2&theater. Accessed September 5, 2016.

National Center for Transgender Equality (2016). Supporting the Transgender People in Your Life: A Guide to Being a Good Ally. http://www.transequality.org/sites/default/files/docs/resources/Ally-Guide-July-2016_0.pdf. Accessed September 5, 2016.

National Center for Transgender Equality (2016). Understanding Non-Binary People: How to Be Respectful and Supportive. http://www.transequality.org/sites/default/files/docs/resources/Understanding-Non-Binary-July-2016_1.pdf. Accessed September 5, 2016.

The Lambda Legal 2010 report found that 21% of transgender and gender nonconforming individuals reported being subjected to hard or abusive language from a health care professional, and almost 8% reported experiencing physically rough or abusive treatment from a proivider.[24] Therefore creating a safe environment conducive to disclosure and healing is paramount. Cultural competency training is necessary at every stage of the health care process; it is not enough for the provider alone to be competent in the care of transgender people. Individuals who work in registration, nursing, medical assisting, janitorial services, medical billing, medical records, radiology, etc. must all learn to create a positive experience for the patient. This will require training and attention. It may also require an assessment of systems of processing patient information, for example—how does your patient records and billing information track gender? Is it distinct from sex assigned at birth? How about legal name versus preferred name? Are patient's pronouns noted? Importantly, many electronic medical records have challenges with certain "sex specific" services. For example, when working with a transgender man who has a gender marker of male, is it possible in your system to still document and bill for a Pap smear? Considering the challenges that patients may face prior to any encounters with transgender patients is critical to ensuring a safe and welcoming environment. Tools for the clinician aiming to evaluate and improve the clinical environment can be found in Box 13.3.

OBTAINING A SEXUAL HISTORY

Once a patient is in the clinical setting with a reproductive health provider, much can be done to enhance patient experience and the quality of information gathered from the patient, such as using language free of gendered assumptions about the patient and or any romantic or sexual relationships.[19] Transgender individuals may have any of a variety of SOs and behavior patterns. One study by Bauer et al. addressed the sexual health of 227 female-to-male transgender individuals and found a diverse array of identities: bisexual/pansexual 24%; gay 10%; lesbian 4.1%; asexual 14.9%; queer 48.2%; straight/heterosexual 34.3%; Two-spirit 3%; Not sure/Questioning 11.9%; and other 5% which did not necessarily correspond with the past-year's partners of whom 10% were trans men, 21.3% were cisgender men, 6.8% were transgender women, 43.6% were cisgender women, and 13.7% were genderqueer persons.[25]

These type of data emphasize the importance of recognizing that that our patient's partners are also multifaceted with respect to their gender, sex assigned at birth, and SO and it may important to also ask: "What are the genders of your sexual partners?" "What was the sex assigned at birth of your sexual partners?" And finally, "What specific sexual acts are you undertaking with examples: penis-in-vagina, vagina-to-vagina, penis-in-anus, mouth-to-anus, etc." With training, providers can also become familiar using language that is more commonly used in the transgender community when describing genitalia and sex acts. For example, "Do you use your frontal opening/back opening for sexual activity?" As language is constantly changing and differs in time, geography, identity, and by individual, using the patient's own language for their gender, sex, genitalia, sexual acts, and partners will help clarify the type of information clinicians are receiving while ensuring patients feel heard and understood. The importance of gathering both identity and specific sex behavior information will help in assessing risk for sexually transmitted infections and contraceptive needs for patients and their partners. Box 13.4 contains information on sexual history taking and suggested resources to help enhance the clinical interview.

BOX 13.3 RESOURCES ON EVALUATING AND ENHANCING CLINICAL ENVIRONMENTS FOR THE SERVICE OF TRANSGENDER PEOPLE

National LGBT Health Education Center (2015). Ten Things: Providing an Inclusive and Affirmative Health Care Environment for LGBT People. http://www.lgbthealtheducation.org/lgbt-education/continuing-education/?y=114. Accessed September 5, 2016.
The Joint Commission (2011). Advancing Effective Communication, Cultural Competence, and Patient- and Family-Centered Care for the Lesbian, Gay, Bisexual, and Transgender (LGBT) Community. https://www.jointcommission.org/assets/1/18/LGBTFieldGuide_WEB_LINKED_VER.pdf. Accessed September 5, 2016.
National LGBT Cancer Network (2012). Best Practices in Creating and Delivery LGBTQ Cultural Competency Trainings for Health and Social Service Agencies. http://www.cancer-network.org/downloads/best_practices.pdf. Accessed September 2016.
Human Rights Campaign. All Children, All Families. http://hrc-assets.s3-website-us-east-1.amazonaws.com//files/assets/resources/HRC_All_Children_All_Families_Benchmarks_2016.pdf. Accessed September 5, 2016.

BOX 13.4 SEXUAL HISTORY TAKING AND KEY QUESTIONS TO ADD TO ENCOUNTER FORMS/CLINICAL INTERVIEWS

Association of American Medical Colleges. Diversity 3.0 Learning Series. Section: LGBT, Gender Nonconforming, and DSD Health. Includes over 20 videos on integrating LGBT health into medical education, interviewing techniques, strategies for teaching learners, development activities, curricular, and health promotion strategies. https://www.aamc.org/initiatives/diversity/learningseries/.
National LGBT Health Education Center (2016). Do Ask, Do Tell! Collecting Data on Sexual Orientation and Gender Identity in Health Centers" http://www.lgbthealtheducation.org/lgbt-education/online-courses/continuing-education/?y=142. Accessed September 5, 2016.
National LGBT Health Education Center (2016). Training Frontline Staff to Collect Data on Sexual Orientation and Gender Identity. http://www.lgbthealtheducation.org/lgbt-education/online-courses/continuing-education/?y=149. Accessed September 5, 2016.
National LGBT Health Education Center (2014). Taking a History of Sexual Health: Opening the Door to Effective HIV and STI Prevention. http://www.lgbthealtheducation.org/lgbt-education/continuing-education/?y=72. Accessed September 5, 2016.
National LGBT Health Education Center (2014). Understanding and Assessing the Sexual Health of Transgender Patient. http://www.lgbthealtheducation.org/lgbt-education/webinars/. Accessed September 5, 2016.
The Fenway Institute (2009). Knowing Your Patients: Taking a History and Providing Risk Reduction Counseling. http://www.lgbthealtheducation.org/wp-content/uploads/Module-2-Knowing-Your-Patients.-Taking-a-History-and-Providing-Risk-Reduction-Counseling.pdf. Accessed September 5, 2016.

TABLE 13.1	Gender-Neutral Language for Use During Pelvic Examinations		
Gendered	**Less Gendered**	**Least Gendered**	
Vulva		External pelvic area Outer parts	
Labia		Outer folds	
Vagina		Genital opening, frontal pelvic opening, internal canal	
Uterus, ovaries	Reproductive organs	Internal organs	
		Internal parts	
Breasts		Chest	
Pap smear	Pap test Cervical cancer	Cancer screening Cancer, HPV-related cancer	
Bra/panties		Underwear	
Pads/tampons		Any absorbent product that works for the patient	
Period/menstruation		Bleeding	

From Potter J, Peitzmeier SM, Bernstein I, et al. Cervical cancer screening for patients on the female-to-male spectrum: a narrative review and guide for clinicians. J Gen Intern Med. 2015;30(12):1857–1864.

THE GYNECOLOGIC EXAM

Another critical moment in the gynecological encounter is the physical exam. Many providers use gendered language during the exam, which can be uncomfortable for many and may worsen dysphoria in some transgender patients. Transgender men are significantly less likely to be up-to-date on Pap smears[26] and often have longer latency between follow-up Pap smears when compared to cisgender women.[27] One explanation for this finding may be poorer access to care, but another more likely reason is the physical and emotional discomfort patients may feel during gynecologic examinations. Potter et al. describe ways in which gendered language is often used during gynecologic exams and the authors offer alternatives that could be very useful in making transmasculine patients feel more comfortable.[28] These terms are presented in Table 13.1 and were derived from narrative reviews of transgender men undergoing gynecologic services. We believe that incorporating this type of language into practice is important and will improve the care received not only by trans individuals but also by people of any gender in the gynecology office.

Gynecologic Care for Transmasculine People

BASICS OF TRANSITION

The concept of "transition"—also known as gender affirmation—will mean different things to different patients. One definition includes "a person's adoption of characteristics that they feel match their gender identity."[29] Though often discussed as a journey that starts with one's sex assigned at birth and a gender congruent with that assigned sex and transitioning to the "other sex" and "other gender," this understanding is limited. Many transgender individuals feel as though their affirmed gender has always been a part of their lives, and so the process is more of a revealing or affirmation than a transition. Additionally, the

idea of moving from "one sex to another sex" is predicated on the notion of a gender binary wherein there are only two options: male or female. In one study, the minority of people reported a linear transition from one sex to another and the authors discovered a diversity of paths and definitions of transition.[30] As part of this diversity, gender is increasingly seen as existing on a spectrum. Thus there is no such thing as "complete transition" as this process can often be very dynamic with each individual having different goals and milestones. Throughout this section of the chapter, the term "transmasculine" will be used to describe people who are assigned female at birth but identify somewhere along the masculine gender spectrum. Conversely the term "transfeminine" will be used for those assigned male at birth but who identify along the feminine gender spectrum. Though imperfect, we believe that these terms allow for a more inclusive discussion of the social/medical/and surgical components of transition and are more inclusive of a myriad of different identities including but not limited to: female-to-male (FTM), trans man, genderqueer/non-binary, gender non-conforming, and masculine of center for those on the masculine spectrum. For those who identify along the feminine spectrum other notable identities include but are not limited to: male-to-female (MTF), trans woman, genderqueer/non-binary, gender non-conforming, and feminine of center (see separate section below). The term "trans" will be used when referring to all communities that fall somewhere within a transgender framework and who are gender nonconforming, inclusive of transmasculine, transfeminine, and genderqueer identities.

It is important to remember that not everyone will identify with or engage in a transition process. For those who do, this may include social transition, or physical transition, which can include medical and or surgical components. Social transition is generally considered disclosing one's GI within social circles. The degree of disclosure will be unique to every individual. This often involves dressing openly in a manner concordant with GI (e.g., modifications of one's gender expression). Some people may change names (casually or legally) and/or pronouns. Transitioning into using gender-segregated spaces (e.g., bathrooms and locker rooms) that align most with one's sense of self may also be a component of social transition. Social transition may not always be possible without medical or surgical components however: 28% of the lesbian, gay, bisexual, and transgender (LGBT) population lives in states that require proof of sex reassignment surgery, court order, and/or amended birth certificate in order to change gender marker.[31]

Social transition may occur at different times with different groups of people, as many trans people may not feel comfortable disclosing their identity to their family, employers, or certain friends or acquaintance groups due to the risk of rejection, loss of employment, being ostracized from communities, or violence. For example, 52% of LGBT people in the United States live in a state that does not prohibit employment discrimination based on GI or SO.[32] In 2011, a large survey of trans people found that 35% of those who expressed their GI between the age of 5 and 18 experienced physical violence.[1] This violence continues throughout life as trans people are murdered at an alarming rate. Recent international research documented 2115 murders of trans people between 2008 and 2016, which is likely a gross underestimation given the underreporting and misidentification of trans people.[33]

Even in the United States, which seems to have a comparative lower rate of murder of trans people than other countries, other policies make social transition dangerous and daunting. In 2016, North Carolina joined many other states in a recent spate of newly emergent restrictive transgender laws, but was the first state in the country mandating that people use the bathroom consistent with the sex designated on their birth certificate by passing House Bill 2 (HB2—Session Law 2016-3).[34] Beyond simple policy that protects majority citizens, the felt effects of these bills are threatening the safety, well-being, and access to public accommodation for trans people—especially those who don't "pass" in their affirmed gender.[35] Beyond mere inconvenience, there are data from over 2300 transgender people suggesting that those who are denied access to bathrooms consistent with their affirmed gender have a significantly higher rate of suicide than those with safe and available bathroom access.[36] Internationally, obtaining legal documentation of affirmed gender may require a statement of mental illness, divorce, and or sterilization.[37] These daunting realities faced by many trans people may profoundly affect someone's ability to disclose their identity and pursue medical or surgical transition. Others may not engage in any form of transition by choice, as they do not feel it a necessary element of their GI or expression.

Physical Transition

There are elements of physical transition that do not include hormones or surgery. For transmasculine people, this may include wearing masculine or "men's" clothing in public and/or getting a more traditionally masculine haircut. Some might engage in chest binding to achieve a flatter contour. This can be done with specific binders designed for these purposes. Others might use a tightly fitting sports bra or, more rarely, an ace bandage or duct tape. The latter is far more uncomfortable and may restrict blood flow or breathing. If a patient is using uncomfortable or unsafe methods of binding, this could be due to financial resources or lack of awareness for different options. There are many cities that have community organizations that help connect people with used binders and many online stores that sell more comfortable and durable products. Binding does not have any known health effects on breast tissue, though we are unaware of any studies in this area. However, it is important to consider the potential for skin breakdown and subsequent infection depending on the method of binding used.

Medical Transition: Hormones

Hormone therapy should be considered a medically necessary intervention.[12] For those transmasculine people who are interested in medical transition, this is done primarily with the administration of testosterone, whereas for transfeminine people this is primarily achieved with estrogen with or without other androgen blockers. As mentioned in prior chapters, the WPATH publishes Standards of Care for the Health of Transsexual, Transgender, and Gender Nonconforming People in 14 languages. In version 7, the most recent version published in 2011, there is a clinical tool to assess "readiness" for hormones.[6] The WPATH provides general guidelines to be used as a framework by providers and individual clinical assessment of the patient is necessary prior to beginning treatment. Determining a contraindication to hormone treatment should be done with great care. Given that the risk of severe depression and suicide attempt in trans people is estimated to be approximately 41%, denying hormone treatment due to concern for clinical side effects must account for the risk of untreated gender dysphoria.[29] Additionally, hormone therapy improves mental health, psychological adjustment, and quality of life.[38–40] One study demonstrated that once estrogen therapy was initiated for transgender women they had decreased anxiety and depression.[41] Therefore as long as the patient has decision-making capacity, they should be provided with hormonal treatment and concurrent treatment for support of mental health concerns or conditions. Furthermore, given the significant barriers to health care commonly experienced by trans people, many patients will present to providers already taking hormones they have procured through their communities, dealers, or online,[42] in which case the assessment of readiness becomes obsolete.

There are a number of different masculinizing hormone regimens used by patients and providers. There have been no controlled clinical trials comparing different hormone regimens in terms of efficacy, safety, or patient satisfaction.[6] For this reason, WPATH does not endorse any specific regimen. Geographic and regional variation of available medications, insurance access and coverage, socioeconomic situation, and patient preference should be considered when choosing between regimens. Protocols for masculinizing hormone therapy and management have been reviewed in Chapter 5, *Hormone Therapy for Adults.*

If a transmasculine patient is not interested in the virilizing effects of testosterone, but would like to achieve amenorrhea, this can be accomplished through a number of hormonal methods. If they do not have any contraindications to combined oral contraceptives, they can be placed on a continuous low-dose regimen for the purpose of suppressing menses. Alternatively, a levonorgestrel intrauterine device (IUD) can be offered for those patients who have contraindications to combined oral contraceptives, do not want to take systemic hormones, or who have breakthrough bleeding with oral regimens. Oral (daily) or injectable (every 3 months) medroxyprogesterone acetate is another alternative that may be preferable for some patients or if menses prove difficult to suppress with combined oral contraceptives or the levonorgestrel IUD. Combined oral contraceptives, the levonorgestrel IUD, and injectable medroxyprogesterone acetate are also effective contraceptive methods if the patient is having penis-in-vagina sex and not desiring to conceive (see section on "contraception").[43]

With virilizing hormone therapy, hair growth tends to occur in a similar distribution experienced by cisgender males during puberty. Darkening and thickening of chest and extremity hair generally develops first. Facial hair growth may begin slowly and take 1 to 4 years to reach full thickness. Overall, hair distribution tends to follow maternal inheritance, as does male pattern baldness. Hair growth is a permanent change, though body hair may thin following cessation of testosterone similar to that of older cisgender men. Hair loss can occur shortly after initiating therapy and occurs as either frontal/temporal recession or more classic male pattern baldness. If troublesome, thinning or balding hair is treated similarly in transmasculine and cisgender men and involves treatment with minoxidil, a 5-alpha-reductase inhibitor, or surgery.[44]

Vocal pitch deepening usually occurs between 6 to 10 weeks after initiation and is a permanent change. It may take up to 1 year for the voice to drop to its permanent pitch. After initiation of testosterone, body fat distribution will change (generally with more abdominal distribution and less subcutaneous) and muscle mass tends to increase. Fat distribution and muscle mass changes are reversible if someone discontinues hormones.[45] Acne is a common side effect of testosterone and is usually worse in the first year of therapy. Treatment is similar to those of cisgender patients with acne and may be helped by dermatologic consultation. Maintaining physiological testosterone dosing and avoiding large peak/trough dosing regimens may help decrease the incidence of acne.[46] Enlargement of clitoral tissue can be expected with testosterone treatment, though the degree of enlargement varies widely by individual. This is a permanent change. Increased libido is generally noted with testosterone treatment and is a reversible change.[45]

Additional metabolic changes can be expected in both short[47] and long-term follow-up,[48,49] and findings suggest overall safety. Overall, it seems that there may be increased cardiometabolic risk, but overall mortality is not increased. The details of these metabolic changes are beyond the scope of this chapter.

Gender Affirmation Surgeries

Surgery may be an element of transition for many transmasculine people. There are a number of different surgeries and many different names of these surgeries within transmasculine communities. "Top surgery" refers to chest reconstruction surgeries that serve to masculinize the chest. Details regarding this procedure are described in Chapter 9, *Breast and Chest Surgery for Transgender Patients*.

"Bottom surgeries" may refer to a number of different procedures. This could include hysterectomy, hysterectomy with bilateral or unilateral salpingo-oophorectomy, or vaginectomy. WPATH recommends 1 year on testosterone prior to proceeding with hysterectomy/bilateral salpingo-oophorectomy.[6] This should be interpreted as a guideline and patients should be considered on an individual basis. Some patients may never be interested in taking testosterone but would like a hysterectomy as part of their gender affirmation or to eliminate the need for suppression of menses. If not on testosterone, ovaries may be retained for the purpose of bone and cardiovascular health, and potentially for overall improved general mortality outcomes until approximately the age of natural menopause or 50.[50] Some transmasculine people may opt to retain one or both ovaries if they would like to retain possible fertility options or might be interested in coming off testosterone and would like the ability to produce endogenous hormones. Removing the ovaries may allow for a decrease in testosterone dose postoperatively; however decreasing the dose routinely after gonadectomy is not advised. If a patient would like to decrease their testosterone dose following oophorectomy, Follicle Stimulating Hormone (FSH)/Luteinizing Hormone (LH) levels should be followed to assure they remain in the premenopausal range.[44] If adhering to the recommendations of 1 year of testosterone treatment (for patients for whom this is relevant), providers should not postpone hysterectomy for patients with other indications for hysterectomy other than gender affirmation. Other gynecological indications for hysterectomy could include: abnormal uterine bleeding unresponsive to medical management, cervical dysplasia, endometrial hyperplasia, symptomatic leiomyomata, or adenomyosis.

With regard to reconstructing external genitalia, there are in general two common procedures: metoidioplasty and phalloplasty. Metoidioplasty involves using native clitoral tissue that has undergone hypertrophy after testosterone therapy. This may or may not include urethral rerouting through the clitoral tissue/phallus. Phalloplasty is a procedure that requires use of flaps or grafts to construct a larger phallus. This is a staged procedure that often involves the use of penile and scrotal implants. Vaginectomy may be performed with either or both of these procedures, but is generally considered necessary if vaginal obliteration is performed concurrently with either of these procedures. Details regarding these procedures can be found in Chapter 11, *Genital Confirmation Surgery for Patients Assigned Female at Birth*.

AMENORRHEA, ABNORMAL BLEEDING, AND PELVIC PAIN
Abnormal Bleeding

Amenorrhea is usually achieved with adequate testosterone treatment; however if breakthrough bleeding occurs or menses cannot be suppressed, other options can be considered as discussed previously. If a transmasculine patient is not on testosterone and is of reproductive age, their menstrual patterns should be evaluated as one would a cisgender woman's. Oligomenorrhea, intermenstrual bleeding, heavy, painful, or irregular bleeding warrants investigation.

Physiologic natal male levels of testosterone should lead to cessation of menses within 6 months of hormone initiation. For those transmasculine patients who had heavy or irregular bleeding prior to beginning testosterone therapy, achieving amenorrhea may prove more difficult.[51] If the patient has risk factors for, or symptoms concerning for, endometrial hyperplasia or cancer, an endometrial biopsy should be performed. This may include a return to menses after a long period of amenorrhea on testosterone, but inquiry into changes of hormonal regimen and use of anticoagulants should also be investigated. Transvaginal ultrasound and/or sonohysterography may be useful if symptoms are consistent with fibroids or polyps. If transvaginal ultrasound is not possible or is distressing to the patient, alternative imaging modalities such as abdominal ultrasound, computerized axial tomography (CT) scan, and magnetic resonance imaging (MRI) may be considered. Diagnosing and treating structural abnormalities will likely aid in the establishment of amenorrhea once testosterone therapy is initiated. Etiologies of oligomenorrhea prior to initiation of testosterone therapy should also be investigated. Pregnancy should be ruled out in patients who are engaging in penis-invagina sexual intercourse with partners who are capable of producing sperm.

Amenorrhea in transgender men after initiation of testosterone ranges from 1 to 13 months.[52–56] Higher and more frequent doses of testosterone have been shown to decrease time to amenorrhea.[53] Therefore one proposed definition of abnormal uterine bleeding in transmasculine patients would be bleeding that occurs after 12 months of physiologic male testosterone levels in the setting of FSH/LH suppression. Body habitus and route of administration may also affect the timing of menstrual suppression. Patients with larger adipose stores will have higher circulating estrogen levels and likely need longer periods of testosterone exposure prior to achieving amenorrhea.[51]

Treatment of abnormal uterine bleeding should be tailored based on etiology. If there are structural lesions present, such as a polyp or submucosal fibroid, resection should be discussed with the patient. Adjusting the testosterone-dosing regimen may also lead to more rapid cessation of menses. Testosterone has been shown to incompletely inhibit ovulation, and should not be considered adequate contraception. Therefore, patient's contraceptive needs should also be considered while discussing treatment of persistent bleeding. As mentioned previously, a levenorgestrel-secreting IUD or implanted, intramuscular, or oral progestogen will likely facilitate amenorrhea while also providing effective birth control for those at risk of pregnancy.[51]

If the patient does not desire fertility but has surgical comorbidities or is not interested in hysterectomy, an endometrial ablation is an option for ongoing bleeding. If the patient has risk factors for endometrial hyperplasia or cancer, an endometrial biopsy should be performed prior. Aromatase inhibitors may also be considered for short-term adjunctive treatment of persistent bleeding.[57–59] As these medications inhibit the peripheral production of estrogen, they will likely be particularly helpful in patients with high body mass index. Weight loss will also decrease the production of peripheral estrogen and likely aid in the cessation of menses.[51]

Pelvic Pain

Pelvic pain for transmasculine patients and cisgender women is a complicated and sometimes debilitating condition that is often multifactorial in origin. Pelvic pain, once chronic, in any individual is generally best treated with a multidisciplinary approach.[60–62] A full pain history should be elicited. A pain diary may be helpful in documenting inciting factors and frequency, as well as pain patterns. The clinical interview should consider gastrointestinal, urological, gynecological, musculoskeletal, and emotional/psychiatric/trauma components. Etiologies may include postsurgical pain or adhesive disease, pelvic floor muscle dysfunction or hypertonicity, infection, endometriosis, constipation, post-traumatic stress disorder (PTSD), or depression.

Etiologies specific to transmasculine patients on testosterone therapy include atrophic changes to the lower genital tract tissues (including the vulva and vagina) and increased risk of vaginitis and cervicitis due to pH changes from testosterone. If patients present with pelvic pain following hysterectomy and have retained one or both gonads, these remaining organs should be evaluated for pathology. Given the increased risk of violence and assault experienced by trans people, a trauma-informed approach to care should be used as gynecologic exams or invasive studies may cause additional trauma or trigger previous experiences.[51]

A thorough exam should be performed assessing for costovertebral angle tenderness, abdominal pain, or tenderness in the pelvic floor muscles. If a speculum exam is needed and the patient does not use their vagina for penetrative sexual activity, consider starting the exam with a pediatric speculum. Evaluate for vestibulodynia prior to performing a speculum exam (if indicated). If vestibulodynia is present, topical lidocaine will help to establish a diagnosis and decrease the discomfort of speculum insertion. With a speculum, evaluate for atrophic changes of the vaginal and cervical tissues and for abnormalities in discharge. Perform a wet prep, pH test, and consider vaginal culture. Screen for gonorrhea and chlamydia if indicated by risk profile or symptoms.

Transvaginal ultrasound should be performed to evaluate for adnexal pathology if gonads are still present. If the patient has undergone vaginectomy, a transrectal approach may allow for visualization. It is critical to take a thorough organ inventory to appropriately direct diagnostic tests. For those on testosterone therapy, understanding when the symptoms began in relation to therapy initiation (and any changes in therapeutic regimen or dose) is critical. If the patient experiences cyclical pain, this may be associated with ovulation and further ovulatory suppression may prove therapeutic. If vestibulodynia is thought to be the primary etiology of pelvic pain, treatment may start with the application of 2% to 5% topical lidocaine.

Testosterone is known to cause atrophy of the genital tract, which can lead to vaginitis and dyspareunia mimicking a postmenopausal state.[63–65] If the patient's symptoms and exam are consistent with atrophic vaginitis or cervicitis, vaginal estrogen (in either cream, tablet, or ring preparations) may help alleviate symptoms.[66] As there is limited systemic absorption of vaginal estrogen, patients should not expect feminizing side effects of treatment or need for adjustment of their testosterone doses.[67,68] Vaginal estrogen in a cream formulation may be applied to external genitalia if patients do not want to place the medication vaginally. If patients are not interested in using estrogen, changing lubrication used during sexual activities (if relevant) or a vaginal moisturizer may also improve their discomfort. Some patients experience pelvic pain immediately following their testosterone dose. The etiology of this is unknown. In addition to the vaginal treatments described above, nonsteroidal antiinflammatories should be considered a mainstay of treatment. Treatment with selective serotonin reuptake inhibitors or tricyclic antidepressants may be considered, though little is known about their efficacy in this particular application.[51]

Treatment of levator myalgia is similar to the treatment recommended for cisgender women, and involves referral to physical therapists specializing in the pelvic floor therapy.[61] It is critical to be aware of the physical therapist's level of experience and knowledge of trans patients so as to not refer the patient to a culturally insensitive provider which could exacerbate any gender dysphoria, sexual or genital trauma, or prior poor experiences with health care providers. If the patient is not comfortable seeing a pelvic floor physical therapist, or finances are prohibitive, instruction on pelvic floor massage can be provided so that the patient may perform therapy on their own, with a tool, or with a partner.

For many patients with pelvic pain, pelvic examinations may prove traumatic. With transmasculine patients, exams may exacerbate gender dysphoria, and transmasculine patients may decline exams.[28] In these cases, less invasive examinations should be primarily initiated (such as abdominal exams and imaging). If an exam is absolutely clinically indicated and the patient does not feel comfortable being examined in the office, exam under anesthesia or with moderate sedation should be offered where resources allow. PTSD and depression are common among transgender people and are often co-occurring disorders with chronic pain conditions.[1,61,69,70] When present, these conditions should be treated by mental health professionals in a collaborative approach to treatment of pelvic pain.[51,60,62]

As hysterectomies are often performed for gender affirmation, this may be considered earlier in the pelvic pain algorithm than with cisgender women. However, fertility plans and pain expectations postoperatively should be discussed with the patient prior to recommending hysterectomy, as pelvic pain may not be improved. The decision to remove gonads simultaneously should also be discussed in the context of planned duration of testosterone therapy, etiology of pelvic pain, and fertility desires.[51]

GYNECOLOGICAL APPROACH TO HEALTH MAINTENANCE AND ROUTINE SCREENING
Chest Health

If a transmasculine patient has not undergone top surgery (chest reconstruction) or has only had a reduction, they need mammogram screening, similar to cisgender women. This begins at age 40 to 50 depending on risk factors, family history, and choice of guideline adherence.[43,71,72] As guidelines vary, risks and benefits should be discussed with patients so that they may make an informed decision. It should be noted that mammography may exacerbate gender dysphoria as mammography centers are generally gendered spaced and many transmasculine patients may not feel comfortable. Anticipatory discussion of the gendered space and potential dysphoric triggers should be included in discussions with patients prior to referral. In referring to a mammography center, it is critical to investigate and then ensure that its providers are capable of delivering culturally sensitive care.

If a transmasculine patient has undergone top surgery, it is important to clarify the extent of surgery performed (mastectomy vs reduction). Chest reconstruction, done for the purpose of gender affirmation, is not usually performed by oncologists and residual breast tissue is left behind for the purpose of contouring the chest. For this reason, it should not be considered a risk reducing procedure. While the incidence of breast cancer in trans men following top surgery is unknown, there are only a few case reports in the literature and it is thought to be exceedingly uncommon.[73,74] While data are limited, it appears cross-sex hormone administration does not place trans people at increased risk for breast cancer. The incidence of breast cancer in both transmasculine and transfeminine people is comparable to the incidence of breast cancer found in cisgender men.[75,76]

Mammography is not possible for most transmasculine people following top surgery. Alternative considerations such as ultrasound, MRI, or annual chest wall exams can be considered but are not firmly recommended.[44] If a transmasculine patient is considering top surgery and has a strong family history of breast or ovarian cancer, they should be referred to a genetic counselor for evaluation. Patients with known mutations (such as BRCA1 or BRCA2) should be referred to a breast cancer surgeon who will ideally be able to perform risk reduction surgery in collaboration with a plastic surgeon capable of performing chest masculinization.

Screening for Gynecological Malignancies

When considering cancer risk in all trans patients, a full organ inventory is critical. Reviewing operative reports, when possible, allows for increased accuracy as patients may not remember or fully understand the procedures they have undergone. A lack of complete understanding may be due to lack of physician communication, varying terminology used amongst community members and providers, and/or patient health literacy.

If a transmasculine patient has not had a hysterectomy and is between the age of 21 and 65, they should undergo cervical cancer screening per the American Society for Colposcopy and Cervical Pathology (ASCCP) guidelines.[77] Again, if a patient has a history of a hysterectomy, it is critical to know whether or not the cervix was removed, and whether there was a clinically significant lesion prior to cervix removal that would require continued screening.

Routine screening for endometrial or ovarian cancer in transgender men on testosterone is not recommended. Generally the histopathological sequelae of testosterone use in transmasculine individuals includes uterine atrophy rather than hyperplasia and very few cases of gynecological malignancy have been reported.[63,78–81] Diagnostic evaluations should be reserved for clinical scenarios in which there is unexplained or irregular bleeding or symptoms, as discussed previously.[44]

Sexually Transmitted Disease/Infection Screening

Screening for sexually transmitted infections in transmasculine patients should be tailored based on sexual history and risk factors. It is critical to take a full sexual history. As discussed previously, GI does not in any way predict sexuality or sexual behavior. The 2015 Centers for Disease Control (CDC) Sexually Transmitted Disease (STD) Screening Guidelines include trans people as a discrete population for the first time but do not give population-specific recommendations other than noting: the few studies that exist suggest that Human Immunodeficiency Virus (HIV) prevalence may be lower in transgender men than transgender women and given the anatomic and behavioral diversity of transmasculine individuals, screening should be individualized for HIV, cervical Human Papillomavirus (HPV), and cervical cancer. However, two small studies suggest that HIV and sexually transmitted infection (STI) burden may be significant among transgender men and thus risk factor assessment and screening in this population should not be overlooked.[82,83] As with all individuals, the CDC recommends assessing for STD risk based on current anatomy, sexual behaviors, IV drug use or other possible exposures, and symptoms.[84]

Contraception

Testosterone alone does *not* serve as reliable contraception. If trans men are engaging in sexual activities that could result in pregnancy (e.g., penis-in-vagina sex) and do not desire to conceive, they should be counseled on the need for contraception.[44] Little data guides contraceptive efficacy and preferences for transgender men. However, anatomic capacity to conceive is retained by many transmasculine people as only 21% undergo hysterectomy[1] and many engage sexually with either cisgender or transgender men.[25] In a study of 41 transgender men who were pregnant and delivered after transitioning, one third of the pregnancies were unplanned.[55] However, it is not clear how many of these unplanned pregnancies occurred in the setting of current testosterone use. As discussed previously, effective contraception can often support other efforts to achieve amenorrhea if patients do not achieve amenorrhea on testosterone alone.

Gynecological Care for Transfeminine People

BASICS OF TRANSITION

The transition processes for transfeminine and transmasculine people are similar in many regards. They both include the elements of social, physical, medical, and surgical transition previously discussed. The complexities of disclosure and safety apply to both transmasculine and transfeminine people.

Physical Transition

For transfeminine people, this may include wearing more traditionally feminine clothing or hairstyles in public or in safe spaces. Some transfeminine people may wear makeup. Some may wax or shave body hair, or have it permanently removed via electrolysis or laser. There are also a number of ways someone might change the contour of their body to give a more traditionally feminine appearance. This includes "tucking," a practice of concealing the external genitalia by replacing testicles into the inguinal canal and repositioning the scrotum and penis along the perineum. This may include using tape or supportive underwear once the genitalia is repositioned to help maintain the "tucked" placement of genitals. People may or may not wear bras and augment with breast forms, prosthetics, or other methods of nonsurgical chest enhancement. The frequency, health benefits, and risks of tucking are understudied and warrant further investigation.

Medical Transition: Hormones

As previously discussed, WPATH provides guidelines to assist providers as they initiate patients on hormonal treatment. Again, these are suggestions rather than definitive rules about who can and cannot have hormones.[6] The prescribing provider should outline which changes are permanent and which changes regress if hormones are stopped. The provider should also assess for future desired fertility and suggest fertility preserving options (e.g., sperm banking) prior to hormone therapy initiation. Fertility counseling is particularly important, as the long-term effects of estrogen and testosterone blockers on fertility are unknown and most transfeminine patients experience markedly decreased spermatogenesis after initiation of hormones.[85]

Similar to transmasculine available regimens, WPATH does not endorse a specific feminizing medication protocol, as there are no randomized controlled trials comparing different regimens.[6] Protocols for feminizing hormone therapy have been reviewed in Chapter 5, *Hormone Therapy for Adults*.

Every patient will have a different process of transition once initiating hormonal treatment. Some patients will choose to use estrogen, progesterone, and an androgen blocker, while others will choose not to use progesterone. There are mixed data on the use of progesterone as an adjunct particularly to support breast development.[86] As transwomen do not have a uterine lining to consider, prescribing unopposed estrogen is thought to be safe.

Transfeminine patients can expect some level of breast development. This usually begins 2 to 3 months following hormone initiation with the maximum effect noted at 2 years.[52,87] With the use of estrogen, skin texture generally softens and facial hair tends to become finer. This effect is generally maximal after 4 months of hormone use. Many transfeminine patients, depending on their gender presentation goals, will proceed to have facial hair removed (via permanent or temporary measures) as hormones alone will not cause already existing hair follicles to stop producing.[52,87] Body fat will tend to redistribute and muscle mass decreases. Hair loss of the scalp will likely be arrested or slowed but new hair will not regrow where it has already been lost. Sexual effects of treatment often include decrease in erectile function and decreased spermatogenesis. Some transfeminine people will lose the ability to ejaculate, which may be viewed as a positive effect or an unwanted side effect depending on the individual patient's goals.[44] Emotional changes can also be expected.

GYNECOLOGICAL APPROACH TO HEALTH MAINTENANCE AND ROUTINE SCREENING
Breast Cancer Screening

There are little data to guide the recommendations for breast cancer screening in transfeminine patients. There have been two retrospective studies that suggest breast cancer incidence in transfeminine patients receiving gender affirming hormone therapy is lower than the general incidence in cisgender women.[75,88] As there is debate as to when breast cancer screening should be initiated in cisgender women, this controversy also applies to transfeminine patients. Given the likely lower incidence of breast cancer among transfeminine people, in the absence of additional risk factors, we often recommended to start screening at age 50 for those patients on hormonal therapies for a minimum of 5 years. Screening can be performed every 2 years.[44] This should be adjusted if the patient has a family history of breast or ovarian cancer or a known oncogene mutation (such as BRCA1 or BRCA2).

Prostate Cancer Screening

As a gynecologist, it is reasonable to consider prostate screening as part of routine gynecological care for transfeminine patients. The decision to screen for prostate abnormalities or neoplasm should be based on the recommendations for cisgender men. The American Urological Association does not recommend prostate cancer screening below the age of 40 or between the ages of 40 to 55 in the absence of risk factors (such as African American heritage or family history). Between the ages of 55 to 69 years of age, it is recommended that the provider have an informed discussion with the patient outlining the number needed to screen to prevent one prostate cancer mortality (1 per 1000) and the morbidity associated with screening and positive screening follow-up procedures.[89] For patients who have undergone vaginoplasty and elect to undergo prostate cancer screening, the prostate can often be palpated vaginally (it lies anterior to the neovagina). Prostate-specific antigen (PSA) may be artificially lowered by antiandrogen therapy (estrogen and or spironolactone) and the upper limit of normal may need to be adjusted to 1.0 ng/mL.[90]

Sexually Transmitted Disease/Infection Screening

Screening for STIs in transfeminine patients is similar to screening in transmasculine patients: it should be based on risk factors, exposures, and sexual activities. For the first time, the 2015 CDC guidelines include transgender people but give few specific guidelines. For transfeminine patients they specifically note the high prevalence of HIV infection, "27.7% among all transgender women and 56.3% among black transgender women in the United States," but acknowledge that these data are based largely on convenience samples and that there is little information about bacterial infections. Therefore risk assessment should be based on current anatomy and sexual behaviors, symptoms consistent with infection, and screening for asymptomatic STIs based on history.[84] While general screening guidelines apply regardless of GI, it is important to consider that transfeminine people may be at an increased risk of HIV acquisition and overall have decreased use and access to medically supported preventative measures such as HIV pre-exposure prophylaxis (PrEP).[91]

Sexual Health Following Vaginoplasty

A neovagina, whether created by colovaginoplasty or penile inversion, does not have the same anatomy or tissue types as a natal vagina. Additionally, neovaginas do not have a cervix, so cervical cancer screening by cytology and/or human papillomavirus (HPV) screening is not indicated. However, both low-risk and high-risk HPV subtypes have been found among transfeminine individuals who have undergone vaginoplasty, but the population prevalence is unknown.[92] Therefore we recommend routine visual inspection to aid in the detection of condylomata or other clinically significant lesions which have been observed in transfeminine people after vaginoplasty.[93,94]

Depending on the type of surgery the patient has, there may be mucosal tissue present that is susceptible to infection with gonorrhea or chlamydia; however the population-based incidence of infection is unknown. Therefore, routine risk-based screening and symptom-based diagnostic techniques should be employed. Inverted penile tissue is keratinized and it is unclear how susceptible this tissue is to common STIs. It is known that infections affecting keratinized tissues in natal penises, such as chancroid, syphilis, and herpes, can also be found in neovaginas.[82,83]

Exam of a neovagina can be performed with either a standard speculum or anoscope (size of speculum will need to be tailored individually, similar to cisgender women). Depending on the anatomy, an anoscope may be a better instrument for visualization. There are no guidelines regarding necessity of routine pelvic exams on transfeminine people with neovaginas. As cancers that affect keratinized skin (basal cell, melanoma, squamous) can occur within a neovagina, annual exams should be considered.[44] While HPV infection has been documented in the neovaginas of transwomen, routine Pap screening is not recommended.[94] Additionally, the microbiome of a neovagina is quite different than that of a natal vagina. For neovaginas created with penile inversion, *Staphylococcus sp.*, *Streptococcus sp.*, *Enterococcus sp.*, *Corynebacterium sp.*, *Mobiluncus sp.*, and *Bacteroides sp.* were found to be the most common in a cohort of 50 transwomen with and without symptoms of discharge. Furthermore, contrary to standard findings in cisgender women, only 1 in 30 transwomen sampled were colonized with *Lactobacilli* and *Candida* was not isolated from any of the study participants.[95] Reports of troublesome discharge in transfeminine patients who have undergone vaginoplasty by penile inversion is likely due to keratin debris, retained lubricant or semen, or sebum.[44]

Unlike natal vaginas, neovaginas do not usually contain mucosa and routine douching is recommended. Douching needs will be based on proximity to surgery and sexual habits. While performing frequent dilation, daily douching will help prevent buildup of retained lubricant and debris. Once a patient no longer needs to dilate as frequently, douching can be performed 2 to 3 times per week.[44] Patients can use soapy water for the majority of douches. In the setting of increased or malodorous discharge, a vinegar douche may be use for 2 to 3 days. If discharge persists, an exam is warranted to evaluate for granulation tissue or other lesions. In the setting of a normal exam but increased discharge, treatment with metronidazole may be helpful for treatment of overgrowth of anaerobic bacteria.[94]

If granulation tissue is encountered on exam, immediate treatment is not necessary as it will often resolve on its own. Generally patients report yellow or blood-tinged vaginal discharge. If granulation tissue is persistent and does not resolve with decreasing dilation (depending on dilation requirements as recommended by their surgeon), it can be treated with silver nitrate. This can be done in the office, but multiple treatments may be required. An alternative to treatment with silver nitrate is the use of medical grade honey or mild strength topical steroid cream or ointment such as triamcinolone acetonide 0.1%, which can be applied to the tip of a dilator prior to use.

While the majority of vaginoplasties are created with penile inversion, some patients undergo construction with the use of intestinal tissue.[93] When evaluating discharge, it is important to understand the patient's surgical history in detail. When intestinal tissue lines the vaginal vault, intestinal mucosal secretions may be copious and consistently present. Bacterial constituency will be different among those who underwent colovaginoplasty compared to those who underwent a penile inversion surgery. The most common type of pathogenic bacterial overgrowth (diversion colitis) presents with a green discharge.[44] When encountered in routine bowel surgery that does not include the creation of a neovagina, the treatment is surgical. When encountered in the setting of postcolovaginoplasty surveillance, referral to the surgeon who performed the patient's vaginoplasty is appropriate to assess for surgical revision. Medical management includes treatment with short-chain fatty acid enemas, topical 5-aminisalicylic acid, and topical glucocorticoids.[44] As the tissue in the vagina is bowel, it is important to consider that bowel-specific diseases (e.g., inflammatory bowel disease, colitis, polyps, and colon cancers) can occur in this tissue. No routine screening is recommended, but yearly exams should be considered and symptom-targeted evaluation should be performed.[44]

Rarely, an increase in malodorous discharge can be a result of a fistula.[96] This can be either a rectovaginal or a vesicovaginal fistula. Patients may present with stool or gas passing through the vagina. They may present with brown discharge that is not immediately recognized as stool or constant leaking of urine from a vesicovaginal source. These patients should be referred back to their initial surgeon or to a urogynecologist or colorectal specialist for surgical repair. The patient may need a diverting colostomy or prolonged treatment with indwelling urinary catheter. Vaginal dilation plans in the context of a fistula need to be carefully considered since patients are usually recommended to have 5 to 12 weeks of pelvic rest following significant pelvic surgery such as a fistula repair.[97] However, 12 weeks without vaginal dilation of the neovagina will likely lead to loss of vaginal length, girth, or agglutination of the neovaginal walls. These considerations need to be discussed with the primary surgeon and the surgeon performing the repair.

Gender Affirmation Surgeries

Similar to transmasculine patients, transfeminine patients may undergo surgical intervention as part of their gender affirmation. Common surgeries include tracheal shave, facial feminization, vaginoplasty (via penile inversion or use of bowel tissue to create a neovagina), orchiectomy (removal of testicles), breast augmentation, silicone injections or fillers, and laser hair removal or electrolysis. Some patients may undergo none, all, some, or one of these surgeries. Everyone's transition is different. This may be influenced by access to competent surgeons, finances, availability of support for postrecovery care, and ability to take time off work. While a number of insurance companies, including many public plans, are expanding their trans coverage, many surgeries are still considered "cosmetic" and patients need to pay out of pocket for wrap-around surgical care including preoperative evaluation, surgery, and hospital stay as well as postoperative surveillance.

Contraception

While most transfeminine people will experience a reduction in spermatogenesis on estrogen and testosterone blockers, some patients may continue to produce enough sperm to result in a pregnancy if they have sexual partners capable of carrying a pregnancy and engage in penis-in-vagina sexual activity.[98] The possibility of contributing to a pregnancy should be discussed with patients on initiation of hormones and appropriate measures taken to ensure adequate contraception and or fertility preservation—as desired.

Reproductive Options for Transgender Patients

REPRODUCTIVE DESIRES AMONG TRANSGENDER PEOPLE

Data are sparse on the reproductive desires and needs of transgender people. One can surmise a desire to reproduce and have genetically related children, but both contemporary and historical ties of sterilization to transition-related processes has obfuscated much of the data on reproductive outcomes. Indeed, in Europe 23 states (13 in the European Union) require sterilization for legal affirmed gender recognition.[37] Nonetheless many lay sources including documentaries, blogs, and online chat groups describe parenting wishes or ongoing parenting by transgender individuals. In addition, two studies by Wierckx et al. and De Sutter et al. describe reproductive wishes among transgender people. In 2002 De Sutter et al. published a survey describing the opinions of transwomen regarding sperm cryopreservation.[99] They found that among the 121 transwomen interviewed, 51% would have cryopreserved sperm had that option been offered to them and 77% believed sperm cryopreservation should be discussed by treating professionals. Furthermore, they found that those who were younger (<40) and identified as lesbian or bisexual women were most likely to be in favor of discussion of cryopreservation. This indicates that the desire for potential future fertility through cryopreservation is there. In another study published by the same authors, of the transwomen given the option to cryopreserve and the financial and institutional supports to do so, only 15% actually completed cryopreservation.[100] Thus even when removing barriers to access to these services, it is unclear how many transgender women are availing themselves of these options and eventually going on to have children once they have started transitioning.

In yet another study by Wierckx et al., the authors examined the reproductive wishes of 50 transgender men who had undergone hormonal and surgical gender affirming procedures. In this single-center cross-sectional study, the majority (54%) of participants desired children.[101] They also found that 22% (11 participants) already had children. Of those with children, 73% (8 participants) achieved parentage by a female partner with donor sperm and 27% (3 participants) had given birth before hormonal and surgical therapy. A little more than one third (37.5%) of those in the study would have frozen eggs had they been given the chance prior to gender affirmation

procedures. This suggests that transgender men are desirous of having children and the support to retain their capacity to have genetically related children in the future remains necessary.

ETHICAL AND LEGAL CONSIDERATIONS

Recent literature describes some controversy about the "appropriateness" of transgender people being parents. There have been questions about the mental health, stability of the parenting role, and outcomes for children of transgender parents.[102–105] This line of thinking, however, is largely superseded by the acknowledgment that the right to parent is a fundamental right for all people, including transgender people. Recently, the American Society of Reproductive Medicine issued a statement that denying fertility and reproductive services to transgender individuals is unjustified.[106] Furthermore, there are data suggesting that there are no adverse outcomes for children raised by transgender individuals when compared with cisgender individuals.[107,108] Additionally, there is no evidence to suggest that having a transgender parent has a deleterious impact on healthy sexuality or gender development among children.[109–111] As such, fertility discussion is considered a fundamental component of pretransition hormonal and or surgical counseling as described by both the WPATH and the Endocrine Society.[6,52]

Legally speaking, prioritization is given to genetic relationships with regard to parental rights.[105] Legal parental rights are also influenced by the processes that are undertaken to produce genetic offspring and the relationship of parties to one another (partnered, married, domestic partners, sexually intimate partners known, or anonymous donors, etc.). Careful consideration must be given to legal implications of generating and planning to raise a genetically related child outside of a cisgender, heterosexual, two-person, married household and so, legal counsel is recommended.[105,112] The legal pressures and primacy of rights in relation to genetic parentage may pose compelling pressures for transgender individuals to prioritize having genetically related children despite the fact that this may be physically, emotionally, and/or fiscally difficult if not impossible.[112–114]

EFFECT OF GENDER AFFIRMING PROCEDURES ON FERTILITY

Though data are limited, expert opinion extrapolated from corresponding hyperestrogenic and hyperandrogenic cisgender people suggests that cross-sex or gender affirming hormones can have deleterious affects on reproduction. Current pathophysiological models include the effect of antiandrogen therapy in cisgender men with prostate cancer and cases of testosterone secreting (e.g., Sertoli-Leydig) tumors in cisgender women. However, it not clear that we can extrapolate findings from these neoplastic processes onto cross-sex hormone therapy in transgender individuals. For example, the minimum dose of estrogen needed to affect sperm quality and function remains unknown. Furthermore, the persistence of the effects on sperm quality and function are also unclear. For transgender men, it remains unclear what testosterone dose and/or exposure time affects ovulation.[115] It also remains unclear whether the pool of potential oocytes—including primordial follicles—are eventually affected by long-term testosterone use or not.[85] Therefore it is with good reason that the WPATH, the Endocrine Society, and the American Psychological Association all recommend counseling about fertility and reproductive options prior to starting gender affirming hormones or treatments.[6,52,116] Current counseling on absolute sterility risk is limited as there is scant evidence to personalize risk considerations among patients.

There is evidence that transgender women exposed to exogenous estrogen see alterations in sperm count, quality, and motility.[98,117–119] A recent paper showed that at the time of gender affirmation procedures, while the majority transwomen on estrogen therapy had poor sperm quality, some still had morphologically normal sperm developing in the testes.[120] There is some anecdotal evidence of siring pregnancies after prolonged estrogen exposure but the likelihood of this occurring and under what conditions remains unclear. What is clear is that orchiectomy will definitively remove biological reproductive potential, making desires for future fertility an important component of presurgical fertility counseling.

For transgender men, even less is known. Clearly hysterectomy and oophorectomy lead to irreversible changes in fertility and future reproductive capacity. However, presurgical fertility preservation as discussed below may allow transgender men to still have genetically related children after gender affirming hormonal and surgical procedures. Amenorrhea in transgender men tends to follow within a few months after initiation of testosterone (ranging from 1 to 13 months).[52,53–58] Pregnancies have been successfully achieved and carried to birth by transgender men even after testosterone exposure. Light et al. performed a cross-sectional survey of 41 transgender men who were pregnant and gave birth after transitioning. Of these patients, 25 had been on testosterone prior to conception, pregnancy, and delivery. They found that transgender men were able to conceive even after being on hormones for more than 10 years.[55] This corroborates findings in two other *in vitro* studies that have demonstrated that the primordial and antral follicles of the ovary do not seem to be irreversibly affected by testosterone therapy.[121,122] It is unclear whether transmasculine individuals have higher rates of polycystic ovarian syndrome (PCOS) and hyperandrogenism at baseline or whether being on testosterone induces a PCOS phenotype with mixed insights.[79,122–124] Increased baseline or therapy-induced PCOS could affect fertility (and other metabolic) considerations for these patients.

There is clearly much more to study and to understand about the impact of gender affirming or "cross-sex hormones" on the physiology and pathology of both the transgender male and female reproductive systems. Best practices support discussing reproductive health issues with transgender people before the initiation of hormone therapy and again before gonadectomy (oophorectomy or orchiectomy) or genital surgery, and providers need to be prepared to discuss assisted reproductive technologies options with their patients.[125]

TRANSGENDER PARENTING

As with all areas of this field, very little is known about transgender people as parents. The most substantial source of data we have comes from the National Transgender Discrimination Survey (NTDS). The NTDS was a cross-sectional study published in 2011 which surveyed 6456 transgender people in the United States. In the NTDS, 38% of the sample were parents,

and parentage was very strongly tied to the age of transition; those who transitioned later were more likely to have children. Latinos had the highest rates of parenting and Asians had the lowest and transgender women were more likely to have been parents (52%) than transgender men (17%). Those who identified as gender nonconforming were less likely than those who identified as transgender to be parents. Sadly, 29% of those with children had their contact with their children limited by an ex-partner, and 13% had courts and legal processes limit or stop relationships with their children. It is unfortunately not uncommon for transgender people to have lost their rights through the transition processes.[126]

REPRODUCTIVE OPTIONS FOR TRANSGENDER INDIVIDUALS

When considering an individual's options for reproduction it is important to consider a nonbinary approach to how individuals identify and with whom they may choose to reproduce. As Dickey et al. notes—"it is important to challenge gender dichotomies about reproduction just as it is with all other aspects of transgender health and health care. This expanded notion will allow an appreciation of the many gender non-conforming individuals who may not identify with or ascribe to identities of transgender maleness or femaleness and yet still desire to create a family."[112] In this section we will use the language that Dickey et al. have published to talk not about transgender men and women exclusively, but rather discuss those who were born with sperm-making capacity (or have sperm) and those who have egg-making capacity and gestational capacity. To support the reader in thinking about what reproductive dyads may look like for transgender people, Table 13.2 can be referenced. This table displays what creation of a genetically related child may look like for pairings between individuals who are at different stages of transition and have different sets of base gametes. We recognize that gender nonconforming individuals and those whose primary relationships are not comprised of two-person dyads may seem less visible in this table, but in general, this table can be used as a reference for navigating different options for reproduction.

METHODS OF REPRODUCTION FOR TRANSGENDER INDIVIDUALS

Where someone is in their gender transition will determine which methods of reproduction are available to them. Therefore we will consider available methods by transition stage, keeping in mind that the principle ingredients necessary to create a child remain the same: sperm, egg, joining of the sperm and egg, and gestation in a uterus.

In addition to considering transition stage, a large part of how one goes about creating a child will depend upon with whom the patient is partnered. There are five exemplar scenarios to consider for transgender men—or those born with ovaries and uterus—and five exemplar scenarios to consider for transgender women—or those with sperm (see Table 13.2). Though these do not encompass all possible scenarios or identities they help elucidate major patterns in reproductive needs.

For transgender men or transmasculine people born with ovaries, uterus, and tubes, the fundamental questions are: (1) Where are they in the gender affirmation process: have they engaged in social, medical, and or surgical transition? As part of that question, it is critical to elicit precisely what procedures have been undertaken as part of the individual's unique gender transition. (2) Does the index patient desire a genetically related child? (3) Assuming that the index patient retains a uterus, ovaries, and tubes—are they interested in carrying a pregnancy?

Additional considerations relate to the patient's partner. For example, if they have a cisgender female partner or a transmasculine partner with uterus, ovaries and tubes, consideration must be given to the source of the oocytes (patient or partner), who will carry (patient and partner), and source of sperm. The sperm contribution may be from a known or anonymous donor. Then consideration must be given to how the sperm and oocyte will be joined, either through coitus or assisted reproductive techniques.

If indeed a transmasculine individual desires fertility, the question becomes one of timing and relationship to any

TABLE 13.2	Reproductive Options for Transgender Individuals and Their Partners by Index Patient Stage of Transition				
Index Patient	*Partner:* Cisgender woman or person born with uterus, ovaries, and fallopian tubes who identifies as a woman	*Partner:* Cisgender man or person born with penis and testes who identifies as a man	*Partner:* Transgender Woman, transfeminine person, or person born with penis and testes	*Partner:* Transgender Man, transmasculine person or person born with uterus, ovaries, and fallopian tubes	*No partner*
Transgender Man, transmasculine person or person born with uterus, ovaries, and fallopian tubes (Social Transition)	*Need:* Sperm *Decide:* Whose oocytes? Whose uterus? Source of sperm (known or unknown donor).	*Need:* None: all gametes (sperm and eggs) and uterus present *Decide:* Will use transgender man oocytes? Will transgender man carry or surrogate?	*Need:* Possibly none. Ostensibly sperm, ovaries, and uterus present. Depending on sperm availability/ viability. *Decide:* Will use transgender man oocytes or egg donor? Will transgender man carry or surrogate? Does transgender woman have viable sperm?	*Need:* Sperm *Decide:* Whose eggs? Whose uterus? Source of sperm (known or unknown donor). Dependent on desires of couple and stage of transition of partner.	*Need:* Sperm *Decide:* Will transgender man use own oocytes? Will transgender man carry? Source of sperm (known or unknown donor).
Transgender Woman, transfeminine person, or person born with penis and testes (Social Transition)	*Need:* None: Gametes (sperm and eggs) and uterus present. *Decide:* Timing of pregnancy and method of insemination (coital vs. ART).	*Need:* Uterus and oocytes. *Decide:* Whose sperm will be used? Surrogate to be used.	*Need:* Uterus and oocytes. *Decide:* Whose sperm will be used (dependent on viability of partner sperm). Surrogate to be used.	*Need:* Possibly none. Ostensibly gametes and uterus present depending on oocyte and uterus availability in partner. *Decide:* Will use transgender man oocytes? Will transgender man carry or surrogate?	*Need:* Oocytes and uterus. *Decide:* Whether to use a surrogate +/– egg donor versus adopting.
Transgender Man, transmasculine person or person born with uterus, ovaries, and fallopian tubes (Hormonal Transition)	*Need:* Sperm *Decide:* Whose oocytes? Whose uterus? Source of sperm (known or unknown donor). *Note:* Transgender man would have to stop testosterone to produce oocytes and/or carry.	*Need:* Possible none: Ostensibly all gametes (sperm and oocytes) and uterus present. *Decide:* Will use transgender man oocytes or egg donor? Will transgender man carry or surrogate? *Note:* Transgender man would have to stop testosterone to produce oocytes and/or carry.	*Need:* Possibly none. Ostensibly all gametes (sperm and oocytes) and uterus present depending on sperm availability and transgender man's feelings about oocyte harvesting/usage and carrying. *Decide:* Will use transgender man oocytes or will use oocyte donor? Will transgender man carry or surrogate? Does transgender woman have viable sperm? Does transgender woman need to come off estrogen to produce sperm? *Note:* Transgender man would have to stop testosterone to produce oocytes and or carry.	*Need:* Sperm (known or unknown donor). *Decide:* Whose eggs? Whose uterus?	*Need:* Sperm *Decide:* Will use transgender man oocytes? Will transgender man carry or surrogate? Source of sperm (known or unknown donor).

TABLE 13.2	Reproductive Options for Transgender Individuals and Their Partners by Index Patient Stage of Transition—cont'd				
Index Patient	*Partner:* **Cisgender woman or person born with uterus, ovaries, and fallopian tubes who identifies as a woman**	*Partner:* **Cisgender man or person born with penis and testes who identifies as a man**	*Partner:* **Transgender Woman, transfeminine person, or person born with penis and testes**	*Partner:* **Transgender Man, transmasculine person or person born with uterus, ovaries, and fallopian tubes**	*No partner*
Transgender Woman, transfeminine person, or person born with penis and testes (Hormonal Transition, assume retention of uterus, ovaries, and tubes)	*Need:* None: Gametes (sperm and oocytes) and uterus ostensibly present. *Decide:* Is there viable sperm from transgender woman? *Note:* Here transgender woman would have to go off estrogen to produce sperm if not cryopreserved. Timing of pregnancy and method of insemination (coital vs. ART).	*Need:* Uterus and oocytes. *Decide:* Whose sperm will be used. Surrogate to be used. *Note:* Here transgender woman would have to go off estrogen to produce sperm if not cryopreserved.	*Need:* Uterus and oocytes. *Decide:* Whose sperm will be used (dependent on availability and viability of both index patient and partner sperm). Surrogate to be used. *Note:* Here transgender woman may have to go off estrogen to produce sperm if not cryopreserved.	*Need:* Possibly none. Ostensibly gametes and uterus present depending on oocyte and uterus availability in partner and sperm viability and availability of index patient. *Decide:* Will use transgender man oocytes or will use an egg donor? Will transgender man carry or surrogate? *Note:* Here transgender woman may have to go off estrogen to produce sperm if not cryopreserved.	*Need:* Oocytes and uterus. *Decide:* Whether to use a surrogate +/− egg donor. *Note:* Here transgender woman may have to go off estrogen to produce sperm if not cryopreserved.
Transgender Man, transmasculine person or person born with uterus, ovaries, and fallopian tubes (Surgical Transition, assume removal of uterus ovaries, and tubes)	*Need:* Sperm. *Decide:* Source of sperm. Method of insemination (coital vs. ART).	*Need:* Uterus and oocytes. *Decide:* Surrogate +/− egg donor. Method of insemination (coital vs. ART).	*Need:* Uterus and oocytes, possibly sperm, depending on sperm availability and viability of partner. *Decide:* Surrogate +/− egg donor. Method of insemination (coital vs. ART). *Note:* Here transgender woman may have to go off estrogen to produce sperm if not cryopreserved.	*Need:* Sperm, possibly uterus and oocytes depending on stage of transition of partner. *Decide:* Is partner going to carry and or be source of oocytes? Versus using a surrogate +/− egg donor? Source of sperm (known vs. donor).	*Need:* Sperm, uterus, and oocytes. *Decide:* Whether to use donor egg, donor sperm, and surrogate, or to adopt.
Transgender Woman, transfeminine person, or person born with penis and testes (Surgical Transition, assume removal of testes)	*Need:* Sperm. *Decide:* Is there viable sperm from transgender woman cryopreserved, if not will need to use donor sperm.	*Need:* Uterus and oocytes. *Decide:* Whose sperm will be used (depending on if cryopreserved sperm from transgender woman or not). Surrogate to be used. Method of insemination of surrogate (coitus vs. ART).	*Need:* Uterus, oocytes, and possibly sperm. *Decide:* Whose sperm will be used (dependent on if cryopresned sperm from index patient and considering availability and viability of sperm of partner. Surrogate to be used.	*Need:* Possibly none depending on oocyte and uterus availability in partner and if cryopreserved sperm availability from index patient. *Decide:* Will use transgender man oocytes or will use an egg donor? Will transgender man carry or surrogate?	*Need:* Oocytes, uterus, and possibly sperm (depending on availability of cryopreserved sperm from index patient). *Decide:* Whether to use a surrogate +/− egg donor +/− sperm donor (versus adopting).

ART: Assisted reproductive technology. This includes but is not limited to: intracervical insemination, intrauterine insemination, in-vitro fertilization. Social Transition: Signifies (adult) individuals who socially identify with their affirmed gender but have not initiated hormones or surgical procedures that would affect fertility. In this table we do not consider modifications stemming from baseline fertility issues (e.g., undiagnosed infertility, or age-related fertility). Hormonal Transition (i.e., use of gender affirming hormones): Signifies (adult) individuals who retain natal anatomy but have undergone medical; also known as hormonal therapies for gender affirmation. Surgical Transition (i.e., use of gender affirming surgical procedures including gonadectomy): Signifies (adult) individuals who have undergone surgical procedures as part of gender affirmation. Note, we delineate adults here because the care and reproductive considerations of youth are handled in a separate section. Additionally, this table assumes that at baseline there is full anatomic and functional fertility. Fertility problems from any partners will augment levels of diagnostic and therapeutic interventions needed. Furthermore, we are approaching options from a functional perspective; different options may have different physiological, emotional, fiscal, and legal implications. Finally, this table is directed towards achieving a genetically related offspring when possible. Other options for family creation are available.

desired gender affirming interventions. Whether to proceed with childbearing prior to transition or at a future date is a personal decision and some providers have noted that patients may actively delay gender affirmation procedures for childbearing and lactation.[127] If fertility in the future is desired, there are options to cryopreserve oocytes and embryos. In 2012 the American Society for Reproductive Medicine (ASRM) declared that oocyte preservation was no longer experimental and had similar age-related live birth outcomes as embryo cryopreservation. Oocytes frozen before the age of 35 have approximately a 50% live birth rate.[128,129] While these data are encouraging and provide options for patients, counseling should also include the cost of these services. Cryopreservation can be expensive with an average of $10,000 per cycle (range $5000 to $15,000) and multiple cycles may be necessary to achieve an appropriate storehouse of oocytes.[130,131] Furthermore, the process can be laborious with daily injections and multiple patient visits over a 4- to 6-week time span. After cryopreservation, maintenance of the frozen specimens until they are ready to be used must also be fiscally accounted for and can cost on average $500 per year.[130,131] It is unknown at this time how many transmasculine individuals are availing themselves of cryopreservation prior to starting gender affirmation processes, though one study reported that 37.5% of respondents would have frozen their eggs had they been given the chance prior to gender affirmation procedures.[101]

If a transmasculine individual has retained his uterus, ovaries, and tubes, insemination can occur. If oocytes are cryopreserved, then one must engage with the process of embryo creation by selecting a sperm source and working with a reproductive endocrinologist. The newly made embryo(s) can then be transferred with assisted techniques. Because these processes are tied to the menstrual cycle and because testosterone is a teratogen, testosterone must be stopped prior to implantation. Menses should resume several months prior to implantation to ensure an appropriate hormonal milieu for gestation. The transmasculine patient may also gestate an embryo produced from a partner or donor. This would also require cessation of testosterone and resumption of menses. Alternatively, the transmasculine patient may have a partner with a uterus who desires to gestate a pregnancy resulting from the patient's oocytes. This process is increasingly used by partners who were both born with gestational capacity and is called "co-IVF" or "reciprocal IVF."

If a transmasculine person has a cisgender male partner or a transfeminine partner who is able to produce sperm, the partner may be able to contribute sperm to produce a pregnancy. This of course will depend on the partner's availability and viability of sperm and the transmasculine patient's desire to carry a pregnancy. If these conditions are met, achieving a pregnancy can occur through sexual activity or through assisted reproduction. Assisted reproduction in this scenario usually begins with either augmented or natural ovulation and either intravaginal, intracervical, or intrauterine insemination. If pregnancy is not achieved through these measures, in vitro fertilization (IVF) is usually the next step—if finances allow. If oocytes or embryos have been frozen prior to surgical or hormonal transition, IVF and/or embryo transfer is needed to achieve pregnancy. If the transmasculine individual has been using testosterone, it must be stopped for all components of this process. It is important to note that IVF is often prohibitively expensive, and it is often not covered by insurance. Given the profound economic disparities present within many trans communities, finances may prove to be the most daunting barrier to fertility care.

Transgender women or transfeminine people may choose to form families in a number of different ways. This will depend on the patient's desire for a genetically related child, if the transfeminine person has a partner, what the partner's reproductive capacity and desires are, and what gender affirming procedures the patient has had. If the individual has cryopreserved sperm the main decision becomes the source of the oocytes and the carrier of the pregnancy. If the transfeminine individual wishes to contribute genetically to a pregnancy but has not preserved sperm before initiating estrogen but still has testes, they can stop cross-sex hormone therapy, allow for resumption of sperm maturation, and production. The exact time needed for this process is unclear. It is important for providers to be supportive of their patients undergoing this process as it can be emotionally, physically, and socially challenging.

If the transfeminine patient has a partner with a uterus, ovaries, and tubes, this may be an option for gestation. If they do not have a partner with a uterus, or their partner is not interested or able to carry a pregnancy, they will need to find a surrogate. They will also need to decide whose oocytes will be used to produce the pregnancy. If they have a partner with ovaries, this could be an option if the partner is interested in going through the process of oocyte harvesting. If a transfeminine person is able to produce sperm, their choice of insemination route depends on which oocytes and uterus will be used, if they are able to ejaculate and have ample sperm count and motility, and what their sexual practices are at baseline. If a transfeminine person is able to produce sperm and has a partner with ovaries and a uterus and is comfortable and able to engage in penetrative sex with their partner, pregnancy may be attempted this way. If their partner has a uterus and ovaries and penetrative sex with ejaculation is not possible, assisted intravaginal, intracervical, or intrauterine insemination with or without augmented ovulation is an option. If a transfeminine person does not have a partner who has a uterus and is interested in gestating, IVF and surrogacy is another option. Surrogacy adds significant expense to an already costly endeavor, so this may be limiting to many individuals.

ADOPTION

If a trans person is not interested in genetically related children or does not have the ability or resources to pursue assisted reproductive technologies, adoption is another option for family building. Adoption can be a very rewarding but also emotionally and fiscally demanding process. There are also documented challenges stemming from bias against transgender people with regard to adopting children.[126,132,133] Furthermore, adoption laws for lesbian, gay, bisexual, transgender, queer/questioning (LGBTQ) people vary from state to state in the United States making uniform strategies or considerations even for one family across time and location challenging.[114] These multiple overlapping challenges may prove to be a barrier for some families.[133]

REPRODUCTIVE OPTIONS FOR TRANSGENDER AND GENDER NONCONFORMING YOUTH

Increasingly there is openness to identifying and facilitating access to care for transgender and gender nonconforming youth. This includes early access to supportive social and medical services, hormone-blocking agents which halt natal puberty, gender affirming hormone therapies, and even surgical processes as appropriate. Positive psychological, social, and physical outcomes have been demonstrated for gender affirming care that provide these components of care to youth.[134,135] For a number of individuals hormone blockade (which may begin at Tanner Stage II) may be followed by initiation of gender affirming (or cross-sex) hormone therapy.[134,135] This prevents individuals from undergoing natal sex puberty and rather encourages pubertal development consistent with an affirmed GI. Though a critical tool in the care and treatment of transgender and gender nonconforming youth, treatment with pubertal blockers until initiation of gender affirming hormones precludes the process of natal gamete development and therefore, given currently available technologies, eliminates the possibility of future reproduction of genetically related children. Some consideration has been given to processes of cryopreservation of prepubertal ovarian and testicular material, but current technologies for delayed or in-vitro maturation of these tissues to produce mature gametes is not yet ready for general clinical use. Developments have up until now been fostered by oncology literature and research working to preserve fertility for young cancer survivors.[136] As these strategies are still considered experimental they are largely out-of-pocket expenditures for transgender youth and their families.

If transgender or gender nonconforming youth undergo natal puberty with or without the start of gender affirming hormones, they would have the same reproductive options available to them as adults who have socially and/or medically transitioned. As Dickey et al. note, although discussion of the fertility implications of hormonal treatments are recommended for all transgender and gender nonconforming individuals prior to initiation of gender affirming procedures, these discussions may not be developmentally appropriate for youth and therefore quite difficult to have in meaningful ways that do not solely rely on parental assignation of significance towards their children's future potential as parents or their role (or loss thereof) as grandparents.[112]

OBSTETRICAL CARE FOR TRANSGENDER PATIENTS

While many transmasculine patients report wanting children,[101] little is known about pregnancy in these patients. We do have data that show that pregnancy poses particular challenges to transmasculine individuals. In a study of eight male or gender variant patients who experienced pregnancy, most demonstrated profound loneliness and reported internal struggles around pregnancy and childbirth and the investigators describe significant "external struggles," or difficulty with how these patients were received or treated by medical providers.[137] This finding was also reported in a larger study by Light et al. which describes the common experience of transmasculine patients unable to access culturally competent providers.[55]

Recently, uterine transplant with subsequent pregnancies and deliveries has been successfully accomplished in a small series of cisgender women with congenital müllerian anomalies.[138,139] As innovations like this continue to evolve, there will be a dialogue about the physical and ethical feasibility of uterine transplantation in the transgender woman so that she some day may be able to gestate and deliver a pregnancy.[140,141] We are still a long way away from this becoming part of the fertility discussion with these patients, but as these surgeries become more common in cisgender women, it is possible that some innovators may begin thinking about additional options for transfeminine patients in the future.

Physical Considerations

The effect of testosterone on fertility is unclear, but its effect on cessation of menstruation is thought to attenuate fertility at least temporarily, even if not absolutely.[142] It is also unclear whether the effect of testosterone on fertility (both in the immediate and long term) is more pronounced in certain populations, at what dose and length of use of testosterone this effect is seen, and whether testosterone effects are reversible. As described in Light et al.'s study, the longer it has been since testosterone was used, the greater the likelihood of achieving pregnancy: 72% of patients conceived within 6 months of attempting pregnancy, 80% resumed menses within 6 months of stopping testosterone, and 20% of individuals conceived while still amenorrheic from testosterone. While discussing family planning and fertility in trans patients, it is important to note that in this study, 24% of those surveyed had an unplanned pregnancy, making it clear that there is a need for contraception counseling in the transmasculine patient population if child bearing is not desired.[55]

Psychosocial Considerations

Pregnancy and delivery experiences are not uniform across transmasculine individuals. For some, pregnancy and delivery may precipitate or worsen baseline gender dysphoria.[55,143] Pregnancy may necessitate disclosure of trans status that had not been previously revealed, which could cause personal trauma or employment instability. In one study of transmasculine individuals looking at lactation and chestfeeding, some participants responded that chest masculinizing surgery helped them with their decision to become pregnant, as some reported that the anticipated dysphoria of "female-appearing mammary tissue" would have been too great to handle: "I don't think I could have navigated this entire process [pregnancy] without having had top surgery."[127] Additionally, experiencing pregnancy with a male GI may be met with a host of logistical challenges such as obtaining insurance coverage for a sex-specific service (pregnancy and birth) or encountering problems with documentation as electronic medical records may not allow for relevant charting.[144] Both emotional and physical changes associated with the cessation of testosterone and experiencing the endogenous hormones of pregnancy may be difficult for some trans patients and this may increase the risk for peri- and postpartum depression.[145] It is important to note, however, that not all individuals experience an increase in dysphoria, with some feeling that "it was relieving to feel comfortable in the body I'd been born with."[55,127,146]

Delivery Considerations

Light et al. found that 36% of the men surveyed who had ever used testosterone delivered by cesarean compared to 19% who had never used testosterone. In this study, the sample size was small and it is therefore unclear if this finding is representative of a true effect that testosterone use may have on a patient's likelihood of achieving a vaginal delivery. Testosterone and estrogen suppression can cause atrophic changes of the vagina.[63,64] In the setting of vaginal atrophy from testosterone use, it is unclear whether this will affect delivery or lead to increased obstetrical trauma as a result of decreased tissue compliance. Vaginal atrophy in the setting of testosterone use can be severe, but it should not an indication for cesarean delivery unless requested by the patient. If the patient had some form of genital reconstruction (such as metoidioplasty without vaginectomy), primary elective cesarean section should be discussed with the patient as a means to avoid trauma to the reconstructed area. However, prior reconstruction should not mandate cesarean section—if the patient desires and is functionally able to achieve vaginal delivery.[147]

Pregnancy Complications

It is unknown whether testosterone use prior to the pregnancy contributes to increased pregnancy complications or neonatal morbidity. Patients are instructed to stop testosterone therapy while attempting to achieve pregnancy and during the pregnancy as it is considered a US Food and Drug Administration (FDA) pregnancy category X drug. Testosterone is considered a teratogen as it affects the fetal sex development pathway.[148] However, the washout period from last testosterone use until initiation of progestational activities is not known. This is an area that warrants future investigation.

Chest/Breastfeeding

Transmasculine people regardless of whether or not they have had previous top surgery may be interested in chestfeeding; however surgical history may make chestfeeding difficult if not impossible.[55,127,143,148] MacDonald et al. looked at 22 trans men, and report that type of procedure seems to the main predetermining factor in ability to chestfeed postpartum.[127] Surgeons who perform top surgery should have a discussion with patients about their fertility goals, specifically their plans with regard to chestfeeding. This is a topic that often gets overlooked in the preoperative consultation, but it remains important. Data show that patients are often afraid to have this discussion with their surgeon fearing that they may be denied the procedure if future considerations of child-bearing and lactation were raised.[127]

Double incision with free nipple grafts (a commonly used technique for top surgery) disrupts milk ducts, making chestfeeding very unlikely. There are other procedures that do not disrupt the neurovascular bundle to the nipple areolar complex and may preserve the opportunity to chestfeed; however data are still lacking. There are also reports of mammary tissue growth/regrowth after surgery during pregnancy and lactation but the extent to which regrowth occurs, how it is influenced by procedure type, and how functional remaining/regrown tissue is for lactation also remains unknown.[127]

Gender dysphoria may be exacerbated with chestfeeding, and for this reason (as well as other logistical, social, medical, or psychological considerations) some transgender men may choose not to chestfeed regardless of their surgical history. For those patients who have undergone chest reconstruction and are unable to lactate but are interested in the experience of chestfeeding, supplemental nursing systems (SNS) are possible. Providers should make sure to increase the awareness of lactation consultants, nurses, and midwives when it comes for caring for this patient population so as to create a supportive infrastructure that is necessary to promote dyad-appropriate feeding for the lactating parent and child.[5,150–152] We encourage all health care providers interacting with pregnant and lactating transmasculine individuals to have open-ended conversations about comprehensive ways to support patients' goals and desires around child feeding.

Little is known about transwomen and their ability to breastfeed, but there are anecdotal reports of initiation of lactation and successful feeding.[152] One protocol that has been used and reported as effective for some individuals is the Newman-Goldfarb protocol, which has been previously used to initiate lactation in adoptive cisgender female parents. This protocol involves oral contraceptive pills for 6 months prior to arrival of the baby. Oral contraceptives are then stopped 6 to 8 weeks prior to the anticipated birth date or adoption day of the infant and domperidone (not available in the United States and not FDA approved) is initiated, combined with physical stimulation and pumping. Hormone doses may need to be adjusted as they can suppress lactation.[148] Spironolactone, often used as an antiandrogen adjunct to testosterone, appears to be safe in breastfeeding.[153]

REFERENCES

1. Grant, Jaime M., Lisa A. Mottet, Justin Tanis, Jack Harrison, Jody L. Herman, and Mara Keisling. *Injustice at Every Turn: A Report of the National Transgender Discrimination Survey*. Washington: National Center for Transgender Equality and National Gay and Lesbian Task Force, 2011.
2. Dutton L, Koenig K, Fennie K. Gynecologic care of the female-to-male transgender man. *J Midwifery Womens Health*. 2008;53 (4):331–337.
3. Erickson-Schroth L, ed. *Trans Bodies, Trans Selves: A Resource for The Transgender Community*. 1st ed. New York, NY: Oxford University Press; 2014.
4. American Congress of Obstetrics and Gynecology. Committee Opinion No. 512: Health Care for Transgender Individuals. *Obstet Gynecol*. 2011;118(6):1454–1458.
5. American College of Nurse Midwives; 2012 http://www.midwife.org/ACNM/files/ ACNMLibraryData/UPLOADFILENAME/ 000000000278/Transgender Gender Variant Position Statement December 2012.pdf. Accessed, December 16, 2018.
6. The World Professional Association for Transgender Health. Standards of care for the health of transsexual, transgender, and gender-nonconforming people. *Int J Transgenderism*. 2011;13(4):165–232.
7. Educational Committee of the Council on Resident Education in Obstetrics and Gynecology. *Educational Objectives: Core Curriculum in Obstetrics and Gynecology*. 10th ed. Washington, DC: American College of Obstetricians and Gynecologists; 2013.
8. Obedin-Maliver J. Time for OBGYNs to care for people of all genders. *J Womens Health*. 2015;24(2):109–111.
9. Grimstad FW, Satterwhite CL, Wieneke CL. Assessing residency program approaches to the transgender health CREOG objective. *Transgend Health*. 2016;1(1):69–74.
10. Unger CA. Care of the transgender patient: a survey of gynecologists' current knowledge and practice. *J Womens Health*. 2015;24(2):114–118.
11. Institute of Medicine Board on the Health of Select P. The National Academies Collection: Reports funded by National Institutes of Health. In: *Collecting Sexual Orientation and Gender Identity Data in Electronic Health Records: Workshop Summary*. Washington, DC: National Academies Press (US) National Academy of Sciences; 2013.
12. Makadon HJ, Mayer KH, Potter J, et al. *Fenway Guide to Lesbian, Gay, Bisexual, and Transgender Health*. 2nd ed. Philadelphia: American College of Physicians; 2015.
13. Cahill SR, Baker K, Deutsch MB, et al. Inclusion of sexual orientation and gender identity in stage 3 meaningful use guidelines: a huge step forward for LGBT health. *LGBT Health*. 2015;3(2):100–102.
14. Federal Registrar: The Daily Journal of The United States Government. "Medicare and Medicaid Programs; Electronic Health Record Incentive Program-Stage 3 and Modifications to Meaningful Use in 2015 Through 2017" National Archives and Records Administration; Washington D.C.; 2015:62761-62995. https://www.federalregister.gov/documents/ 2015/10/16/2015-25595/medicare-and-medicaid-programs-electronic-health-record-incentive-program-stage-3-and-modifications. Accessed: December 16, 2018.
15. Cahill S, Singal R, Grasso C, et al. Do ask, do tell: high levels of acceptability by patients of routine collection of sexual orientation and gender identity data in four diverse American community health centers. *PLoS One*. 2014;9 (9). e107104.

16. Sexual Minority Assessment Research Team (SMART). Best practices for asking questions about sexual orientation on surveys. The Williams Institute. Los Angeles, CA. 2009.

17. The Gender Identity in U.S. Surveillance (GenIUSS) Group. Best practices for asking questions to identify transgender and other gender minority respondents on population-based surveys. *The Williams Institute*: 2014 Los Angeles, CA.

18. Sausa LA, Sevelius J, Keatley J, et al. *Policy Recommendations for Inclusive Data Collection of Trans People in HIV Prevention, Care, & Services*. San Francisco, CA: Center of Excellence for Transgender HIV Prevention, University of California, San Francisco; 2009.

19. Bradford J, Cahill S, Grasso C, et al. *Policy Focus: How to Gather Data on Sexual Orientation and Gender Identity in Clinical Settings*. Boston, MA: The Fenway Institute; 2011.

20. Case P, Austin SB, Hunter DJ, et al. Disclosure of sexual orientation and behavior in the Nurses' Health Study II: results from a pilot study. *J Homosex*. 2006;51(1):13–31.

21. Cahill S, Makadon H. Sexual orientation and gender identity data collection in clinical settings and in electronic health records: a key to ending LGBT health disparities. *LGBT Health*. 2014;1(1):34–41.

22. McNair R, Hegarty K, Taft A. Disclosure for same-sex attracted women enhancing the quality of the patient-doctor relationship in general practice. *Aust Fam Physician*. 2015;44 (8):573–578.

23. Bernstein KT, Liu KL, Begier EM, et al. Same-sex attraction disclosure to health care providers among New York City men who have sex with men: implications for HIV testing approaches. *Arch Intern Med*. 2008;168(13): 1458–1464.

24. When Health Care Isn't Caring: Lamdba Legal's Survey on Discrimination Against LGBT People and People Living with HIV. New York; 2010.

25. Bauer GR, Redman N, Bradley K, et al. Sexual health of trans men who are gay, bisexual, or who have sex with men: results from Ontario, Canada. *Int J Transgend*. 2013;14(2):66–74.

26. Peitzmeier SM, Khullar K, Reisner SL, et al. Pap test use is lower among female-to-male patients than non-transgender women. *Am J Prev Med*. 2014;47(6):808–812.

27. Peitzmeier SM, Reisner SL, Harigopal P, et al. Female-to-male patients have high prevalence of unsatisfactory Paps compared to non-transgender females: implications for cervical cancer screening. *J Gen Intern Med*. 2014;29 (5):778–784.

28. Potter J, Peitzmeier SM, Bernstein I, et al. Cervical cancer screening for patients on the female-to-male spectrum: a narrative review and guide for clinicians. *J Gen Intern Med*. 2015;30(12):1857–1864.

29. Winter S, Diamond M, Green J, et al. Transgender people: health at the margins of society. *Lancet*. 2016;388(10042):390–400.

30. Scheim AI, Bauer GR. Sex and gender diversity among transgender persons in Ontario, Canada: results from a respondent-driven sampling survey. *J Sex Res*. 2014;1–14.

31. Movement Advancement Project (MAP). Equality Maps; Identity document laws and policies; 2016. http://www.lgbtmap.org/equality-maps/identity_document_laws; 2016. Accessed 30 August 2018.

32. Movement Advancement Project (MAP). Equality Maps; Non-Discrimination Laws. http://www.lgbtmap.org/equality-maps/non_discrimination_laws; 2016. Accessed 30 August 2016.

33. International Day Against Homophobia, Transphobia & Biphobia (IDAHOT). 2016 Press Release—Trans Murder Monitoring Update. In: *Transgender Europe*: 2016.

34. House Bill 2. An Act to Provide for Single-Sex Multiple Occupancy Bathroom and Changing Facilities in Schools and Public Agencies and to Create Statewide Consistency in Regulation of Employment and Public Accomodations. In: *General Assembly of North Carolina*, ed. Session Law 2016-3, House Bill 2; 2016.

35. Pearce M. *What it's like to live under North Carolina's bathroom law if you're transgender*. Los Angeles, CA: *LA Times*; 2016.

36. Seelman KL. Transgender adults' access to college bathrooms and housing and the relationship to suicidality. *J Homosex*. 2016;1–22.

37. Transgender Europe - Trans Rights Europe Index, 2018. Produced by: The International Lesbian, Gay, Bisexual, Trans & Intersex Association (ILGA) Europe. Ed Burssels, Belgium. 2018. https://tgeu.org/wp-content/uploads/2018/05/SideB_TGEU2018_Print.pdf. Accessed December 17, 2018.

38. Feldman J, Spencer K. Medical and surgical management of the transgender patient: what the primary care clinician needs to know. In: Makadon HMK, Potter J, Goldhammer H, eds. *Fenway Guide to Lesbian, Gay, Bisexual and Transgender Health*. 2nd ed. Philadelphia: American College of Physicians; 2015:479–511.

39. Newfield E, Hart S, Dibble S, et al. Female-to-male transgender quality of life. *Qual Life Res*. 2006;15(9):1447–1457.

40. White Hughto JM, Reisner SL. A systematic review of the effects of hormone therapy on psychological functioning and quality of life in transgender individuals. *Transgend Health*. 2016;1(1):21–31.

41. Gomez-Gil E, Gomez A, Canizares S, et al. Clinical utility of the Bem Sex Role Inventory (BSRI) in the Spanish transsexual and non-transsexual population. *J Pers Assess*. 2012;94 (3):304–309.

42. de Haan G, Santos GM, Arayasirikul S, et al. Non-prescribed hormone use and barriers to care for transgender women in San Francisco. *LGBT Health*. 2015;2(4):313–323.

43. American College of Obstetricians and Gynecologists (ACOG) Practice Bulletin No.110. Noncontraceptive uses of hormonal contraceptives. *Obstet Gynecol*. 2010;115:206–218.

44. Deutsch MB, ed. *Guidelines for the Primary and Gender-Affirming Care of Transgender and Gender Nonbinary People*. 2nd ed. San Francisco: Center of Excellence for Transgender Health—University of California; 2016.

45. Steinle K. Hormonal management of the female-to-male transgender patient. *J Midwifery Womens Health*. 2011;56(3):293–302.

46. Wierckx K, Van de Peer F, Verhaeghe E, et al. Short- and long-term clinical skin effects of testosterone treatment in trans men. *J Sex Med*. 2014;11(1):222–229.

47. Wierckx K, Van Caenegem E, Schreiner T, et al. Cross-sex hormone therapy in trans persons is safe and effective at short-time follow-up: results from the European network for the investigation of gender incongruence. *J Sex Med*. 2014;11(8):1999–2011.

48. van Kesteren PJ, Asscheman H, Megens JA, et al. Mortality and morbidity in transsexual subjects treated with cross-sex hormones. *Clin Endocrinol*. 1997;47(3):337–342.

49. Gooren LJ, Giltay EJ. Review of studies of androgen treatment of female-to-male transsexuals: effects and risks of administration of androgens to females. *J Sex Med*. 2008;5 (4):765–776.

50. American College of Obstetricians and Gynecologists (ACOG). Practice Bulletin No. 89: Elective and Risk-Reducing Salpingo-oophorectomy. *Obstet Gynecol*. 2008;111: 231–241.

51. Obedin-Maliver J. Pelvic pain and persistent menses in transgender men. In: Deutsch MB, ed. *Guidelines for the Primary and Gender-Affirming Care of Transgender and Gender Nonbinary People*. 2nd ed. San Francisco: Center of Excellence for Transgender Health, Department of Family and Community Medicine, University of California San Francisco; 2016.

52. Hembree WC, Cohen-Kettenis P, Delemarre-van de Waal HA, et al. Endocrine treatment of transsexual persons: an Endocrine Society clinical practice guideline. *J Clin Endocrinol Metab*. 2009;94(9):3132–3154.

53. Nakamura A, Watanabe M, Sugimoto M, et al. Dose-response analysis of testosterone replacement therapy in patients with female to male gender identity disorder. *Endocr J*. 2013;60 (3):275–281.

54. Pelusi C, Costantino A, Martelli V, et al. Effects of three different testosterone formulations in female-to-male transsexual persons. *J Sex Med*. 2014;11(12):3002–3011.

55. Light AD, Obedin-Maliver J, Sevelius JM, et al. Transgender men who experienced pregnancy after female-to-male gender transitioning. *Obstet Gynecol*. 2014;124(6):1120–1127.

56. Deutsch MB, Bhakri V, Kubicek K. Effects of cross-sex hormone treatment on transgender women and men. *Obstet Gynecol*. 2015;125 (3):605–610.

57. Ferrero S, Gillott DJ, Venturini PL, et al. Use of aromatase inhibitors to treat endometriosis-related pain symptoms: a systematic review. *Reprod Biol Endocrinol*. 2011;9:89.

58. Amsterdam LL, Gentry W, Jobanputra S, et al. Anastrazole and oral contraceptives: a novel treatment for endometriosis. *Fertil Steril*. 2005;84(2):300–304.

59. Ailawadi RK, Jobanputra S, Kataria M, et al. Treatment of endometriosis and chronic pelvic pain with letrozole and norethindrone acetate: a pilot study. *Fertil Steril*. 2004;81(2):290–296.

60. Jarrell JF, Vilos GA, Allaire C, et al. Consensus guidelines for the management of chronic pelvic pain. *J Obstet Gynaecol Can*. 2005;27(9): 869–910.

61. Abercrombie PD, Learman LA. Providing holistic care for women with chronic pelvic pain. *J Obstet Gynecol Neonatal Nurs*. 2012;41 (5):668–679.

62. Miller-Matero LR, Saulino C, Clark S, et al. When treating the pain is not enough: a multi-disciplinary approach for chronic pelvic pain. *Arch Womens Ment Health*. 2015;.

63. Miller N, Bedard YC, Cooter NB, et al. Histological changes in the genital tract in transsexual women following androgen therapy. *Histopathology*. 1986;10(7):661–669.

64. Perrone AM, Cerpolini S, Maria Salfi NC, et al. Effect of long-term testosterone administration on the endometrium of female-to-male (FtM) transsexuals. *J Sex Med.* 2009;6(11):3193–3200.

65. Kao A, Binik YM, Kapuscinski A, et al. Dyspareunia in postmenopausal women: a critical review. *Pain Res Manag.* 2008;13(3):243–254.

66. Weber MA, Kleijn MH, Langendam M, et al. Local oestrogen for pelvic floor disorders: a systematic review. *PLoS One.* 2015;10(9). e0136265.

67. Dorr MB, Nelson AL, Mayer PR, et al. Plasma estrogen concentrations after oral and vaginal estrogen administration in women with atrophic vaginitis. *Fertil Steril.* 2010;94(6): 2365–2368.

68. Santen RJ. Vaginal administration of estradiol: effects of dose, preparation and timing on plasma estradiol levels. *Climacteric.* 2015;18 (2):121–134.

69. Cochran BN, Balsam K, Flentje A, et al. Mental health characteristics of sexual minority veterans. *J Homosex.* 2013;60(2–3):419–435.

70. Shipherd JC, Maguen S, Skidmore WC, et al. Potentially traumatic events in a transgender sample. Frequency and associated symptoms. *Traumatology.* 2011;17:56–67.

71. Gooren LJ. Clinical practice. Care of transsexual persons. *N Engl J Med.* 2011;364 (13):1251–1257.

72. Spade D. Medical therapy and health maintenance for transgender men: a guide for health care providers. In: Gorton NBJ, ed. *Lyon-Martin Women's Health Services* 2005:89. San Francisco.

73. Nikolic DV, Djordjevic ML, Granic M, et al. Importance of revealing a rare case of breast cancer in a female to male transsexual after bilateral mastectomy. *World J Surg Oncol.* 2012;10:280.

74. Gooren L, Bowers M, Lips P, et al. Five new cases of breast cancer in transsexual persons. *Andrologia.* 2015;47(10):1202–1205.

75. Gooren LJ, van Trotsenburg MA, Giltay EJ, et al. Breast cancer development in transsexual subjects receiving cross-sex hormone treatment. *J Sex Med.* 2013;10(12):3129–3134.

76. Mueller A, Gooren L. Hormone-related tumors in transsexuals receiving treatment with cross-sex hormones. *Eur J Endocrinol.* 2008;159 (3):197–202.

77. Massad LS, Einstein MH, Huh WK, et al. 2012 updated consensus guidelines for the management of abnormal cervical cancer screening tests and cancer precursors. *J Low Genit Tract Dis.* 2013;17(5 Suppl 1):S1–S27.

78. Grynberg M, Fanchin R, Dubost G, et al. Histology of genital tract and breast tissue after long-term testosterone administration in a female-to-male transsexual population. *Reprod Biomed Online.* 2010;20(4):553–558.

79. Dizon DS, Tejada-Berges T, Koelliker S, et al. Ovarian cancer associated with testosterone supplementation in a female-to-male transsexual patient. *Gynecol Obstet Invest.* 2006;62 (4):226–228.

80. Hage JJ, Dekker JJ, Karim RB, et al. Ovarian cancer in female-to-male transsexuals: report of two cases. *Gynecol Oncol.* 2000;76(3):413–415.

81. Urban RR, Teng NN, Kapp DS. Gynecologic malignancies in female-to-male transgender patients: the need of original gender surveillance. *Am J Obstet Gynecol.* 2011;204(5): e9–e12.

82. Green N, Hoenigl M, Morris S. Risk behavior and sexually transmitted infections among transgender women and men undergoing community-based screening for acute and early HIV infection in San Diego. *Medicine.* 2015;94 (41). e1830.

83. Stephens SC, Bernstein KT, Philip SS. Male to female and female to male transgender persons have different sexual risk behaviors yet similar rates of STDs and HIV. *AIDS Behav.* 2011;15 (3):683–686.

84. Centers for Disease Control and Prevention. Sexually transmitted diseases treatment guidelines. *MMWR Recomm Rep.* 2015;64(RR-03):1–137.

85. Jones CA, Reiter L, Greenblatt E. Fertility preservation in transgender patients. *Int J Transgenderism.* 2016;0(0):1–7.

86. Wierckx K, Gooren L, T'Sjoen G. Clinical review: breast development in trans women receiving cross-sex hormones. *J Sex Med.* 2014;11(5):1240–1247.

87. Seal LJ. A review of the physical and metabolic effects of cross-sex hormonal therapy in the treatment of gender dysphoria. *Ann Clin Biochem.* 2016;53(Pt 1):10–20.

88. Brown GR, Jones KT. Incidence of breast cancer in a cohort of 5,135 transgender veterans. *Breast Cancer Res Treat.* 2015;149(1):191–198.

89. Carter HB, Albertsen PC, Barry MJ, et al. Early Detection of Prostate Cancer: American Urological Association (AUA) Guideline. *Am Urol Assoc.* 2013;1–28.

90. Trum HW, Hoebeke P, Gooren LJ. Sex reassignment of transsexual people from a gynecologist's and urologist's perspective. *Acta Obstet Gynecol Scand.* 2015;94(6):563–567.

91. Deutsch MB, Glidden DV, Sevelius J, et al. HIV pre-exposure prophylaxis in transgender women: a subgroup analysis of the iPrEx trial. *Lancet HIV.* 2015;2(12):e512–e519.

92. Loverro G, Di Naro E, Caringella AM, et al. Prevalence of human papillomavirus infection in a clinic sample of transsexuals in Italy. *Sex Transm Infect.* 2016;92(1):67–69.

93. Unger CA. Care of the transgender patient: the role of the gynecologist. *Am J Obstet Gynecol.* 2014;210(1):16–26.

94. Weyers S, De Sutter P, Hoebeke S, et al. Gynaecological aspects of the treatment and follow-up of transsexual men and women. *Facts Views Vis Obgyn.* 2010;2(1):35–54.

95. Weyers S, Verstraelen H, Gerris J, et al. Microflora of the penile skin-lined neovagina of transsexual women. *BMC Microbiol.* 2009;9:102.

96. Horbach SE, Bouman MB, Smit JM, et al. Outcome of vaginoplasty in male-to-female transgenders: a systematic review of surgical techniques. *J Sex Med.* 2015;12(6):1499–1512.

97. Nygaard IE, Hamad NM, Shaw JM. Activity restrictions after gynecologic surgery: is there evidence? *Int Urogynecol J.* 2013;24(5): 719–724.

98. Lubbert H, Leo-Rossberg I, Hammerstein J. Effects of ethinyl estradiol on semen quality and various hormonal parameters in a eugonadal male. *Fertil Steril.* 1992;58(3):603–608.

99. De Sutter P. The desire to have children and the preservation of fertility in transsexual women: a survey. *Int J Transgenderism.* 2002;6(3).

100. Wierckx K, Stuyver I, Weyers S, et al. Sperm freezing in transsexual women. *Arch Sex Behav.* 2012;41(5):1069–1071.

101. Wierckx K, Van Caenegem E, Pennings G, et al. Reproductive wish in transsexual men. *Hum Reprod.* 2012;27(2):483–487.

102. Brothers D, Ford WC. Gender reassignment and assisted reproduction: an ethical analysis. Bristol Centre for Reproductive Medicine Ethics Advisory Committee. *Hum Reprod.* 2000;15(4):737–738.

103. Murphy TF. The ethics of fertility preservation in transgender body modifications. *J Bioeth Inq.* 2012;9(3):311–316.

104. Murphy TF. The ethics of helping transgender men and women have children. *Perspect Biol Med.* 2010;53(1):46–60.

105. Minter SM, Wald DH. "Protecting parental rights." In: Transgender Family Law: A Guide to Effective Advocacy. Eds. Levi, Jennifer L. and Monnin-Browder, Elizabeth E.

106. Ethics Committee of the American Society for Reproductive Medicine. Access to fertility services by transgender persons: an Ethics Committee opinion. *Fertil Steril.* 2015;104(5): 1111–1115.

107. White T, Ettner R. Disclosure, risks and protective factors for children whose parents are undergoing a gender transformation. *J Gay Lesbian Psychotherapy.* 2004;8:129–147.

108. White T, Ettner R. Adaptation and adjustment in children of transsexual parents. *Eur Child Adolesc Psychiatry.* 2007;16(4):215–221.

109. Freedman D, Tasker F, Di Ceglie D. Children and adolescents with transsexual parents referred to a specialist gender identity development service: A brief report of key development features. *Clin Child Psychol Psychiatry.* 2002;7:423–432.

110. Green R. Transsexuals' children. *Int J Transgenderism.* 1988;2(4).

111. Green R. Sexual identity of 37 children raised by homosexual or transsexual parents. *Am J Psychiatry.* 1978;135(6):692–697.

112. Dickey LM, Ducheny KM, Ehrbar ED. Family creation options for transgender and gender nonconforming people. *Pyschobiol Sex Orientat Gend Divers.* 2016;3(2):173–179.

113. Erickson-Schroth L, ed. *Trans Bodies, Trans Selves: A Resource for the Transgender Community.* 1st ed. New York: Oxford University Press; 2014.

114. Levi JL, Monnin-Browder EE, eds. *Transgender Family Law: A Guide to Effective Advocacy.* Bloomington, IN: Authorhouse; 2012.

115. Caanen MR, Soleman RS, Kuijper EA, et al. Antimullerian hormone levels decrease in female-to-male transsexuals using testosterone as cross-sex therapy. *Fertil Steril.* 2015;103 (5):1340–1345.

116. American Psychological Association. Guidelines for psychological practice with transgender and gender nonconforming people. *Am Psychol.* 2015;70:832–864.

117. Schulze C. Response of the human testis to long-term estrogen treatment: morphology of Sertoli cells, Leydig cells and spermatogonial stem cells. *Cell Tissue Res.* 1988;251(1):31–43.

118. De Roo C, Tilleman K, T'Sjoen G, De Sutter P. Fertility options in transgender people, International Review of Psychiatry. *Int Rev Psychiatry.* 2016;28(1):112–119.

119. De Sutter P. Gender reassignment and assisted reproduction: present and future reproductive options for transsexual people. *Hum Reprod.* 2001;16(4):612–614.

120. Hamada A, Kingsberg S, Wierckx K, et al. Semen characteristics of transwomen referred

for sperm banking before sex transition: a case series. *Andrologia*. 2015;47(7):832–838.

121. Van Den Broecke R, Van Der Elst J, Liu J, et al. The female-to-male transsexual patient: a source of human ovarian cortical tissue for experimental use. *Hum Reprod*. 2001;16(1): 145–147.

122. Ikeda K, Baba T, Noguchi H, et al. Excessive androgen exposure in female-to-male transsexual persons of reproductive age induces hyperplasia of the ovarian cortex and stroma but not polycystic ovary morphology. *Hum Reprod*. 2013;28(2):453–461.

123. Pache TD, Chadha S, Gooren LJ, et al. Ovarian morphology in long-term androgen-treated female to male transsexuals. A human model for the study of polycystic ovarian syndrome? *Histopathology*. 1991;19(5):445–452.

124. Chadha S, Pache TD, Huikeshoven JM, et al. Androgen receptor expression in human ovarian and uterine tissue of long-term androgen-treated transsexual women. *Hum Pathol*. 1994;25(11):1198–1204.

125. Wallace SA, Blough KL, Kondapalli LA. Fertility preservation in the transgender patient: expanding oncofertility care beyond cancer. *Gynecol Endocrinol*. 2014;1–4.

126. Movement Advancement Project (MAP). Equality Maps: Foster and Adoption Laws. http://www.lgbtmap.org/equality-maps/foster_and_adoption_laws; 2016. Accessed 19 July 2016.

127. MacDonald T, Noel-Weiss J, West D, et al. Transmasculine individuals' experiences with lactation, chest feeding, and gender identity: a qualitative study. *BMC Pregnancy Childbirth*. 2016;16:106.

128. Practice Committees of American Society for Reproductive Medicine—Society for Assisted Reproductive Technology. Mature oocyte cryopreservation: a guideline. *Fertil Steril*. 2013;99 (1):37–43.

129. Borini A, Levi Setti PE, Anserini P, et al. Multicenter observational study on slow-cooling oocyte cryopreservation: clinical outcome. *Fertil Steril*. 2010;94(5):1662–1668.

130. Neighmond P. Women Can Freeze their Eggs for the Future, But at a Cost. Shots: Health News from National Public Radio. All Things Considered. National Public Radio; 2014.

131. Polly K, Polly RG. Parenting. In: Erickson-Schroth L, ed. *Trans Bodies, Trans Selves: A Resource for the Transgender Community*. New York: Oxford University Press; 2014: 390–408.

132. U.S. Case Law. Supreme Count of Nevada Decisions—1986: Daly v. Daly. http://law.justia.com/cases/nevada/supreme-court/1986/15423-1.html; 1986. Accessed 9 September 2016.

133. LGBTQ. *Parenting Network. Transgender Parents and Ontario Family Law: Parenting Through Transition, Together or Apart*. Toronto, Canada.

134. Olson J, Forbes C, Belzer M. Management of the transgender adolescent. *Arch Pediatr Adolesc Med*. 2011;165(2):171–176.

135. Rosenthal SM. Approach to the patient: transgender youth: endocrine considerations. *J Clin Endocrinol Metab*. 2014;99(12):4379–4389.

136. Practice Committee of American Society for Reproductive Medicine. Ovarian tissue cryopreservation: a committee opinion. *Fertil Steril*. 2014;101(5):1237–1243.

137. Ellis SA, Wojnar DM, Pettinato M. Conception, pregnancy, and birth experiences of male and gender variant gestational parents: it's how we could have a family. *J Midwifery Womens Health*. 2015;60(1):62–69.

138. Brannstrom M, Johannesson L, Bokstrom H, et al. Livebirth after uterus transplantation. *Lancet*. 2015;385(9968):607–616.

139. Brannstrom M, Johannesson L, Dahm-Kahler P, et al. First clinical uterus transplantation trial: a six-month report. *Fertil Steril*. 2014;101(5):1228–1236.

140. De Roo C, Tilleman K, T'Sjoen G, et al. Fertility options in transgender people. *Int Rev Psychiatry*. 2016;28(1):112–119.

141. Murphy TF. Assisted gestation and transgender women. *Bioethics*. 2015;29(6):389–397.

142. Obedin-Maliver J, Makadon H. Transgender men and pregnancy. *Obstet Med*. 2016;9(1): 4–8.

143. Ellis SA, Wojnar DM, Pettinato M. Conception, pregnancy, and birth experiences of male and gender variant gestational parents: it's how we could have a family. *J Midwifery Womens Health*. 2014;60(1):62–69.

144. Berger AP, Shutters CM, Imorek KL. Pregnant transmen and barriers to high quality healthcare. *Proc Obstet Gynecol*. 2015;5(2):12.

145. Reisner SL, Katz-Wise SL, Gordon AR, et al. Social epidemiology of depression and anxiety by gender identity. *J Adolesc Health*. 2016;59 (2):203–208.

146. Hempel J. My brother's pregnancy and the making of a new American family. *TIME*; September 9, 2016.

147. LactMed: *A TOXNET Database [Internet]: Testosterone*. Toxnet: Toxicology Data Network: National Institutes of Health—United States National Library of Medicine; 2016.

148. MacDonald T. http://www.milkjunkies.net/2012/03/tips-for-transgender-breastfeeders-and.html; 2012. Accessed 9 July 2015.

149. Farrow A. Lactation support and the LGBTQI community. *J Hum Lact*. 2015;31(1):26–28.

150. Wolfe-Roubatis E, Spatz DL. Transgender men and lactation: what nurses need to know. *MCN Am J Matern Child Nurs*. 2015;40(1):32–38.

151. Adams ED. If transmen can have babies, how will perinatal nursing adapt? *Am J Matern Child Nurs*. 2010;35(1):26–32.

152. MacDonald T. http://www.milkjunkies.net/2013/05/trans-women-and-breastfeeding-personal.html; 2013. Accessed 9 May 2013.

153. LactMed. *A TOXNET Database [Internet]: Spironolactone*. Bethesda (MD): National Institutes of Health—United States National Library of Medicine; 2016.

Hysterectomy for the Transgender Man

MATTHEW SIEDHOFF | PARISA SAMIMI | CHERIE MARFORI

Introduction

The World Professional Association for Transgender Health (WPATH) considers hysterectomy with or without salpingectomy and/or oophorectomy a medically necessary gender-affirming surgery for trans men interested in the procedure.[1] The reasons for surgery are diverse: a sense of organs feeling incongruent with one's gender identify, to promote further masculinization, to assist with changing legal documents, avoiding gynecology visits and prevention of gynecologic problems, or for specific gynecologic issues such as pelvic pain, cramping, bleeding, tumors, cysts, or endometriosis.[2]

The psychological benefits of gender-affirming surgery are well-documented.[3] Cases of regret are rare. In cases of female-to-male gender-affirming surgery, sexual function appears to improve.[4] Over half of all transgender men surveyed desire hysterectomy in the future, with approximately 21% having had the procedure already.[5]

Mistrust and mistreatment between the transgender community and the health-care system are well-established.[5] Approximately half of transgender persons can recall having to educate their providers regarding care, with 19% surveyed being refused care altogether. Given the experience of discrimination and the lack of appropriate providers, many have avoided the health-care system. By understanding the experiences of transgender patients in the health-care system, providers can better understand their reasons for requesting gender-affirming surgery. In this chapter, we will review various perioperative considerations for surgeons performing hysterectomy in the transgender man (Table 14.1).

Preoperative Considerations

As with cisgender patients, preoperative counseling is critical in the transitioning patient. A thorough preoperative assessment should include a discussion about the mode and extent of surgery, coordination with other health-care providers, review of postoperative care and expectations, and assessment of the patient's support system.

WORLD PROFESSIONAL ASSOCIATION FOR TRANSGENDER HEALTH CRITERIA

Several criteria for genital surgery exist, but most surgeons follow those put forth by the WPATH.[6] Patients are candidates for surgery if they meet the following criteria: well-documented gender dysphoria, capacity to give informed consent, age of majority in the patient's country, well-controlled medical and/or mental health concerns, and 12 months of hormonal therapy when able (Table 14.2). They also recommend preoperative evaluation and letters of support for the surgery by two separate mental health professionals trained in transgender care. This so-called requirement has been contended by some as of late, as many see a second letter as unnecessary and overly burdensome for patients. This recommendation may change in the future. WPATH also recommends starting hormonal therapy prior to genital surgery to "introduce a period of reversible estrogen or testosterone suppression, before the patient undergoes an irreversible surgical intervention."[6] They also affirm that living in their self-identified gender role will allow the transgender man to experience a number of various life events and establish a support system. Surgeons may find themselves using these guidelines a as a framework only and adapting them based on their working relationship with the patient, as well as the extent of the surgery being considered.

GENITAL SURGERY

Genital surgery can include hysterectomy, salpingectomy, oophorectomy, metoidioplasty, vaginectomy, scrotoplasty, and implantation of prostheses. The role of hysterectomy, with concomitant salpingectomy, and/or oophorectomy, will be reviewed in this chapter. These procedures can be performed through an open, laparoscopic/robotic, or vaginal approach, with minimally invasive strategies being preferable. A total hysterectomy (as opposed to subtotal or supracervical) with salpingectomy is superior, to avoid additional future procedures, as well as complications related to leaving the fallopian tubes in situ. Bilateral oophorectomy is performed in the majority of cases where fertility preservation isn't desired. Additional concomitant reconstructive surgery (metoidioplasty, phalloplasty) may be considered for those patients seeking complete genital surgery.

Elective appendectomy can be safely performed during gynecologic surgery.[7] The procedure is easy to perform, low-risk, may simplify the differential for acute exacerbations of chronic pain, and has the potential to avoid future imaging and surgical procedures. The benefit is greatest for patients less than 35 years of age,[8] making this procedure relevant for many trans men having hysterectomies in early adulthood. This vulnerable population may want to avoid needing future emergent care from unfamiliar providers with varying levels of cultural sensitivity.

Preoperative testing for the transgender male should include age-appropriate and risk-appropriate screening. Transgender patients are at increased risk for misuse of drugs and alcohol, avoidance of the health-care system due to discrimination and/or lack of insurance, and attempts at self-harm and suicide.[5] Transgender patients report HIV infection at four times the national average.[5] Surgeons should individualize sexually transmitted infection screening according to the risk profile of the particular patient considering hysterectomy.

Patients should be counseled regarding cervix cancer screening, and PAP testing should generally be performed according

TABLE 14.1	Perioperative Considerations for Hysterectomy in the Transgender Man

- Consideration of concomitant procedures
  - Bilateral salpingectomy and/or salpingo-oophorectomy
  - Metoidioplasty
  - Vaginectomy
  - Scrotoplasty
  - Implantation of prostheses
  - Appendectomy
- Cervix cancer screening
- Discussion of future fertility
  - Consideration of oocyte or embryo cryopreservation
- Preoperative testing according to ASA guidelines
- Optimization of hemoglobin/hematocrit, lipids, blood pressure
- Diabetes screening
- Thromboembolism and antibiotic prophylaxis
- Creating a safe and welcoming environment/staff training
- Enhanced Recovery After Surgery protocols with same-day discharge if possible
- Minimally invasive route for surgery (vaginal or endoscopic)

ASA, American Society of this Anesthesiologists.

TABLE 14.2	World Professional Association for Transgender Health Criteria for Undergoing Genital Surgery in the Transgender Patient

- Well-documented gender dysphoria
- Capacity to give informed consent
- Age of majority in the patient's country
- Well-controlled medical and/or mental health concerns
- Preoperative evaluation by two separate mental health professionals
- 12 months of hormonal therapy when able

to the most recent American Society for Colposcopy and Cervical Pathology (ASCCP) guidelines.[9] Female-to-male patients have a higher rate of inadequate PAP smears as well as longer time to follow-up,[10] thought secondary to both provider and patient discomfort during pelvic examination, as well as the atrophic and cellular changes that can occur with testosterone therapy. Recommendations for making pelvic exams in trans men more comfortable are outlined in the University of California San Francisco's (UCSF) Center of Excellence for Transgender Health website.[11] Although there are no data to support this approach, some have deferred speculum exams for cervix dysplasia screening after evaluating history of sexual practices and potential symptoms of cervix cancer, since the only condition that would change the planned procedure from simple hysterectomy would be an invasive carcinoma greater than stage 1A2. Routine screening for ovarian cancer or endometrial cancer in the asymptomatic patient is not recommended. While there is a theoretical concern for the conversion of exogenous testosterone to estrogen, there is currently no strong evidence that trans men are at increased risk for endometrial cancer compared with the general population.

Plans for future fertility should always be considered during discussions of genital gender-affirming surgery. There has historically been an unwillingness to offer reproductive services to transgender persons, due to concern for offspring, the patient, or outright discrimination. American Congress of Obstetricians and Gynecologists (ACOG) has addressed the latter issue, firmly opposing any discrimination of transgender persons based on

the principle of justice.[12] Similarly, the American Society for Reproductive Medicine released a statement indicating that "denial of access to fertility services is not justified."[13] Review of available studies do not show evidence for psychological injury to the offspring of transgender persons, with the American Academy of Pediatrics pointing out lack of evidence to support such claims.[14]

A discussion of fertility plans with a trans man considering hysterectomy (and his partner, if applicable) is similar to preoperative counseling with a cisgender woman who is considering surgical removal of her reproductive organs for benign or malignant reasons. For more in-depth discussions or procedures such as preoperative oocyte or embryo cryopreservation, transgender men should be referred to reproductive endocrinologists, preferably with experience treating trans patients. Patients should be informed that fertility treatment involves temporary cessation of exogenous testosterone in order to achieve ovulation induction. Data are scant regarding ovarian function recovery after testosterone therapy, but extrapolating from case reports and from patients with polycystic ovarian syndrome, it seems that recovery of the functional gonadal tissues is possible.[15,16] Discussing fertility with the prepubertal patient requires a particularly careful approach, given that young patients may feel unprepared to make decisions regarding their future fertility. These conversations should be held with the patient's clinician, a mental health professional, and the patient's parents or supportive persons when possible. Many patients will choose to delay puberty with GnRH analogs. While spontaneous ovulation should theoretically occur following cessation of these suppressive medications, there are few data to support the response and timing of return to ovulation.[17] The Endocrine Society suggests deferring genital gender-affirming surgery until an individual is at least 18 years of age.[17]

Perioperative Management

There are currently no specific guidelines on the perioperative care of transgender men undergoing hysterectomy; however, planning is necessary, and there are some nuances in this patient population that should be considered before proceeding to the operating room. Preoperative testing including laboratory studies, cardiac evaluation, and pulmonary function tests should be performed according to standard American Society of Anesthesiologists (ASA) guidelines,[18] taking into account the patient's comorbid medical conditions.

Testosterone therapy is associated with an increased risk of hyperlipidemia, hypertension, and polycythemia,[19] and it is best to have these health conditions optimized prior to surgery, either through titration of testosterone dosing or independent treatment. These conditions, however, are common even in the general population, and are not a contraindication to "elective" hysterectomy in general, and should not be considered as such for trans men. Most trans men on testosterone therapy have some degree of polycythemia. There is no evidence that secondary polycythemia is an independent risk factor for venous thromboembolism (VTE),[20] so standard prophylaxis with sequential compression devices is reasonable. If the patient is also obese or has other risk factors (prior VTE, malignancy, etc.), adding pharmacologic prophylaxis is indicated. Smoking or obstructive sleep apnea are important ventilatory issues as laparoscopic hysterectomy is performed in the Trendelenburg position. The effect of testosterone on weight isn't completely understood, but may cause fat redistribution from a subcutaneous location to a visceral one, which is relevant to patient positioning and feasibility of performing the procedure. Some studies show increased insulin resistance and fasting blood glucose associated with testosterone use,[21–23] so if not already done, screening for diabetes mellitus should be performed, so that the postoperative period may include glycemic control if appropriate. No studies have demonstrated an increased risk of cardiovascular events such as myocardial infarction, VTE, or stroke among transgender men on hormone therapy; therefore, cardiac testing should follow standard risk assessment.[24–26] Standard antibiotic prophylaxis should be administered according to Surgical Care Improvement Project (SCIP) guidelines.[27]

It is important to create a safe and welcoming medical environment for transgender patients, a population already at risk for avoiding care due to discrimination or disrespect. Guidelines can be found at the UCSF Center of Excellence website that include recommendations for cultural humility, gender-neutral bathrooms, staff training, and so on.[28] This is especially true for men who are being seen by a gynecologic surgeon who almost exclusively treats cisgender women. Providing advance notice to front-line staff that a transgender patient is on the schedule can avoid awkward misunderstandings at clinic visits and in the operating room. Preparing as many people as possible is wise, especially if the electronic medical record (EMR) does not capture the patient's identity well due to its own limitations or for insurance reasons.

Most minimally invasive hysterectomies are now outpatient procedures, and the ability to discharge a posthysterectomy patient on the same day as surgery is especially important for transgender patients, as it reduces the chance of an insensitive encounter or an inadvertent admission to a gynecology floor occupied by women. Scheduling earlier in the day is associated with greater success for same-day discharge,[29] so making these surgeries first-start cases is helpful. Implementation of Enhanced Recovery After Surgery (ERAS) pathways such as pre-emptive analgesia, prevention of postoperative nausea/vomiting, in operating room (OR) catheter removal, early resumption of normal diet, and so on are similarly important.[30] Surgeons should be mindful of loved ones who accompany the patient on surgery day and ask the patient in private if they are aware of the procedure specifics and if he would like the surgeon to provide them with an update after surgery.

Liberal introduction of activity is generally warranted after gynecologic laparoscopy, but opening of the vaginal cuff (dehiscence) occurs more commonly after laparoscopic hysterectomy compared with other modalities,[31] and isn't necessarily associated with penetrative vaginal intercourse,[32] so avoiding strenuous activity for several weeks following hysterectomy is warranted. If a patient doesn't use the vagina for sex and hasn't experienced bleeding following surgery, a speculum exam can be safely deferred at the postoperative visit. Vaginal PAP tests are needed in future visits only if a patient has had a history of severe cervix dysplasia within the last two decades.[9] There is no recommended ovarian cancer screening for those who retain ovaries, but future providers should keep in mind that ovarian pathology is possible if oophorectomy is not performed at the time of hysterectomy, and constitutional symptoms suggesting pelvic disease should be evaluated in a standard fashion. Although rare, primary peritoneal cancer can still occur in patients after the ovaries are removed; thus trans men with symptoms should be assessed.[33]

Route of Surgery, Technique

As with any hysterectomy, the goal in trans men is to provide the safest, most efficient, and cost-effective procedure possible. The ACOG and the American Association of Gynecologic Laparoscopists (AAGL) provide consensus statements supporting a minimally invasive approach to hysterectomy for benign conditions whenever possible.[34,35] This should represent the vast majority of cases, and referral to a specialist is warranted if the surgeon is not experienced with these evidenced-based approaches to surgery. These opinions are further bolstered by a Cochrane review that includes 47 randomized trials.[36] As previously mentioned, minimally invasive surgery is especially important for the transgender patient when diminishing time spent in the hospital is relevant.

For patients without health insurance or for those who have a policy that excludes hysterectomy for the indication of gender dysphoria, knowledge of costs associated with the route of hysterectomy is crucial. We know that vaginal hysterectomy is the most cost-effective route of hysterectomy,[37,38] and case series demonstrate the feasibility of vaginal hysterectomy for gender-affirming surgery,[39,40] including concurrent oophorectomy. One of these series reported on the success of combined hysterectomy with vaginectomy.[39]

Laparoscopic hysterectomy may be preferable in most patients, as there are technical challenges associated with testosterone-driven vaginal atrophy, common nulliparity, lack of uterine descensus, and infrequent or no vaginal intercourse resulting in a narrowed vagina.[41–44] Robotic, multiport laparoscopic, minilaparoscopic, and laparoendoscopic single site surgery seem to have similar outcomes when considering OR time, pain scores, and complications.[45] The single site approach could be particularly applicable for transgender hysterectomy where pelvic or uterine pathology is less likely to be encountered.

Role of Concurrent Bilateral Salpingo-Oophorectomy and Vaginectomy

BILATERAL SALPINGO-OOPHORECTOMY

Gender-affirming surgery is a step some men choose *not* to perform, since they can successfully live in their preferred gender role without untoward symptoms. As such, it should not be assumed that every transgender man will want a hysterectomy and/or removal of the ovaries. There are some patients who PAP tests desire only a bilateral salpingo-oophorectomy (BSO) without an accompanying hysterectomy, or vice versa. When no bothersome pelvic pathology exists and the patient is willing to continue screening pelvic exams, this is a reasonable choice.

A BSO can typically be performed easily and safely at the time of hysterectomy or on its own as a gender-affirming surgery. Performing a BSO will eliminate the concern for future ovarian and tubal pathology (both benign and malignant) and, when performed with a hysterectomy, obviates the need for "routine" pelvic exams in the future. This is an important consideration in this often marginalized and vulnerable population, who may be uncomfortable as males seeking gynecologic care, or for those who are unable to find providers capable of providing such care.

Polycystic ovarian syndrome appears to be more common in transgender men, both before and during testosterone therapy.[15,16] This should be taken into consideration when evaluating irregular uterine bleeding and cardiovascular health. There is some concern that, analogous to cisgender women who have disorders resulting in elevated androgen levels, testosterone therapy in transgender men may increase the risk of ovarian cancer.[6] However, there are no data that support this hypothesis,[17,46] and as such, no screening recommendations exist. The long-term effect of exogenous testosterone on ovarian function is uncertain.

Removing the ovaries eliminates the possibility of having biologic offspring. Patients should be offered options of oocyte and embryo cryopreservation prior to oophorectomy and ideally prior to the initiation of testosterone therapy. Greater than 50% of surveyed transgender men report a desire to have children,[25] and over one-third would have cryopreserved oocytes if it had been offered and made possible for them prior to undergoing BSO. The risk of sterility regret has not been extensively studied in this population, and care should be taken to ensure that all patients, especially teens or young adults, seriously consider cryopreservation. Patients on testosterone therapy will have to temporarily stop their cross-sex hormone therapy in order to undergo ovulation stimulation. Alternatively, ovarian tissue cryopreservation may become a promising alternative to this process, but it still remains experimental. In vitro maturation techniques to obtain gametes would remove the need for reimplantation and hormonal interruption, and could even allow prepubertal ovarian tissue preservation.

A serious consequence of oophorectomy in premenopausal natal females is premature osteoporosis. The long-term risks in the transgender man are still being studied, but short-term studies show that testosterone therapy preserves or even increases bone mineral density (BMD) in the first 3 years of use.[6] Transgender men after BSO who continue testosterone maintain their larger bone radius, increased muscle mass, and stable bone density.[46] Therefore continued adequate dosing of testosterone is important to maintain bone, mass after BSO. Fracture data, however, in transgender men are not available. The Endocrine Society recommends BMD testing at baseline if risk factors for osteoporotic fracture are present (e.g., previous fragility fracture, family history, glucocorticoid use, prolonged hypogonadism). In individuals at low risk, screening for osteoporosis should be initiated at age 60 and in those patients who do not remain compliant with hormone therapy.

The need to remove the ovaries may become a factor in deciding which route of surgery to offer a patient when planning a concurrent hysterectomy. As discussed in the preceding section, the vaginal route is feasible for BSO, but many surgeons who perform these surgeries routinely argue that there are factors relevant to trans men that make laparoscopy a less technically challenging approach for this patient population.

Procedures should be individualized based on a patient's anatomy, the surgeon's skill, and consideration of cost, efficiency, and safety.

While ovarian preservation may be relevant for the patient wishing to preserve his fertility, there is no downside to universal opportunistic bilateral salpingectomy, and this has been supported by ACOG.[47] The leading theory of ovarian carcinogenesis suggests that most ovarian cancers arise in the fallopian tube rather than primarily in the ovary,[48–51] and thus salpingectomy at the time of hysterectomy is thought to be a cost-effective strategy in ovarian cancer prevention.[52]

VAGINECTOMY

Vaginectomy is a procedure undertaken by a minority of transgender men to either resect or obliterate the vaginal canal, either at the time of hysterectomy or as a stand-alone procedure.[53] Full-thickness resection of either the entire or upper vagina can be performed. Alternatively, obliterative procedures such as colpocleisis can also be offered and may be associated with less morbidity than actual resection. Vaginectomy is usually performed at the time of reconstructive external genitalia surgery or "bottom surgery," and in some cases, a portion of the excised anterior vaginal epithelium can be used as a vaginal flap and can be used to lengthen the urethra in the creation of a neophallus.[39,42,43,54–57]

Both laparoscopic[42] and vaginal[39] approaches have been described for vaginectomy. With laparoscopy, the procedure begins with hysterectomy, BSO, and then vaginectomy. Creation of a vaginal flap for the neourethra is performed in the same setting and stored and cultivated in a groin incision. A phalloplasty can then be completed 3 months later. With the vaginal route, a complete mucosal vaginectomy first provides the graft for a neourethra, and subsequently, the vaginal hysterectomy, BSO, and vaginal closure are performed.

Many transgender men do not undergo a vaginectomy and/or phalloplasty as part of their gender transition. Some trans men enjoy and engage in vaginal intercourse. Risks associated with vaginectomy may outweigh the actual benefits for some patients, and this should be considered, especially since the vagina typically harbors minimal risk of pathology. Resection vaginectomy is associated with high rates of complications such as fistulae, voiding and defecatory dysfunction, and hemorrhage. Access to surgeons who have expertise in these procedures can also be a limiting factor for many patients. Genital reconstruction is often a multistage process and can be cost-prohibitive, as many insurers still do not consider the surgery medically necessary. Lastly, the search for a procedure that can successfully create a sensate, cosmetically pleasing, and functional neophallus capable of penetrative intercourse and standing micturition is ongoing. Current techniques typically sacrifice one or more of these desired factors and can be associated with significant morbidity.

REFERENCES

1. Position Statement on Medical Necessity of Treatment, Sex Reassignment, and Insurance Coverage in the USA. http://www.wpath.org/site_page.cfm?pk_association_webpage_menu=1352&pk_association_webpage=3947; 2016. Accessed 5 January 2017.
2. Rachlin K, Hansbury G, Pardo ST. Hysterectomy and oophorectomy experiences of female-to-male transgender individuals. *Int J Transgenderism*. 2010;12:155–166.
3. Gijs L, Brewaeys A. Surgical treatment of gender dysphoria in adults and adolescents: recent developments, effectiveness, and challenges. *Ann Rev Sex Res*. 2007;18:178–224.
4. Klein C, Gorzalka BB. Sexual functioning in transsexuals following hormone therapy and genital surgery: a review. *J Sex Med*. 2009;6:2922–2939 quiz. 40–41.
5. Grant JM, Mottet LA, Tanis J. *Injustice at Every Turn: A Report of the National Transgender Discrimination Survey*. Washington, DC: National Center for Transgender Equality and National Gay and Lesbian Task Force; 2011.

6. World Professional Association for Transgender Health (WPATH). Standards of Care for the Health of Transsexual, Transgender, and Gender Nonconforming People, 7th ed.; 2011. http://www.wpath.org/site_page.cfm?pk_association_webpage_menu=1351. Accessed 5 January 2017.

7. Nezhat C, Nezhat F. Incidental appendectomy during videolaseroscopy. *Am J Obstet Gynecol.* 1991;165:559–564.

8. Snyder TE, Selanders JR. Incidental appendectomy—yes or no? A retrospective case study and review of the literature. *Infect Dis Obstet Gynecol.* 1998;6:30–37.

9. Committee on Practice Bulletins—Gynecology. Practice Bulletin No. 168: Cervical cancer screening and prevention. *Obstet Gynecol.* 2016;128:e111–e130.

10. Peitzmeier SM, Reisner SL, Harigopal P, et al. Female-to-male patients have high prevalence of unsatisfactory Paps compared to non-transgender females: implications for cervical cancer screening. *J Gen Intern Med.* 2014;29:778–784.

11. Transgender patients and the physical examination. http://transhealth.ucsf.edu/trans?page=guidelines-physical-examination; 2016. Accessed 5 January 2017.

12. Committee Opinion No. 500 ACOG. Professional responsibilities in obstetric-gynecologic medical education and training. *Obstet Gynecol.* 2011;118:400–404.

13. Ethics Committee of the American Society for Reproductive Medicine. Access to fertility services by transgender persons: an Ethics Committee opinion. *Fertil Steril.* 2015;104:1111–1115.

14. Perrin EC, Siegel BS. Promoting the well-being of children whose parents are gay or lesbian. *Pediatrics.* 2013;131:e1374–e1383.

15. Spinder T, Spijkstra JJ, van den Tweel JG, et al. The effects of long term testosterone administration on pulsatile luteinizing hormone secretion and on ovarian histology in eugonadal female to male transsexual subjects. *J Clin Endocrinol Metab.* 1989;69:151–157.

16. Baba T, Endo T, Honnma H, et al. Association between polycystic ovary syndrome and female-to-male transsexuality. *Hum Reprod.* 2007;22:1011–1016.

17. Hembree WC, Cohen-Kettenis P, Delemarre-van de Waal HA, et al. Endocrine treatment of transsexual persons: an Endocrine Society clinical practice guideline. *J Clin Endocrinol Metabol.* 2009;94:3132–3154.

18. Apfelbaum JL, Connis RT, Nickinovich DG, et al. Practice advisory for preanesthesia evaluation: an updated report by the American Society of Anesthesiologists Task Force on Preanesthesia Evaluation. *Anesthesiology.* 2012;116:522–538.

19. Callen-Lorde Community Health Center. Protocols for the provision of hormone therapy. New York, NY: Callen-Lorde; 2014.

20. Nadeem O, Gui J, Ornstein DL. Prevalence of venous thromboembolism in patients with secondary polycythemia. *Clin Appl Thromb Hemost.* 2013;19:363–366.

21. Weinand JD, Safer JD. Hormone therapy in transgender adults is safe with provider supervision; a review of hormone therapy sequelae for transgender individuals. *J Clin Transl Endocrinol.* 2015;2:55–60.

22. Gooren LJ, Giltay EJ, Bunck MC. Long-term treatment of transsexuals with cross-sex hormones: extensive personal experience. *J Clin Endocrinol Metab.* 2008;93:19–25.

23. Polderman KH, Gooren LJ, Asscheman H, et al. Induction of insulin resistance by androgens and estrogens. *J Clin Endocrinol Metab.* 1994;79:265–271.

24. Wierckx K, Elaut E, Van Caenegem E, et al. Sexual desire in female-to-male transsexual persons: exploration of the role of testosterone administration. *Eur J Endocrinol.* 2011;165:331–337.

25. Wierckx K, Mueller S, Weyers S, et al. Long-term evaluation of cross-sex hormone treatment in transsexual persons. *J Sex Med.* 2012;9:2641–2651.

26. Asscheman H, T'Sjoen G, Lemaire A, et al. Venous thrombo-embolism as a complication of cross-sex hormone treatment of male-to-female transsexual subjects: a review. *Andrologia.* 2014;46:791–795.

27. Munday GS, Deveaux P, Roberts H, et al. Impact of implementation of the surgical care improvement project and future strategies for improving quality in surgery. *Am J Surg.* 2014;208:835–840.

28. Guidelines for the Primary and Gender-Affirming Care of Transgender and Gender Nonbinary People. http://transhealth.ucsf.edu/trans?page=guidelines-clinic-environment; 2016. Accessed 5 January 2017.

29. Korsholm M, Mogensen O, Jeppesen MM, et al. Systematic review of same-day discharge after minimally invasive hysterectomy. *Int J Gynaecol Obstet.* 2017;136:128–137.

30. Kalogera E, Dowdy SC. Enhanced recovery pathway in gynecologic surgery: improving outcomes through evidence-based medicine. *Obstet Gynecol Clin North Am.* 2016;43:551–573.

31. Uccella S, Ceccaroni M, Cromi A, et al. Vaginal cuff dehiscence in a series of 12,398 hysterectomies: effect of different types of colpotomy and vaginal closure. *Obstet Gynecol.* 2012;120:516–523.

32. Siedhoff MT, Yunker AC, Steege JF. Decreased incidence of vaginal cuff dehiscence after laparoscopic closure with bidirectional barbed suture. *J Minim Invasive Gynecol.* 2011;18:218–223.

33. Schmeler KM, Daniels MS, Soliman PT, et al. Primary peritoneal cancer after bilateral salpingo-oophorectomy in two patients with Lynch syndrome. *Obstet Gynecol.* 2010;115:432–434.

34. Committee Opinion No. 444 ACOG. choosing the route of hysterectomy for benign disease. *Obstet Gynecol.* 2009;114:1156–1158.

35. AAGL position statement. route of hysterectomy to treat benign uterine disease. *J Minim Invasive Gynecol.* 2011;18:1–3.

36. Aarts JW, Nieboer TE, Johnson N, et al. Surgical approach to hysterectomy for benign gynaecological disease. *Cochrane Database Syst Rev.* 2015. Cd003677.

37. Dorsey JH, Holtz PM, Griffiths RI, et al. Costs and charges associated with three alternative techniques of hysterectomy. *N Eng J Med.* 1996;335:476–482.

38. Sculpher M, Manca A, Abbott J, et al. Cost effectiveness analysis of laparoscopic hysterectomy compared with standard hysterectomy: results from a randomised trial. *BMJ.* 2004;328:134.

39. Kaiser C, Stoll I, Ataseven B, et al. Vaginal hysterectomy and bilateral adnexectomy for female to male transsexuals in an interdisciplinary concepts. *Handchirurgie, Mikrochirurgie, plastische Chirurgie: Organ der Deutschsprachigen Arbeitsgemeinschaft fur Handchirurgie: Organ der Deutschsprachigen Arbeitsgemeinschaft fur Mikrochirurgie der Peripheren Nerven und Gefasse.* 2011;43:240–245.

40. Obedin-Maliver J, Light A, de Haan G, et al. Feasibility of vaginal hysterectomy for female-to-male transgender men. *Obstetrics Gynecol.* 2017;129:457–463.

41. O'Hanlan KA, Dibble SL, Young-Spint M. Total laparoscopic hysterectomy for female-to-male transsexuals. *Obstetrics Gynecol.* 2007;110:1096–1101.

42. Gomes da Costa A, Valentim-Lourenco A, Santos-Ribeiro S, et al. Laparoscopic vaginal-assisted hysterectomy with complete vaginectomy for female-to-male genital reassignment surgery. *J Minim Invasive Gynecol.* 2016;23:404–409.

43. Weyers S, Monstrey S, Hoebeke P, De Cuypere G, Gerris J. Laparoscopic hysterectomy as the method of choice for hysterectomy in female-to-male gender dysphoric individuals. *J Gynecol Surg.* 2008;5:269.

44. Bogliolo S, Cassani C, Babilonti L, et al. Robotic single-site surgery for female-to-male transsexuals: preliminary experience. *Sci World J.* 2014;2014:674579.

45. Ridgeway BM, Buechel M, Nutter B, et al. Minimally invasive hysterectomy: an analysis of different techniques. *Clin Obstet Gynecol.* 2015;58:732–739.

46. Van Caenegem E, Wierckx K, Taes Y, et al. Bone mass, bone geometry, and body composition in female-to-male transsexual persons after long-term cross-sex hormonal therapy. *J Clin Endocrinol Metab.* 2012;97:2503–2511.

47. Committee Opinion No. 620 ACOG. Salpingectomy for ovarian cancer prevention. *Obstet Gynecol.* 2015;125:279–281.

48. Salvador S, Gilks B, Kobel M, Huntsman D, Rosen B, Miller D. The fallopian tube: primary site of most pelvic high-grade serous carcinomas. *Int J Gynecol Cancer.* 2009;19:58–64.

49. Przybycin CG, Kurman RJ, Ronnett BM, Shih Ie M, Vang R. Are all pelvic (nonuterine) serous carcinomas of tubal origin? *Am J Surg Pathol.* 2010;34:1407–1416.

50. Kindelberger DW, Lee Y, Miron A, et al. Intraepithelial carcinoma of the fimbria and pelvic serous carcinoma: evidence for a causal relationship. *Am J Surg Pathol.* 2007;31:161–169.

51. Piek JM, van Diest PJ, Zweemer RP, et al. Dysplastic changes in prophylactically removed Fallopian tubes of women predisposed to developing ovarian cancer. *J Pathol.* 2001;195:451–456.

52. Kwon JS, McAlpine JN, Hanley GE, et al. Costs and benefits of opportunistic salpingectomy as an ovarian cancer prevention strategy. *Obstetrics Gynecol.* 2015;125:338–345.

53. Ergeneli MH, Duran EH, Ozcan G, et al. Vaginectomy and laparoscopically assisted vaginal hysterectomy as adjunctive surgery for female-to-male transsexual reassignment: preliminary report. *Eur J Obstet Gynecol Reprod Biol.* 1999;87:35–37.

54. Frey JD, Poudrier G, Chiodo MV, et al. An update on genital reconstruction options for the female-to-male transgender patient: a review of the literature. *Plast Reconstr Surg.* 2017;139:728–737.

55. Meyer R, Daverio PJ, Dequesne J. One-stage phalloplasty in transsexuals. *Ann Plast Surg.* 1986;16:472–479.

56. Rohrmann D, Jakse G. Urethroplasty in female-to-male transsexuals. *Eur Urol.* 2003;44:611–614.

57. Monstrey SJ, Ceulemans P, Hoebeke P. Sex reassignment surgery in the female-to-male transsexual. *Semin Plast Surg.* 2011;25:229–244.

INDEX

Note: Page numbers followed by *f* indicate figures, *t* indicate tables, and *b* indicate boxes.

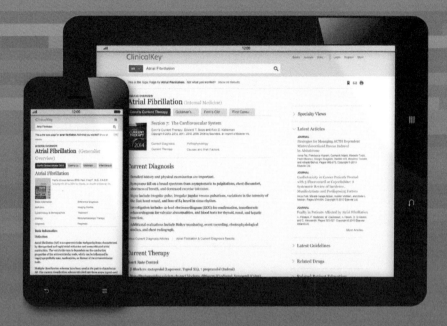

Printed and bound by CPI Group (UK) Ltd, Croydon, CR0 4YY

03/10/2024

01040303-0009